Betty Crocker's
Healthy Home
Cooking

More Than 400 Fast
and Flavorful Recipes

Material in this book has previously been published by Macmillan Publishing USA as *Betty Crocker's Healthy New Choices* (© 1998 by General Mills, Inc.) and by IDG Books Worldwide, Inc. as *Betty Crocker's Eat and Lose Weight* (© 2000 by General Mills, Inc.)

Basic 4, BETTY CROCKER, Bisquick, Cheerios, FiberOne and Potato Buds are registered trademarks of General Mills, Inc.

Printed in the United States of America

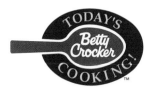

GENERAL MILLS, INC.
Betty Crocker Kitchens
Manager, Publishing: Lois Tlusty
Recipe Development: Betty Crocker Kitchens Home Economists
Food Stylists: Betty Crocker Kitchens Food Stylists
Photography: Photographic Services Department

Cover Designer: Christina Gaugler

Library of Congress Cataloging-in-Publication Data

Crocker, Betty.
    [Betty Crocker's healthy new choices]
    Betty Crocker's healthy home cooking : more than 400 fast and flavorful recipes.
        p.   cm.
    "Previously been published by Macmillan Publishing USA as Betty Crocker's Healthy New Choices in 1998."
    Includes index.
    ISBN-13 978–1–57954–581–9 hardcover
    ISBN-10 1–57954–581–5 hardcover
    1. Reducing diets—Recipes.   2. Low-fat diet—Recipes.   3. Nutrition.   I. Title: Healthy home cooking.   II. Title.
RM222.2 .C7495   2002
613.2'5—dc21   2002004587

Manufactured in the United States of America
10 9 8 7 6 5 4   hardcover

Cover photos: Zesty Autumn Pork Stew (page 430), Rosemary Lemon Chicken (page 235), Savory Currant Wedges (page 440), Creamy Raspberry-Filled Angel Cake (page 402)

For more great ideas visit www.bettycrocker.com.

INTRODUCTION

Ready, set—GO! With BETTY CROCKER'S HEALTHY HOME COOKING you are on your way to health! Combine great recipes and easy lifestyle changes, and you have a can-do package that will help you enjoy life more. Everything is geared for today's busy lifestyle—recipes that can be made quickly, and that use common ingredients—no searching for hard-to-find foods. Do you think all the material available on health and diet is one big maze? Betty Crocker has sorted through the recent research findings and dietary guidelines and put the science into terms that are easy to understand and simple to use.

Once you have mastered the basics of eating well, you'll want to turn to our chapter on wellness. Explore the connection between diet and health and learn how to reduce your risk of developing some common diseases. You'll also want to check out the information on alternative or "complementary" medicine. These are practices you've heard about, or maybe even tried yourself, such as meditation and yoga. We have taken out the mystery, and left the facts, so you can decide for yourself which approaches will be useful for you or your family.

To help you plan meals using your new *Healthy Home Cooking* strategies, refer to our special chapter of slimming menus. There you'll find an entire week's worth of menus to start you on your way to a deliciously healthy lifestyle.

But let's cut to the chase. The recipes taste great and your family will love them! Try our Pineapple-Orange Colada smoothie, or fresh Tomato Bruschetta with Basil Spread when you want a snack. What can you serve for dinner that's healthy and delicious? Take your pick! Explore Asian Noodle Salad, Risotto with Shrimp, Wild Mushroom Pizza, Crunchy Garlic Chicken, Creamy Crab Au Gratin, Saucy Italian Steak—even Bacon Cheeseburgers.

Really busy? There's a whole chapter just for you: Main Dish Express. These to-the-rescue recipes can be made in a flash, and help you have dinner on the table in thirty minutes, or less. Sample Turkey with Roasted Peppers and Couscous, Shrimp Carbonara with White Cheddar Sauce or Chuck Wagon Chili.

Have a sweet tooth and don't know how to fit it into a healthy eating plan? Simple, just serve Quick Praline Bars, Brownie Trifle, Cherry-Chocolate Fruit Decadence or homey Chocolate Chip Cookies, and dig in!

Enjoy the world of healthy eating and wellness with Betty Crocker!

Betty Crocker

CONTENTS

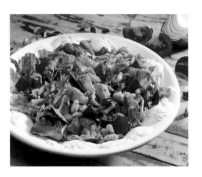

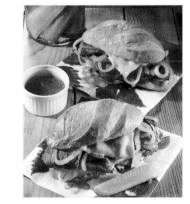

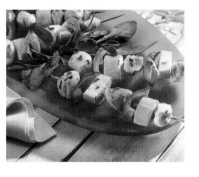

References

EATING WELL

Welcome to health! Let us help you understand why being healthy is important and how to achieve health and wellness—for you and the people you love. All it takes is *Healthy Home Cooking.*

Healthy home cooking begins with nutritious food and healthy lifestyle practices that minimize your risks of developing disease, regardless of your family history. These choices open you to exploring the link between your mind and body as you embark on your journey to health and wellness. Here's to healthy home cooking and a healthy new you.

Eating Well

In this introductory chapter, we'll take a look at why you should eat well and which building blocks will help you do so. We'll highlight the Food Guide Pyramid and provide other guides for eating and snacking to help you make smart food choices.

Eating well means enjoying food. Eating well also means keeping your body healthy through the foods you choose to eat. Can enjoying food and having a healthy body go together? Absolutely! All it takes is a little planning. Is it worth the effort? Without question.

The link between diet and health is strong and continues to grow stronger with each new study published. Consider the following:

➤ The American Cancer Society estimates that about 35 percent of all cancers are related to diet.

➤ Eating a healthy diet can lower your cholesterol level by 10 to 15 percent.

➤ More than half of all neural tube defects, such as spina bifida, might be eliminated if women ate diets rich in folic acid.

In addition to affecting physical health, food plays a part in your mental health and well-being—it can influence your mood. Foods affect your energy level, how well you sleep and how well you think. Studies suggest that certain vitamins and minerals may be helpful in treating depression, premenstrual syndrome and seasonal affective disorder.

Research also indicates that what we eat may impact what medications we need, as well as how much we need and how often we need to take them. We may even be able to stall the onset of certain long-term or chronic diseases by changing what we eat. So is eating well worth it? Maybe the better question is, is *not* eating well worth it?

Legendary tales about food live on—you can call them myths or mistakes. The myths, if believed, can often sabotage your efforts to eat well. To keep you on the track toward good health, let the truth be told.

Myth

Fat-free and low-fat foods are low in calories.

Truth

Not necessarily. Just because fat has been removed from a food doesn't mean the calories have been reduced. When food manufacturers remove fat, other components, usually carbohydrates, are added to improve taste and texture of a fat-reduced food. Check the Nutrition Facts for the truth.

MAKING THE SWITCH TO HEALTHIER FOODS

Nearly all people know that what they eat affects their health, yet only four in ten Americans say they are doing all they can to eat well. Most people say they hedge on eating well because they're afraid they'll have to give up the foods they like. But according to nutrition experts, giving up favorite foods isn't necessary—taste and nutrition can go hand in hand.

Making the switch to healthier foods requires a positive attitude and commitment. Making the switch also takes time; it is a gradual process. Chances are you already have some heart-healthy, bodybuilding behaviors; you just need to add to the list and build on your previous successes.

Here's how:

➤ Decide what's important to you.

Do you have a family history of heart disease, cancer, high blood pressure (hypertension) or osteoporosis? If so, making changes that may lower your risk for a specific disease can be a good place to start.

➤ Key into changes with the greatest effect on your health.

If colon cancer runs in your family, you may be able to lower your risk by filling up on fiber. Eating more fruits, vegetables, whole wheat breads and whole-grain cereals is a terrific place to start.

➤ Break down the changes into practical, doable steps.

If fiber is your focus, commit to eating five fruits or vegetables every day. Try a sliced banana on top of your cereal plus a bowl of berries for breakfast, raisins at lunch, carrot sticks for a snack and a wedge of melon at dinner.

➤ Forget perfection, and remember your goal.

Nobody eats perfectly all the time. If you have a blip in your healthy-eating efforts, remember that it's just a blip. Stay focused on your goal, and pick up where you left off.

➤ Recognize your successes.

Pat yourself on the back for your accomplishments. Adopt an "I-can-do-it" attitude. It will serve you well as you attack your next healthy-eating goal.

BUILDING BLOCKS FOR EATING WELL

Your body needs fuel. The fuel your body needs comes from calories, and calories come from carbohydrates, protein and fat. The amounts you choose to eat from these different fuel sources determine, in part, whether you are eating well.

Myth

Reduced-fat foods are healthier than regular foods.

Truth

Foods with less fat often appear to be better choices than their regular counterparts. However, as fat is removed, so is flavor. To make up for the lost flavor, calories, sugar and sodium may be added to boost taste. Read the labels on packages to be sure.

PERCENT OF CALORIES FROM BUILDING BLOCKS

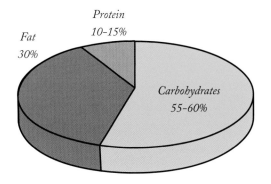

Protein 10-15%

Fat 30%

Carbohydrates 55-60%

Carbohydrates

Carbohydrates are your body's favorite fuel source. They are the foundation of a healthy diet and should comprise the largest percentage of the calories you eat. Your brain uses carbohydrates for thinking, and your muscles use carbohydrates for quick energy. At four calories per gram, carbohydrates are an economical energy source.

Most adults eat about 45 percent of their calories as carbohydrates. Experts say 55 to 60 percent is a healthier amount. Half of the carbohydrates Americans eat come in the form of "simple" carbohydrates, so named because of their simple chemical structure. The other half, called "complex" carbohydrates, have a more complicated chemical structure. Both provide the same amount of energy, but the more complex carbohydrates you eat, the better. They offer an advantage over some of the simple carbohydrates.

Simple carbohydrates, also called *simple sugars,* are found in sugar, honey, corn syrup, desserts and fruit. They are digested quickly and provide a surge of quick energy. Complex carbohydrates, found in breads, cereals, pasta, rice and potatoes, take longer for your body to digest and therefore leave you feeling full longer. The energy from complex carbohydrates stays with you longer, too.

Complex carbohydrates, particularly less-processed varieties such as whole-grain bread, whole wheat pastas, brown rice and even vegetables, are also an excellent source of fiber.

Protein

Protein is responsible for all sorts of activities in your body. Protein helps to build new cells, make the hormones and enzymes that keep your body functioning and make antibodies that fight off infection and disease. Unlike carbohydrates that most people need to eat more of, the protein in our diets is plentiful, and Americans tend to eat more protein than they need.

Protein is found primarily in animal foods, such as meats, fish, poultry and dairy products. Beans, such as kidney beans and black beans, vegetables and grains, such as rice and pasta, also are sources of protein.

When Considering Calories, Are All Foods Created Equal?

We use grams as a way to figure calories. Gram for gram, some foods are more concentrated sources of calories than others. Keep your portions in proportion.

ENERGY SOURCE	CALORIES PER GRAM
Carbohydrates	4
Protein	4
Fat	9

Myth

Eating pasta, potatoes and bread is fattening.

Truth

Far from it. Complex carbohydrates such as pasta, potatoes and bread do not make people fat. There is no evidence that these foods increase your appetite and lead to more fat being stored in your body. Choosing whole-grain varieties of pasta and bread may actually help you feel full faster, thereby reducing the number of calories you eat. To keep these naturally low-fat foods low in fat, use toppers such as vegetable sauces, fruits and low-fat spreads.

Fat

Some fat is important for your body. We need fat for building new cells. Fat shuttles certain vitamins around in your body, and it helps make some of the hormone-like substances your body needs to regulate your blood pressure and other vital functions. Fat's good qualities can fit into a tablespoon of vegetable oil—literally—and any more fat than that amount is not needed by the body.

Health experts recommend you eat 30 percent or fewer of your calories as fat. To eat well, try trading in some of your fat calories in favor of calories from complex carbohydrates.

What Type of Fat Is Best?

There are several different kinds of fat. Though some fats are heralded as being healthier than others, too much of any kind of fat is bad news for your weight and your health. To eat well, eat a diet that is low in all types of fat.

MORE BUILDING BLOCKS

Cholesterol, vitamins, minerals, fiber and water are as important to your plan for eating well as are carbohydrates, protein and fat.

Cholesterol

The cholesterol in the foods we eat is called *dietary cholesterol*. The cholesterol in our bloodstream comes from two sources: the foods we eat and the body's own manufacturing process. Dietary cholesterol is found only in animal foods such as shellfish, meats and milk.

You may have heard about two other types of cholesterol. "Bad" cholesterol, officially known as low-density lipoproteins (LDL), is so called because it deposits cholesterol on blood vessel walls. "Good" cholesterol, or high-density lipoproteins (HDL), helps remove cholesterol from body tissues and blood, so the cholesterol can be recycled and used again. Together, LDL and HDL make up your blood cholesterol.

For most of us, dietary cholesterol seems to have only a small influence on blood cholesterol because the body controls how much cholesterol it makes. Our intake of fat, particularly saturated fat, affects blood cholesterol levels the most. That's why limiting our intake of saturated fat is important.

The Many Faces of Fat

Several different kinds of fat are outlined below. Though some fats, such as monounsaturated and polyunsaturated fats, may be "better" than others for your health, the best advice for eating well is to eat a diet low in all types of fat.

SATURATED FAT

Found primarily in animal foods, such as beef, chicken, turkey and pork. It is also in some dairy foods, such as cheese, whole milk and butter. This type of fat tends to be solid at room temperature, with the exception of certain oils, such as palm and coconut oils, which are highly saturated fats.

POLYUNSATURATED FAT

Found in vegetable oils, such as sunflower oil and corn oil. These fats are usually liquid at room temperature. Omega-3 fats (also known as *fish oils*) are considered polyunsaturated fats.

MONOUNSATURATED FAT

Found mostly in plant foods, such as olive oil, peanut oil, nuts and avocados. These fats are usually liquid at room temperature.

TRANS FATTY ACIDS

Another kind of fat formed when a vegetable oil, such as corn oil, goes through a process called *hydrogenation* to turn it into a solid. Stick margarine and vegetable shortening are examples of foods containing trans fatty acids.

Major Minerals You Need

MAJOR MINERALS	GOOD SOURCES	FUNCTIONS
Calcium	Yogurt, milk, cheese, spinach, broccoli	Keeps bones and teeth strong. Aids in nerve and muscle function and immunity.
Chloride	Salt	Vital for water balance
Magnesium	Peanut butter, spinach, legumes	Helps in energy release from foods. Aids in nerve and muscle function.
Phosphorus	Milk, yogurt, cereal, chicken	Helps build strong bones. Aids in muscle function.
Potassium	Potatoes, yogurt, bananas, tomatoes	Vital for water balance and nerve and muscle function.
Sodium	Salt, soy sauce, soup, pickles	Vital for water balance.
Sulfur	Beef, pork, fish, chicken	Helps with acid-base balance.

Sources of Vitamins

Vitamin	Good Sources	Functions
Vitamin A	Sweet potatoes, carrots, spinach, apricots, broccoli	Vital for proper eyesight, healthy hair and skin. May reduce risk of certain cancers.
Thiamin (B_1)	Pork, cereal, peanuts, peas, wheat bread	Keeps nervous system healthy. Important for energy release from foods.
Riboflavin (B_2)	Milk, cereal, eggs, spinach, Cheddar cheese	Important for energy release from foods. Vital for healthy eyes, mouth and skin.
Niacin (B_3)	Tuna, chicken, salmon, peanuts, beef	Important for energy release from foods. Vital for healthy mouth, skin and nervous system. Sometimes used to lower blood cholesterol.
B_6	Bananas, chicken, pork, beef, salmon	Vital for breaking down protein. Keeps nerves and muscles working. May protect against some birth defects.
B_{12}	Salmon, beef, pork, milk, Cheddar cheese	Necessary for all cells to function. May protect against heart disease and nerve damage.
Folic Acid	Spinach, orange juice, peanuts, cereal, broccoli	Necessary for all cells to function. Helps protect against some birth defects.
Biotin	Soybeans, liver, nuts, eggs	Vital for energy release from foods.
Pantothenic Acid	Cereal, salmon, chicken, milk, peas	Vital for energy release from foods. Helps make certain hormones.
Vitamin C	Kiwifruit, bell peppers, orange juice, broccoli, cantaloupe	Keeps blood vessels, bones, gums and teeth healthy. Promotes healing. May reduce the risk of cancer and heart disease.
Vitamin D	Herring, salmon, margarine, milk, shrimp	Helps build calcium and phosphorus into bones and teeth. Helps prevent osteoporosis.
Vitamin E	Sunflower nuts, peanuts, margarine, oil, eggs	Protects the cells from damage. May reduce the risk of heart attack.
Vitamin K	Spinach, broccoli, asparagus, eggs, strawberries	Aids in blood clotting. May help in cancer prevention.

Vitamins

Vitamins control much of what goes on in your body. They help release the energy in carbohydrates, protein and fat. They are important to your vision, the health of your skin and hair, how strong your bones are, how well your heart and muscles function and how well your nervous system works.

Your body needs thirteen different vitamins that come from a variety of different food sources (see table on facing page). The more diversity in the kinds of foods you choose to eat, the more likely you are to get all of the vitamins your body needs.

Minerals

Your body needs many different minerals, and like vitamins, minerals are responsible for many different processes beneath your skin, such as carrying oxygen to all your cells, building bones and teeth and regulating your heartbeat.

Your body requires both "major" minerals, which are those needed in larger amounts, and "trace" minerals, those needed in very small amounts. As with vitamins, the greater the variety of foods you eat, the greater your chances for getting enough minerals.

Fiber

Another building block to eating well is fiber. Fiber is roughage. It's the skins, seeds and hulls found in plant foods, such as fruits, vegetables and grains. Your body does not digest fiber, yet fiber offers a multitude of health benefits while it passes through your system.

1. *Fiber fills you up without filling you out.*

   Fiber is bulk, giving you a sense of fullness without any calories. Foods high in fiber tend to be low in fat and calories.

2. *Fiber moves foods through your digestive system.*

   Think of fiber as a shuttle service. It helps keep food moving through your digestive tract. The more fiber you eat, the better shape your digestive system is in and the more smoothly foods move through your body.

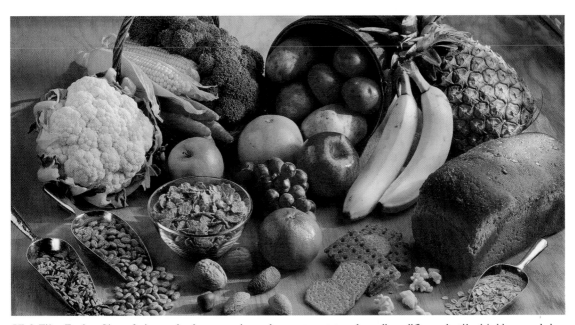

High Fiber Foods—Citrus fruits, apples, bananas, pineapple, carrots, potatoes, broccoli, cauliflower, lentils, dried beans, whole grains, corn on the cob, popcorn, whole-grain breads and whole-grain crackers.

3. *Fiber is a disease fighter.*

Several studies have shown that fiber may lower the risk for some cancers, including colon cancer, perhaps by binding with potential cancer-causing agents and removing them from the body. Fiber has also shown promise in reducing the risk for heart disease by helping lower cholesterol levels. Some research has found that eating a diet high in fiber may help diabetics keep their blood sugar in better control, too.

Fiber-Full Foods

Foods containing 6 or more grams of fiber:

1 cup cooked kidney, black or baked beans

1 cup bran cereal

5 dried figs

1 cup raspberries

2 ounces uncooked whole wheat spaghetti

Foods containing 4 to 5 grams of fiber:

1 pear

1 large apple

1 medium baked potato with skin

3 dried prunes

1 medium avocado

1 orange

Foods containing 2 to 3 grams of fiber:

1 ounce peanuts

1/3 cup raisins

1/2 cup cooked brown rice

1 medium sweet potato

1/2 cup corn

2/3 cup flake or oat cereals

Who Needs Supplements?

Many people take supplements as insurance towards eating well. Pills alone cannot turn a poor diet into a healthy one. Food contains too many substances to fit into a pill, so nutrition experts recommend choosing foods first. For some people, however, a supplement may be beneficial.

PREGNANT WOMEN
When pregnant, women need at least 15 to 50 percent more vitamins each day than when not pregnant. Some women are able to meet their increased needs by the foods they eat, and others need some help. Check with your doctor.

SMOKERS
People who smoke use up vitamin C in their bodies faster than do nonsmokers. Some researchers believe smokers need more folic acid and B_{12}, too.

OLDER ADULTS
The inability to eat enough food or a wide enough variety of foods can put some elderly people at risk for not getting all the nutrients they need. Medications can decrease the absorption of certain nutrients or cause nutrients to be lost. Check with your doctor.

HEAVY DRINKERS
Alcohol can increase the loss of B vitamins and vitamin C.

VEGETARIANS
People who avoid certain food groups for any reason risk not getting all the nutrients they need. For example, eliminating the meat group means iron, zinc, protein and copper may be in short supply.

Trace Minerals You Need

TRACE MINERALS	GOOD SOURCES	FUNCTIONS
Chromium	Whole grains, root vegetables	Helps in energy release from foods.
Copper	Whole grains, carrots, potatoes	Aids in cardiovascular function. Helps in energy release from foods.
Fluoride	Water, tea	Vital in tooth structure. Helps prevent tooth decay.
Iodine	Iodized salt, seafood, milk, grains	Vital for thyroid hormones that affect growth and development.
Iron	Cereal, spinach, beef	Important for oxygen transfer. Prevents anemia.
Manganese	Whole grains, carrots, potatoes	Helps in energy release from foods.
Molybdenum	Whole grains, carrots, potatoes	Helps in energy release from foods.
Selenium	Grains, beef, chicken	Helps prevent cell damage. May protect against cancer.
Zinc	Cereal, beef, chicken, wheat bread	Vital for growth, healing, and our ability to taste.

How Much Fiber Do You Need?

Experts say for good health, eat at least 25 to 30 grams of fiber each day. That's twice as much as most Americans eat. Good sources of fiber are whole fruits and vegetables, legumes such as pinto beans, whole-grain breads and cereals, brown rice and whole wheat pasta.

Drink more fluids as you increase the amount of fiber you eat. Fiber acts like a sponge in your body, absorbing many times its weight in water. Add a few extra glasses of milk, fruit juice or water to your eating-well plan.

Water

Water is critical to your health, yet it is often forgotten in discussions about eating well. Water is the most abundant substance in your body. For example:

➤ 83 percent of your blood is water

➤ 75 percent of your brain and muscles is water

➤ 22 percent of your bones is water

Water moves nutrients through your body. It is also responsible for removing any waste products your body generates. Water cools your body when you get hot and serves as a cushion for your joints and organs.

You lose about ten cups of water a day, all of which needs to be replaced. Water, juices, herbal teas and milk are excellent thirst quenchers. Coffee, tea, colas and alcohol are not. Caffeine and alcohol actually act as diuretics, meaning they pull water out of your body.

Can You Wait Until You're Thirsty to Drink?

Definitely not—you may be fairly dehydrated by then. By the time your brain registers thirst, your

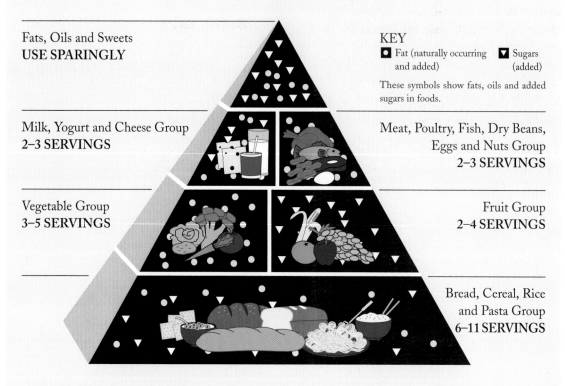

FOOD GUIDE PYRAMID
A Guide to Daily Food Choices

Fats, Oils and Sweets
USE SPARINGLY

KEY
□ Fat (naturally occurring   ▼ Sugars
and added)   (added)

These symbols show fats, oils and added sugars in foods.

Milk, Yogurt and Cheese Group
2–3 SERVINGS

Meat, Poultry, Fish, Dry Beans,
Eggs and Nuts Group
2–3 SERVINGS

Vegetable Group
3–5 SERVINGS

Fruit Group
2–4 SERVINGS

Bread, Cereal, Rice
and Pasta Group
6–11 SERVINGS

Source: U.S. Department of Agriculture, U.S. Department of Health and Human Services

body may have already lost up to four cups of water. Strive to drink eight cups of fluid a day—not counting alcohol and caffeine.

PUTTING IT ALL TOGETHER

The building blocks we just discussed are the ingredients for eating well. The next step is to understand how to use these ingredients. Enter the Food Guide Pyramid.

The Food Guide Pyramid is the road map for eating well. It emphasizes variety in your food choices from the five major food groups and shows you the pro-

portions in which to eat them. For example, at the bottom of the pyramid is the Bread, Cereal, Rice and Pasta Group. Most of the foods you eat in a day should come from this group. It has the largest number of recommended servings compared to the other food groups. To eat well, you want to start at the bottom of the pyramid and work your way up.

At the very top of the pyramid is the Fats, Oils and Sweets Group. That this group represents the smallest proportion of what you should eat is no surprise. Note the space allotted for the other food groups compared to the space allotted for fats, oils and sweets.

The recommended number of servings can be confusing, and knowing which number in the serving range is right for you can be difficult. Smaller adults and children, who need fewer calories, generally should use the smaller number, such as the six servings in the range of six to eleven servings for the Bread, Cereal, Rice and Pasta Group. Those who need more calories, such as men and active women, generally should use the larger number in the serving range. Others fit somewhere in the middle.

Dietary Guidelines: Partner to the Food Guide Pyramid

Seven guidelines, called the Dietary Guidelines for Americans, accompany the Food Guide Pyramid in providing directions for eating well. The Food Guide Pyramid is the illustration; the Dietary Guidelines tell the story.

Guideline 1: *Eat a variety of foods.*

No one food contains all the nutrients you need for good health. The greater the variety of foods you eat, the better for your body.

Guideline 2: *Maintain a healthy weight.*

Keeping your weight in line reduces your chances for several diseases, including heart disease, diabetes and stroke. Eating according to the Food Guide Pyramid is a super start to keeping calories in line.

What Counts as a Serving?

Food Groups		
Bread, Cereal, Rice and Pasta		
1 slice bread	1 ounce ready-to-eat cereal	1/2 cup cooked cereal, rice or pasta
Vegetable		
1 cup raw leafy vegetables	1/2 cup other vegetables, cooked or chopped raw	3/4 cup vegetable juice
Fruit		
1 medium apple, banana or orange	1/2 cup chopped, cooked or canned fruit	3/4 cup fruit juice
Milk, Yogurt and Cheese		
1 cup milk or yogurt	1 1/2 ounces natural cheese	2 ounces processed cheese
Meat, Poultry, Fish, Dry Beans, Eggs and Nuts		
2 to 3 ounces cooked lean meat, poultry or fish	1/2 cup cooked dry beans 1 egg or 2 tablespoons peanut butter count as 1 ounce lean meat	

Guideline 3: *Choose a diet low in fat, saturated fat and cholesterol.*

If you do so, you reduce your risk for all sorts of diseases. Keeping fat down is the quickest way to keep calories in line and your weight where you want it to be.

Guideline 4: *Choose a diet with plenty of vegetables, fruits and grain products.*

These foods provide the vitamins, minerals and fiber essential for good health, plus they contain certain substances, such as phytochemicals, that may significantly lower your risk for cancer and other illnesses (see pages 45–46).

Guideline 5: *Use sugars only in moderation.*

In and of itself, sugar really does not cause health problems. In excess, however, sugar can contribute unnecessary calories. Too much sugar also can lead to tooth decay.

Guideline 6: *Use salt and sodium only in moderation.*

Eating too much sodium may increase your risk for high blood pressure. Some studies suggest that too much sodium may also be bad for your bones because it may increase the amount of calcium lost from your body.

Guideline 7: *If you drink alcoholic beverages, do so in moderation.*

Alcohol contains calories but not much else. Some studies have indicated it may be good for your heart; recommendations are for moderation (not more than one or two drinks per day).

TROUBLESHOOTING KEY NUTRIENTS

Equipped with the Food Guide Pyramid and the seven Dietary Guidelines for Americans, you can build a healthy eating plan at any age. However, at different times in our lives, we tend to miss some important nutrients. The table below highlights the age groups at risk for inadequate intake of certain nutrients. Check the tables in the mineral section on pages 11–13 to find food sources to address the special concerns for you and your family.

Physiological changes, such as a growth spurt, or a change in eating habits, can lead to nutritional shortfalls. Use the Vitamin and Mineral Pyramid on the top of page 19 to help you fill in your vitamin and mineral blanks.

Special Nutrient Concerns

AGE GROUP	NUTRIENT
Infants to age 2	Iron, fluoride, fat, vitamin D
Children (2–12 years)	Calcium
Teenagers (13–18 years)	Calcium, iron, magnesium, vitamin B_6
Adult Women (19–50)	Calcium, iron, magnesium, folic acid, zinc
Adult Men (19–50)	Calcium, magnesium, zinc
Pregnant women	Calcium, iron, folic acid
Older adults (51+)	Calcium, magnesium, zinc, vitamin D

VITAMIN AND MINERAL PYRAMID

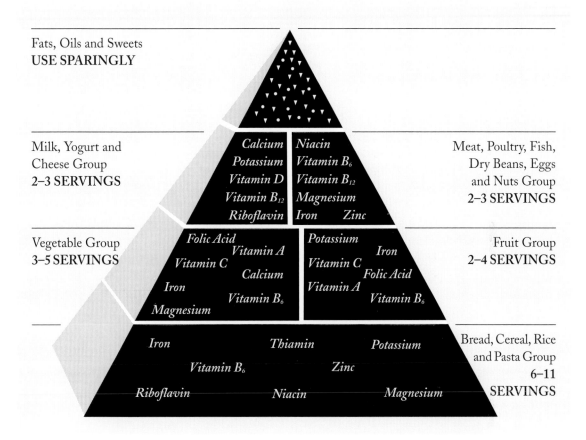

Fats, Oils and Sweets
USE SPARINGLY

Milk, Yogurt and
Cheese Group
2–3 SERVINGS

Calcium
Potassium
Vitamin D
Vitamin B₁₂
Riboflavin

Niacin
Vitamin B₆
Vitamin B₁₂
Magnesium
Iron   Zinc

Meat, Poultry, Fish,
Dry Beans, Eggs
and Nuts Group
2–3 SERVINGS

Vegetable Group
3–5 SERVINGS

Folic Acid
Vitamin A
Vitamin C
Calcium
Iron
Vitamin B₆
Magnesium

Potassium
Iron
Vitamin C
Folic Acid
Vitamin A
Vitamin B₆

Fruit Group
2–4 SERVINGS

Iron   *Thiamin*   *Potassium*

Vitamin B₆   *Zinc*

Riboflavin   *Niacin*   *Magnesium*

Bread, Cereal, Rice
and Pasta Group
**6–11
SERVINGS**

FIND OUT ABOUT YOUR FOOD

Another tool in your commitment to eating well is the Nutrition Facts label of food packages. The Food Guide Pyramid and Dietary Guidelines for Americans offer the big picture, and the Nutrition Facts label provides the details. Nutrition Facts labels give you a wealth of information about what a particular food has to offer in terms of the building blocks: carbohydrates, protein, fat, cholesterol, vitamins, minerals and fiber.

Understanding what kind of information is on the Nutrition Facts label and what certain claims such as "low-fat" mean is helpful. Get acquainted with the Nutrition Facts and the claims that can accompany them on pages 20 and 21.

BOTTOM LINE: Eating well is well worth the effort. With the right tools, such as the Food Guide Pyramid, the Dietary Guidelines for Americans and Nutrition Facts labels, eating well is not much effort at all. To eat well, select a variety of foods from all the food groups, and remember to top it off with several tall glasses of cool water.

Reading a Nutrition Label

The Nutrition Facts Label can be found on food packages in your supermarket. Reading the label tells you more about the food and the nutrients it supplies. The nutrition and ingredient information you see on the food label is required by the government.

Some food packages have a short or abbreviated nutrition label. These foods contain only a few of the nutrients required on the standard label and can use a short label format. What's on the label depends on what's in the food. Small and medium-sized packages with very little label space also may use a short label format. Here's what the label looks like with an explanation of its new features.

NUTRITION FACTS TITLE
The new title "Nutrition Facts" signals the new label.

SERVING SIZE
Serving sizes are standardized based on amounts people actually eat. Now similar food products have similar serving sizes making it easier to compare foods in the same category.

NEW LABEL INFORMATION
Some label information may not be familiar to you. The nutrient list covers those nutrients most important to your health. You may have seen this information on some old labels, but now it is required by the government and must appear on all food labels.

VITAMINS AND MINERALS
The Percent Daily Value replaces the Percent U.S. RDA for vitamins and minerals. The levels are the same. Only vitamin A, vitamin C, calcium, iron, and fortified nutrients are required on the new label: Additional vitamins and minerals can be listed voluntarily.

LABEL NUMBERS
Numbers on the nutrition label may be rounded for labeling.

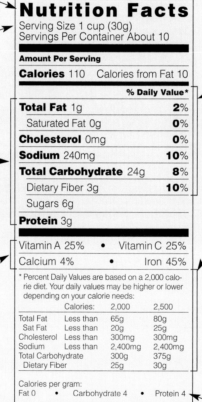

% DAILY VALUE
The Percent Daily Value shows how a food fits into a 2,000 calorie reference diet. These levels are based on dietary recommendations for most healthy people. Percent Daily Values help you judge whether a food contains "a lot" or "a little" of key nutrients important to health.

DAILY VALUES FOOTNOTE
Daily Values are the new label reference numbers. These numbers are set by the government and are based on current nutrition recommendations. Some labels list Daily Values for a diet of 2,000 and 2,500 calories per day. Your own nutrient needs may be less than or more than the Daily Values on the label.

CALORIES PER GRAM FOOTNOTE
Some labels tell the appropriate number of calories in a gram of fat, carbohydrate, and protein. (One gram is about the weight of a regular paperclip.) This information helps you calculate the percentage of calories from these nutrients.

Label Nutrition Claims

Label Claim	Definition Per Serving
Low Calorie	40 calories or fewer
Light (or Lite)	$\frac{1}{3}$ fewer calories *or* 50 percent less fat than the original product; if more than half the calories are from fat, fat content must be reduced by 50 percent or more
Light in Sodium	50 percent less sodium
Fat Free	Less than 0.5 gram of fat
Low Fat	3 grams of fat or fewer
Cholesterol Free	Fewer than 2 milligrams of cholesterol and 2 grams or fewer of saturated fat
Low Cholesterol	20 milligrams or fewer of cholesterol and 2 grams or fewer of saturated fat
Sodium Free	Fewer than 5 milligrams of sodium
Very Low Sodium	35 milligrams or fewer of sodium
Low Sodium	140 milligrams or fewer of sodium
High Fiber	5 grams or more of fiber

Label Health Claims

A Diet That Is:	May Help To Reduce The Risk Of:
High in calcium	Osteoporosis (bone-thinning disease)
High in fiber-containing grain products, fruits and vegetables	Cancer
High in fruits or vegetables (high in dietary fiber or vitamins A or C)	Cancer
High in fiber from fruits, vegetables and grain products	Heart disease
Low in fat	Cancer
Low in saturated fat and cholesterol	Heart disease
Low in sodium	High blood pressure (hypertension)
Low in saturated fat and cholesterol and high in soluble fiber from oats or psyllium	Heart disease
Adequate in folate from grain products, fruits and vegetables	Birth defects of brain and spinal cord (neural tube)

Smart Food Choices

Food Category	Choose More	Choose Less
Breads, Cereals	Whole-grain, whole wheat, pumpernickel and rye breads; breadsticks, English muffins, bagels, rice cakes, pita breads	Croissants, butter rolls
	Oat bran, oatmeal, whole-grain cereals	Presweetened cereals
	Saltines,* pretzels,* zwieback, plain popcorn	Cheese crackers, butter crackers
Rice, Pasta	Rice, pasta	Egg noodles
Baked Goods	Angel food cake	Frosted cakes, sweet rolls, pastries, doughnuts
Fruits	Fresh, frozen or dried fruits	Fruit pies
Vegetables	Fresh or frozen vegetables	Vegetables prepared with butter, cream or cheese sauces
Meat, Poultry, Fish	Lean meats, skinless poultry, fish, shellfish	Fatty meats, organ meats, cold cuts, sausages, hot dogs
Beans, Peas	Split peas, kidney beans, navy beans, lentils, soybeans, tofu	
Eggs	Egg whites, fat-free cholesterol-free egg substitute	Egg yolks
Milk, Cream	Skim milk, 1% milk, low-fat or fat-free buttermilk	Whole milk, 2% milk, half-and-half, whipped toppings, most nondairy creamers, sour cream
Cheese	Fat-free or low-fat cottage cheese, fat-free or low-fat cheeses, farmer cheese	Whole-milk cottage cheese, hard cheeses, cream cheese
Yogurt	Fat-free or low-fat yogurt	Whole-milk yogurt
Frozen Desserts	Ice milk, sherbet, fat-free or low-fat frozen yogurt	Ice cream
Fats, Oils	Polyunsaturated or monounsaturated vegetable oils: sunflower, corn, soybean, olive, safflower, sesame, canola, cottonseed	Saturated fats: coconut oil, palm oil, palm kernel oil, lard, bacon fat
Spreads	Margarine or shortening made with polyunsaturated fat	Butter
Chocolate	Cocoa	Chocolate

*Reduced-sodium varieties

Source: Adapted from *The American Heart Association Diet: An Eating Plan for Healthy Americans,* American Heart Association.

Smart Food Choices

Eating well means eating smart. And that means making smart food choices. Just about every food has some nutritional merit, but some foods have more than others. Certain foods are packed with vitamins and minerals, and they supply more or less, depending on the nutrient. These foods are nutrition stars, also know as "smart choices." (See the chart on facing page.)

TOP 10 FOODS FOR HEALTH

Top 10 lists have become a standard for delivering messages. The *Healthy Home Cooking* message is "eat well," and with that in mind, take a look at the Top 10 list of healthy foods for eating well. The criteria for making the list: Foods must be low in fat and big on nutrition—vitamins, minerals and other health-promoting ingredients.

1. WATER It's been called the forgotten nutrient. For good health, you need to remember to drink lots of water. About 50 to 60 percent of your body is made up of water. It is essential for healthy skin, it keeps your joints, eyes and lungs lubricated and it helps change the food you eat into energy.

   HEALTH TIP *Drink at least 8 cups of water, juice or caffeine-free drinks each day.*

2. CEREAL Ready-to-eat cereals are terrific sources of fiber, vitamins and minerals, including folic acid, vitamin B_6 and iron. Oatmeal and instant oatmeal rank high in nutrition, too.

   HEALTH TIP *To add more fiber to your diet, choose cereals with four or more grams of fiber in a serving. Make a healthy snack by substituting your favorite dry cereal for the usual bag of chips.*

3. DARK GREEN VEGGIES Broccoli, Brussels sprouts, spinach, romaine lettuce and asparagus are a few of the dark green nutrition starlets. These veggies contain lots of vitamins and minerals, including folic acid, vitamin C, calcium and iron. They are also good sources of fiber and contain phytochemicals, substances that may lower your risk for cancer.

   HEALTH TIP *Choose only dark leafy greens for your salads. Nutritionally, they are "heads" and shoulders above iceberg lettuce.*

4. ORANGE and RED VEGGIES Like dark green veggies, orange and red veggies are stacked with nutritional benefits. Carrots, sweet potatoes and winter squash are great sources of beta-carotene. tomatoes are tops, too. They are high in beta-carotene, vitamin C and lycopene, a phytochemical that may have significant cancer-preventing properties.

   HEALTH TIP *Instead of white potatoes for dinner, give sweet potatoes or winter squash the starring role.*

5. ORANGE-COLORED FRUITS Fruits that are orange in color are rich in beta-carotene and are often a good source of folic acid. Cantaloupe, apricots, papaya and peaches grab the honors here.

   HEALTH TIP *Add a little color to your snacks. Try dried apricots mixed with nuts or pretzels.*

6. CITRUS FRUITS and BERRIES Oranges, grapefruit, strawberries and blueberries are high on the list of important fruits to eat. Citrus fruits and strawberries are excellent sources of vitamin C. Berries and citrus fruits are also right sources of antioxidants, which studies show may lower the risk for heart disease and cancer.

   HEALTH TIP *Start every morning with two servings of fruit. Try a 6-ounce glass of fruit juice, and top your high-fiber cereal with ½ cup sliced strawberries.*

7. LEGUMES Get to know your beans. Lentils, black beans, kidney beans and baked beans all are good sources of protein, B vitamins including folic acid, iron and zinc. Beans are known for their fiber content, plus the fiber found in beans may lower cholesterol. Soybeans are becoming a headline grabber for their possible role in reducing the risk for heart disease and several cancers.

   HEALTH TIP *Take your favorite ground-beef casserole recipe, and substitute kidney, black or pinto beans for the beef.*

8. FISH Fish can be an excellent low-fat source of protein. Some fish, such as salmon, tuna and mackerel, are also good sources of omega-3 fatty acids, a type of fat that some studies suggest may help to lower your cholesterol, your risk for certain cancers and even your blood pressure.

   HEALTH TIP *Plan two meals each week that feature fish. For ease, prepare fish in the microwave or on the grill.*

9. MILK and YOGURT About 75 percent of the calcium people get in their diets comes from milk products, yet most Americans—young and old—are not getting all the calcium they need to build strong bones. One cup of milk or yogurt gives you one-fourth of the calcium you need daily.

   HEALTH TIP *Mix 1/8 teaspoon ground cinnamon into 1 cup low-fat vanilla yogurt. Add some chunks of pineapple, pear or nectarine, and you have a super breakfast in a snap.*

10. LEAN BEEF, PORK, CHICKEN and TURKEY They are big on protein, vitamins and minerals. Lean choices are key, however, because meat can be a major source of fat in the diet.

    HEALTH TIP *Choose cuts of meat that have "loin" in their name, such as tenderloin or sirloin. Keep*

portions at 3 ounces or less (about the size of a deck of cards).

HEALTHY SNACKING

Is snacking bad news? Not necessarily. It's a common misconception that snacking is a bad habit. In reality, snacking is part of eating well.

As many as eight out of ten adults snack daily. Research shows that snacks can play an important role in the American diet. Snacks provide energy in the form of calories and carbohydrates, and they provide many other vitamins and minerals we need for well-being.

Snacks supply as much as 11 percent of our daily calories. The rest comes from regular meals. For someone who eats about 2,000 calories a day, snacks may provide as many as 220 calories and supply a host of other nutrients as well. If we don't eat regular meals due to busy schedules or an active lifestyle, snacks may be the only way to round out our eating.

Unfortunately, many snacks go overboard on fat and calories, and sometimes they don't provide much else. Unhealthy snacks like these put us at greater risk for developing disease. To achieve balance in eating means making great snack choices—ones that are low in fat and loaded with nutrients such as calcium, iron and vitamins A and C. Select snacks that provide whole grains, choosing from foods that make up the foundation of the Food Guide Pyramid. Load up on fruits and vegetables, either fresh, frozen, canned or dried. Choose ready-to-eat cereals or pretzels when you're on the run.

Adventurous Tips to Healthy Snacking

➤ *Try something new.* Pick a brand-new snack once a month for variety.

➤ *Put a twist on new forms of old favorites.* Choose a bar or snack mix made from breakfast cereals.

➤ *Create your own.* Mix and match combinations of foods. Select from dried fruits, pretzels, cereal, popcorn, seeds, low-fat chips, imitation bacon bits, sun-dried tomatoes and baked corn snacks.

➤ *Tempt yourself with new toppers.* Sprinkle grated Parmesan cheese, crushed red pepper, basil, oregano, dry mustard, garlic and onion powders or balsamic vinegar on salads or popcorn. For a sweet treat, try ground cinnamon, nutmeg or cloves on applesauce, yogurt, frozen yogurt or pudding. Or top a graham cracker with marshmallow creme.

➤ *Devise a dip for veggies.* Start with fat-free yogurt or fat-free sour cream, and stir in a combination of herbs and spices that suit your fancy.

   ➤ Mix oregano, basil and crushed red pepper for a zesty Italian flavor.

   ➤ Blend in grated carrot and dill weed for a cool veggie-style dip.

   ➤ Stir in salsa—mild, medium or hot—for a south-of-the-border taste.

The sky's the limit when it comes to snacking. Remember that eating well means making great choices.

DINING OUT

Eating in a restaurant used to be a special treat reserved for events such as birthdays, Mother's Day and holidays. Because it was a special occasion, it was also a good excuse for digressing from an otherwise healthy eating plan.

Times have changed. Today, going out to eat is a part of life. Surveys show most Americans eat out several times a week. In fact, one in four people consider restaurant food essential to their way of life. Because the excuse of a "special occasion" no longer applies, we need to find ways to eat well while eating out. Fortunately, good taste and good health have come together on restaurant menus in the last few years.

According to the National Restaurant Association, at least 75 percent of restaurants offer healthier menu items. Some establishments help you out by flagging those dishes that are low in fat or low in sodium; others leave it up to you to figure out how to put together a healthy meal.

To eat out healthily, follow these general tips:

➤ *Choose your restaurants wisely.* Plan where you want to eat. Consider your health goals as you pick the restaurant. Feel free to make special requests for how you want your meal prepared and presented to you. Because the restaurant business is a competitive one, if you cannot find success at one restaurant, you can always try another. Many restaurants are very happy to meet their customers' needs.

➤ *Become assertive by asking for what you want.* Ask how foods are prepared. Then ask for any necessary adjustments, such as using less oil or butter in preparation. Ask for substitutions, such as au jus (plain meat juices) or salsa for your baked potato instead of sour cream. Ask your server to bring your dressings and sauces on the side.

➤ *Size up the portion sizes.* Many restaurants serve very large portions. Ask your server about serving sizes. Look for "petite" servings. If the food served is more than you want or need, ask if they will provide a lunch-size or half-portion. You can split a regular-size entrée with your companion, or before you start in on your meal, box up a portion of it to bring home. Consider having an appetizer as your main meal. Learn to feel comfortable leaving food on your plate.

➤ *Become fluent in "menu-ese."* Being able to spot "healthy" menu terms can save you time when ordering. Though it is always a good idea to verify the way a food is prepared with your server, there are a few key words to guide you in eating well. Choose menu items with these descriptors:

Baked	*Charbroiled*
Barbecued	*Grilled*
Blackened	*Poached*
Braised	*Roasted*
Broiled	*Steamed*

➤ *Stick with the same principles you use at home.* Meals that feature vegetables, pasta (in vegetable sauces), rice or beans can be excellent choices if they're prepared with broth, wine or a minimal amount of oil, such as in stir-fry dishes. Chicken, fish, lean red meats and lean pork can also be winners if they're prepared without fat.

➤ *Move the basket of chips and dip to the other side of the table.* Choose an unbuttered roll, or if you're really hungry, ask that a salad or cup of broth be brought right away.

➤ *Get salad-bar savvy.* Pick the smallest plate available when going through the salad bar. (You can always go back for seconds.) Load up on the fresh veggies, and lighten up on accessory items such as cheese, bacon bits, croutons, creamy salads and diced eggs. Choose vinegar-based dressings over thick, creamy ones, and use a light hand.

➤ *Make sure alcoholic drinks and dessert do not sabotage your otherwise healthy meal.* Drinks and dessert can tack on calories and fat quite quickly. Try drinking a glass of water before ordering an alcoholic drink. Water quenches your thirst without adding calories. When you've finished eating, wait several minutes before ordering dessert. Chances are your appetite for dessert will disappear. If you still have a sweet tooth, split a dessert or try a sweetened coffee drink.

BEYOND RESTAURANTS

No matter where your appetite takes you, there are strategies you can use to eat well when eating out. For example, the next time you make an airline reservation, request a special meal at the same time. Most carriers offer vegetarian, low-fat and low-calorie foods.

Whether you are traveling by car, bus, train or plane, get in the habit of taking dried fruit, ready-to-eat cereal, a bagel or some other heart-healthy snack along for the ride. These foods are easy to pack, they travel well and they are a welcome sight compared to the high-fat foods usually available when you're on the road.

BOTTOM LINE: Many restaurants are ready, willing and able to help you meet your eating-well goals—sometimes they just need a little guidance from you. Know what you want, and ask for it. Stick with your healthy-eating goals, and you can dine out to your heart's content.

WELLNESS

Take responsibility for your health; choose nutritious food and lifestyle practices as the tools for wellness. In the previous section, we talked about eating well and what that means. In this section, we explore the diet and health connection and give you the information you need to enhance your health and reduce your risk for developing some of the major illnesses common today. Learn how lifestyle components such as a healthy body weight, getting enough exercise and not smoking can help to prevent disease and keep you well.

We also explore the link between your mind and body and examine some of the many complementary or alternative medical approaches now available. All together, these are the tools for wellness.

A reminder to our readers: This cookbook provides general information that may help some people enhance their health or reduce their risk of certain diseases. It is not designed to replace the individualized care or advice of your doctor but rather to supplement it. For more information about any of the topics discussed here or other related issues not addressed in this book, please consult your doctor.

Diet and Health Connection

The link between diet and health grows stronger each year as studies show the impact food has on the body. Consider the following:

➤ The American Cancer Society estimates that about 35 percent of all cancers are related to diet, and many believe this is a conservative figure.

➤ Researchers estimate that one out of every four new cases of diabetes could be avoided if people avoided weight gain.

➤ Obesity more than doubles your chances of developing high blood pressure.

You can't change the genes you're born with, but you can make changes in your diet and lifestyle based on what's important to you. If heart disease is common on one side of the family, you can't change your predisposition toward developing the disease, but you can take steps to reduce your risk, thereby enhancing your health.

You may be able to stall the onset of disease, stop taking medications or avoid surgery because of your diet and your lifestyle—factors you can choose to control. You can select what you eat, you have influence on how much you weigh and you can determine how active you are. You also have control over some of your other habits, such as smoking or consuming alcohol. Let's take a closer look at the links between diet and health to help you on your path to wellness.

HEALTHY WEIGHT

Over time, your weight can change for all sorts of reasons. Eating habits may change, your physical activity level may change and of course your age changes. Sometimes these factors can result in a gradual increase in your weight, a gradual tightening of your belt. Extra pounds on your body

Body Mass Index (BMI)

BMI	19	20	21	22	23	24	25	26	27	28	29	30	35	40
HEIGHT*							WEIGHT (LBS)**							
4'10"	91	96	100	105	110	115	119	124	129	134	138	143	167	191
4'11"	94	99	104	109	114	119	124	128	133	138	143	148	173	198
5'0"	97	102	107	112	118	123	128	133	138	143	148	153	179	204
5'1"	100	106	111	116	122	127	132	137	143	148	153	158	185	211
5'2"	104	109	115	120	126	131	136	142	147	153	158	163	191	218
5'3"	107	113	118	124	130	135	141	146	152	158	163	169	197	225
5'4"	110	116	122	128	134	140	145	151	157	163	169	174	204	232
5'5"	114	120	126	132	138	144	150	156	162	168	174	180	210	240
5'6"	118	124	130	136	142	148	155	161	167	173	180	186	216	247
5'7"	121	127	134	140	146	153	159	166	172	178	185	191	223	255
5'8"	125	131	138	144	151	158	164	171	177	184	190	197	230	262
5'9"	128	135	142	149	156	162	169	176	182	189	196	203	236	270
5'10"	132	139	146	153	160	167	174	181	188	195	202	209	243	278
5'11"	136	143	150	157	165	172	179	186	193	200	208	215	250	286
6'0"	140	147	154	162	169	177	184	191	199	206	213	221	258	294
6'1"	144	151	159	166	174	182	189	197	204	212	219	227	265	302
6'2"	148	155	163	171	179	186	194	202	210	218	225	233	272	311
6'3"	152	160	168	176	184	192	200	208	216	224	232	240	279	319
6'4"	156	164	172	180	189	197	205	213	221	230	238	246	287	328

*without shoes   **without clothes

Source: George A. Bray, M.D.

translate into greater risk for health problems, such as heart disease, high blood pressure and diabetes.

Years ago, you were told to "go on a diet" to lose any extra pounds. Today many experts favor educating people on healthy lifestyle habits that include eating well and exercising regularly.

Studies show that together these two habits are a winning combination. People who eat well and lead an active lifestyle are more apt to achieve and—most importantly—maintain a healthy weight.

What Is a Healthy Weight?

A healthy weight goes beyond the numbers on your scale. A scale tells you how many pounds you weigh, but it doesn't tell you how much of that weight is fat. It also doesn't take into account where fat is on your body. Fairly new research suggests that you may be at greater risk for certain diseases depending on where you carry your fat.

Besides your bathroom scale, two calculations can help you figure your figure's health risk. They are the Body Mass Index and Waist-to-Hip Ratio. Body Mass Index (BMI) estimates how much mass, including fat, you have. It relates your weight to the health risks of being overweight better than a scale can. See the table on facing page to find your BMI.

A BMI between 19 and 25 is considered healthy. A BMI between 27 and 30 means you're moderately overweight. A BMI above 30 indicates that you are seriously overweight. BMIs over 27 are associated with a greater risk for weight-related health problems, including heart disease, hypertension and diabetes.

The calculation for Waist-to-Hip Ratio helps to pinpoint where you carry most of your fat. You may have heard references to apple and pear body shapes. "Apples" carry their weight in the stomach area (the potbelly or spare tire look), whereas "pears" carry their weight in the hip and thigh area. Research shows that apple shapes may be at a greater risk for

heart disease, diabetes and cancer than pear-shaped people, partially because the fat in apple shapes surrounds many of the body's organs. Usually a quick look in the mirror will tell you whether you are an apple or a pear, but if you need a more definitive answer, simply take a couple of measurements:

STEP 1: Measure your waist at your navel.

STEP 2: Measure your hips at their widest point (over your buttocks).

STEP 3: Divide your hip measurement into your waist measurement.

Example: If you have a 30-inch waist and 38-inch hips, divide 38 into 30; your Waist-to-Hip Ratio is 0.79.

For women, a healthy ratio is below 0.80. For men, a healthy ratio is below 1.0. Ratios above these numbers may put you at greater risk for health problems.

A Healthy Commitment to a Healthy Weight

Eating well and exercising regularly are the key ingredients for achieving a healthy weight. Several studies have tracked successful "dieters" and asked them how they lost their weight and kept it off. Topping the list of recurring answers is reducing the amount of fat in the diet and becoming more physically active.

Eating Well

Diets are big business—nearly $33 billion a year is spent on weight-loss products and services. But to date, no weight-loss product, program or diet that dramatically changes eating and exercise habits has kept Americans' weight off over the long haul. Only 5 to 10 percent of people who use these strategies succeed.

To achieve and maintain a healthy weight, you need to look for lifestyle changes—ones you are willing

ACTIVITY PYRAMID

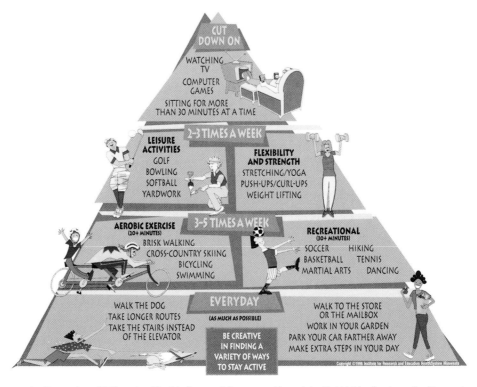

Source: Institute for Research and Education Health System Minnesota. Copyright © 1997 by Institute for Research and Education. Reprinted with permission.

to commit to for a lifetime. The previous section is full of ideas to help you eat well. Next we discuss how exercise can help you maintain a healthy weight and promote a healthy life.

Exercising Often

For exercise, "regular" is what reaps the results. Research repeatedly shows that people who participate in regular physical activity are healthier and more likely to keep their weight at a healthy level. What's your activity level? You can size yourself up using the Activity Pyramid above.

Both men and women lose about a third of a pound of muscle each year after they reach age forty. Because muscle is what burns the calories you eat, less muscle means fewer calories are being

burned. What is not burned is stored as fat. Part of the secret to keeping weight in check is to keep as much muscle as you possibly can. Exercise helps you keep your muscle.

What Kind of Exercise Is Best?

Without question, whatever exercise you enjoy and are willing to do on a regular basis is what's best for you. If you want the specifics on which exercises will help keep your muscle mass and help you maintain a healthy weight, keep reading.

Strength and endurance exercises are considered cornerstones of a healthy body. Strength exercises, meaning working your muscles with weights, keep muscles intact and can reduce the amount of muscle loss that is normally associated with aging. For best results at maintaining muscle mass, work weights with your large muscle groups, such as those in your back, abdomen and thighs. Strength-building exercises also help keep calcium in your bones, which in turn keeps your bones strong, healthy and able to support the activities you enjoy.

Endurance exercises strengthen your heart and the other muscles in your body. Endurance activities, such as swimming, walking and dancing, help increase how efficiently blood and oxygen are pumped by your heart to all the different cells in your body. Endurance exercises use your fat stores for energy.

How Much Exercise Is Enough?

Experts recommend strength-training exercises be done at least twice a week for 15 minutes or more. You can build your muscles by using large machines, or you can do it by using inexpensive hand and leg weights, doing old-fashioned calisthenics or even by lifting cans of food. A trainer or an exercise text can help you get started.

For endurance activities, experts recommend you aim to burn 300 calories a day. At this level of activity, you can lose body fat and keep it off. Three hundred calories translates into 30 minutes of cross-country skiing or aerobics or 45 minutes of biking, swimming or walking.

Carving out 30 minutes or more each day for physical activity goes a long way toward helping you achieve and maintain a healthy weight. You can tag on some "extra-credit" activity by making small changes in your daily schedule, such as taking the stairs instead of the escalator or parking far away from your destination and walking the extra distance. For other exercise ideas, see the Exercise Extra Credit list below—and remember, every little bit helps.

Exercise Extra Credit

Making time, even in small amounts, to move your body will help you feel better about yourself. Try some of these, or add your own exercises:

- Take the stairs whenever possible instead of the escalator or elevator.
- Park your car at the end of a row of spaces or farther from the entrance.
- Use idle time (airport layovers, waiting for medical appointments, waiting to be seated in a restaurant) to take a walk.
- Walk, bike or in-line skate to work rather than driving or busing.
- Schedule walk dates instead of lunch dates.
- Mow the lawn or do yard work.
- Walk around the entire shopping center instead of just select stores.
- Wash the car by hand.
- Carry your own groceries.
- Walk the dog.
- Make more than one trip, such as when carrying laundry, or the like.
- Do housework to music.
- Avoid shortcuts.

BOTTOM LINE: Your healthy weight goes beyond the numbers on the scale. Check your "healthy" status using the formulas provided. Eat well by including fruits, vegetables, and whole grains such as breads, rice and pasta, and become physically active.

ENHANCING HEALTH AND WELLNESS

You've just read about the importance of having a healthy weight and the commitment it takes to achieve and maintain it. Keeping those principles in mind, we look now at some of the major diseases affecting Americans today and what we can do to enhance health and wellness by minimizing risk.

> ## Myth
>
> A quick way to drop a few pounds is to skip eating breakfast.
>
> ## Truth
>
> Some studies show just the opposite. One study found that women who ate breakfast had diets that contained 28 percent of calories as fat, and women who skipped breakfast had diets that contained 40 percent of calories as fat. Skipping breakfast can often lead to overeating later in the day.

Obesity

Did you know that for every five pounds you lose, your total blood cholesterol could drop seven points? Losing just ten pounds could eliminate your need for medication for high blood pressure.

What Is Obesity?

Although many of us think of obesity as excess weight, the term actually means excess body fat. You can weigh more than standard height/weight charts and still have an acceptable amount of body fat. But most Americans who weigh more than is recommended do so because of excess body fat, not muscle.

As a result, when someone weighs 20 percent more than is recommended (one of the simplest measures of obesity), he or she is technically obese. You've already heard the warning, but here it is again: Obese people run the risk of developing chronic diseases, such as diabetes, high blood pressure and stroke, heart disease, some types of cancer and gallbladder disease.

What Causes Obesity?

It's complicated, but lifestyle and genetics play important roles. More than one-fourth of American adults are obese. And although there seems to be a genetic link to the tendency for some people to become obese, lifestyle is a key factor in the condition as well.

We eat too much, exercise too little and expect too much. Regular exercise aids in losing weight and plays a vital role in maintaining it. But effective weight management also depends on realistic and healthy goals. In other words, is the weight you consider desirable really a healthy weight for you? (See Healthy Weight on page 28.) Unhealthy weight goals may lead to eating disorders or repeated weight loss and regain, which may be harmful to you.

How to Avoid Obesity

Eat well, but eat fewer calories. For weight loss to occur, you must eat fewer calories than you use in daily activities. Generally, a deficit of 3,500 calories is required to lose one pound. That means you have to eat 250 fewer calories (a candy bar or 12-ounce soft drink) each day to lose one pound per week. But don't drop below 1,200 calories daily; getting enough of some of the necessary nutrients is difficult if calorie levels are too low.

Change eating behaviors. Pay attention to behaviors that lead to overeating and weight gain. If you regularly skip breakfast or other meals thinking you can "save" calories only to eat voraciously at subsequent meals, you may be setting yourself up for obesity-prone behaviors. Experts recommend spacing out your meals throughout the day, sometimes eating six smaller meals instead of three larger ones or choosing sensible snacks such as fruits, popcorn or pretzels. (See Healthy Snacking, page 24.) Eat more food early in the day, such as at breakfast, and cut back later on at dinnertime.

Exercise more for endurance and strength. Start with 10 to 15 minutes of a low to moderate intensity level that gets your heart beating but doesn't exceed 108 beats per minute. Eventually, aim for more vigorous physical activity every day for at least 30 minutes each time. Try activities you already know, such as walking, swimming, cycling, dancing or gardening. And don't forget about strength training to firm up and tone your muscles. (See Exercising Often on page 30 for more details.)

Present children with positive messages. Weight-loss diets are generally not recommended for children. Experts advise feeding an obese child less food than he or she would normally eat but not less than what a normal-weight child would eat. Try to present positive messages to children, such as "be more active" instead of the more negative "eat less food." Encourage children to increase physical activity and eat healthily to assure they get all the nutrients needed to grow and develop normally. And talk to the child's pediatrician about your concerns.

BOTTOM LINE: Eat well. Achieve and maintain a healthy weight. (See page 29 for more information.) Exercise regularly for both endurance and strength. Monitor your habits, and try to eliminate eating from boredom, stress or excessive hunger. Eat more food at breakfast and less at dinnertime.

Cancer

The small units of life in all living things are called *cells.* An average adult contains more than a trillion cells of many types that grow and help our body tissues function. Sometimes, for reasons that scientists do not fully understand, some of our cells change and become cancerous.

What Is Cancer?
Cancer encompasses more than a hundred different diseases affecting many different body tissues. It affects people of all ages, sizes, shapes and colors. Regardless of the body tissue that is affected, cancer is an uncontrolled growth and spread of abnormal cells. Although you can develop cancer at any age, you're more likely to do so as you grow older. Estimates indicate that one in every five Americans dies from cancer.

Is Cancer Related to Diet?
About 35 percent of cancers may be related to diet. Too much fat has been associated with cancers of the breast, colon, rectum and prostate, and possibly pancreas, uterus and ovary. Too much alcohol is linked with cancers of the mouth and throat, esophagus, liver, colon, breast, head and neck. Smoking and lung cancer are connected.

How to Prevent Cancer
Eat a low-fat, low-cholesterol diet with lots of fiber. Guidelines for total fat intake include no more than 30 percent of calories from fat. Recommendations for fiber intake range from 20 to 30 grams daily, about twice the amount an average American consumes today. A diet high in whole grains and fiber may help reduce risk for cancers of the colon and rectum.

Avoid obesity and limit alcohol consumption. The Dietary Guidelines for Americans recommend no more than two drinks a day for men and one for women. (One drink is measured as 12 ounces of regular beer, 5 ounces of wine or 1½ ounces of 80-proof distilled spirits.) See the section on Obesity (page 32), and read What Is a Healthy Weight? (page 29).

Limit consumption of smoked and cured foods. The American Cancer Society recommends we eat less bacon, ham, hot dogs and sausage. Cancers of the esophagus and stomach are common in countries where these foods are eaten in large quantities.

Be sure to get enough exercise—daily. There is strong scientific evidence in support of physical activity reducing risk for both breast and colon cancer.

Managing Cancer
Check with your doctor or dietitian. Eating to manage existing cancers can be quite different from the guidelines here. The dietary concerns of people who have cancer are very individual. It's impossible to make general recommendations.

BOTTOM LINE: Eat well. Choose at least five servings of fruits and vegetables daily. Include citrus fruits or cruciferous vegetables, such as cabbage, broccoli and cauliflower, at each meal. These vegetables may protect against colorectal, stomach and respiratory cancers. Get enough fiber by including whole-grain breads and cereals with bran as part of each meal. And be sure to get enough daily exercise.

Coronary Heart Disease

The heart is the center of life. About once each second, your heart pumps and sends oxygen- and nutrient-filled blood through arteries to your tissues. When everything is working properly, the heart keeps us alive and well. Sometimes, conditions can develop where the functions of the heart and blood vessels become impaired. Coronary heart disease, often called CHD, is one of those conditions.

What Is CHD?

CHD is a buildup of fatty, cholesterol-filled deposits in the arteries. These deposits can become thick, clogging arteries and blocking the flow of blood, ultimately causing a heart attack. Since 1984, we've seen more than a 29 percent drop in deaths from CHD. But even today, CHD remains the number-one killer of both men and women in the United States.

What Causes CHD?

CHD is caused by a variety of factors, and unfortunately, some are beyond our control. For example, your risks for CHD are greater if you have a family history of CHD, are male or are older. The risks also have an additive effect. If you're male *and* over age fifty *and* one of your parents or a sibling suffers from the disease, your chances for developing CHD become even greater.

Other factors that cause CHD are things we can control or modify. Generally, these are lifestyle factors such as not smoking, getting enough exercise and eating well, to name a few. Other modifiable risk factors include high blood pressure, high blood cholesterol and obesity.

> ## Myth
>
> Eating red meat (beef) is bad for you.
>
> ## Truth
>
> Red meat can be high in saturated fat, depending on which cuts of meat you choose. Eating a diet high in saturated fat raises your cholesterol and risk for heart disease. Too much saturated fat may also increase your risk for certain cancers. However, lean cuts of red meat, such as sirloin, round and tenderloin, are low in saturated fat and important sources of iron and other nutrients. Meats can easily be part of a healthy diet.

How to Prevent CHD

Stop smoking. Cigarette smoking is the most significant modifiable risk that's within your control. Smokers can greatly decrease their chances of developing CHD merely by quitting.

Eat a low-fat, low-cholesterol diet. That shouldn't be a surprise. It's in the news daily. Your daily diet shouldn't exceed 30 percent of calories from fat, with no more than 10 percent of those calories coming from saturated fat. Limit cholesterol intake to no more than 300 milligrams per day, as well. And don't eat more calories than you need, to avoid excessive weight gain and obesity.

Get regular physical activity. If you haven't been active recently or have heart disease, check with your doctor first. Start gradually with light to moderate activity for 10 to 15 minutes, and work your way up to at least 30 minutes daily. Try things you already know, such as walking, swimming, cycling, dancing or gardening. (See Exercising Often on page 30.)

Aim for more vigorous daily physical activity, such as jogging or running, lap swimming, cycling, ice skating, in-line skating, rowing or jumping rope, that really keeps you moving.

BOTTOM LINE: Eat well. Exercise regularly for endurance and strength. Stop smoking. Have your blood cholesterol checked if you're over age twenty. If it's in the desirable range of under 200 mg/dl,* have it rechecked every five years. If it's outside the desirable range, check with your doctor.

*milligrams of cholesterol/deciliter of blood

Diabetes

Nearly eight million people in the United States suffer from diabetes mellitus. Another five million Americans may have diabetes but not yet know it. Where do you fit?

What Is Diabetes?
Diabetes is a chronic disease that results in abnormally high levels of glucose (sugar from breaking down carbohydrates) and fats (including cholesterol and triglycerides) in the blood. If left untreated, diabetes can cause other health problems, including nerve damage, poor blood circulation, impaired vision, kidney disease and atherosclerosis (fatty deposits in the arteries). More than a half-million Americans are diagnosed with this disorder each year.

What Causes Diabetes?
Diabetes is caused by a malfunction. Either there's a lack of insulin, the substance necessary to break down carbohydrate sugars called *glucose,* or the systems necessary to use insulin aren't functioning properly. Sometimes, diabetes can be caused by a combination of these two reasons.

Are There Different Kinds of Diabetes?
Yes, there are two types of diabetes based on the specifics of the malfunction. One kind is called in-sulin-dependent, or Type 1 diabetes, and the other is non-insulin-dependent, or Type 2 diabetes.

In Type 1 diabetes, the body either produces no insulin or not enough to meet its needs. Type 1 diabetes tends to start abruptly, and it generally occurs in children and young adults under age thirty. There is no known means of preventing the disease, and we often cannot predict who will develop it. We do know that roughly two-thirds of those who develop diabetes have a family history of the disease.

Type 2 diabetes develops when the body produces enough insulin but isn't able to use the insulin effectively. About 90 percent of those with diabetes have Type 2. This form of the disease is most common in people over age forty and develops gradually, often preceded by obesity.

Managing Diabetes
Dietary strategies for both types of diabetes are similar. People with Type 1 diabetes may require daily injections of insulin to help them manage the disease. Proper diet and exercise can help manage Type 2 diabetes and also can help to prevent it, to the extent that excess weight and obesity are avoided. It is well known that with weight reduction alone, normal blood glucose levels can be reestablished in people with Type 2 diabetes. In addition, people with Type 2 diabetes sometimes need insulin to manage the disease, but weight reduction often alleviates that need.

BOTTOM LINE: Eat well. Maintain a healthy weight. Exercise regularly. Learn to use diet exchanges on packaged foods and recipes and how they can help you make appropriate food choices (page 20). Use sparingly sources of concentrated sweets, such as table sugar, candies and honey. Avoid desserts with more than 350 calories per serving.

High Blood Pressure

High blood pressure, or hypertension, affects approximately fifty-eight million people in the

United States today. Although it's a disease that develops more frequently as we grow older, well over half of the Americans who suffer from it are under the age of sixty-five.

What Is High Blood Pressure?

Technically, high blood pressure is when blood pressure is equal to or greater than 140/90 millimeters of mercury. High blood pressure triples the risk for developing coronary heart disease and increases the risk of stroke by as much as seven times.

Unfortunately, many people do not even realize they have high blood pressure: one-third of Americans afflicted may be unaware of their own elevated blood pressure. This not knowing makes high blood pressure a "silent killer." And because there are no general symptoms associated with high blood pressure, you can't tell when your blood pressure is high, even if you think you can.

The only way to really know whether or not your blood pressure is high is by having it measured. Because blood pressure can vary daily and throughout the day, elevated blood pressure should be measured on at least two separate occasions before a diagnosis is made.

What Causes High Blood Pressure?

The exact cause is generally unknown. Whether you will develop high blood pressure or not seems to depend on a combination of factors. Your chances for developing high blood pressure are greater if the disease affects others in your family. Lifestyle factors such as obesity, a habitually high alcohol intake (more than two drinks per day), a sedentary lifestyle and various dietary factors are usually present, as well.

What about Limiting Sodium Intake?

Experts suggest limiting sodium, but views are mixed. There has been a great amount of investigation into the impact of sodium on high blood pressure. And people with high blood pressure are generally advised to limit their intake of sodium.

Whether people without high blood pressure need to limit sodium is controversial. The controversy centers on the concept of sodium sensitivity. Some people are able to maintain normal blood pressures regardless of the amount of sodium they consume, yet others are more sensitive to the amount they are consuming. Those who are sensitive can develop elevated blood pressure when eating a diet high in sodium.

Whether you will develop high blood pressure or be among the sodium sensitive is currently impossible to tell. As a result, many experts suggest most people limit sodium.

Consume no more than 3,300 milligrams of sodium daily, according to the recommendations for healthy Americans by the National Heart, Lung and Blood Institute. Americans consume an average of 4,000 to 5,800 milligrams of sodium daily. (A teaspoon of salt contains about 2,400 milligrams of sodium.)

BOTTOM LINE: If you have high blood pressure, limit sodium even if your blood pressure is not sodium sensitive. Limit the salt in cooking and at the table, and avoid salty snacks. Low-sodium intakes may enhance the effectiveness of any medications you take to treat high blood pressure. Your doctor can advise you about how much sodium you should consume.

Osteoporosis

Make no bones about it, calcium is important to your body. Without it, osteoporosis is certain to cause harm.

What Is Osteoporosis?

Osteoporosis, meaning literally "porous bone," is a complex disorder that results from a gradual and

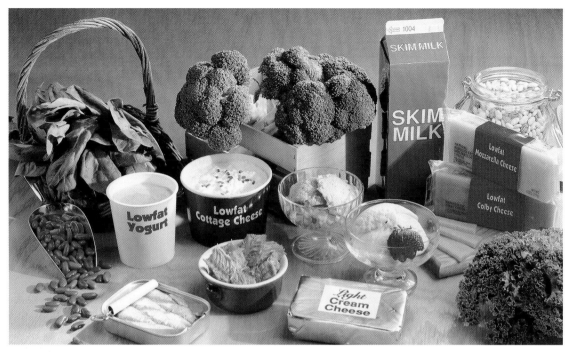

High Calcium Foods—Low-fat dairy products (including cheese, milks, yogurts, frozen yogurt and ice milk), spinach, kale, collard greens, broccoli, dried beans and canned salmon and sardines (with bones).

continual loss of bone mass. Our bones are constantly being rebuilt. Even though they appear to us to be unchanged, they are actually involved in quite a dynamic process.

As we grow older, we all lose bone mass; our bones become less dense and more fragile. A person with osteoporosis loses bone at such a rapid rate that the bones become extremely fragile and prone to fracture. As the disease progresses, its victims frequently become shorter and develop a "dowager's hump," or humped back.

Who Gets Osteoporosis?
Women do. Of the many risks that multiply the chances of developing osteoporosis, one of the greatest is being female. Women have smaller and less-dense bones than men do. In addition, women tend to live longer than men, and osteoporosis is a disease that comes with aging.

Approximately one-half of American women over the age of forty-five and 90 percent of women over age seventy-five have osteoporosis. Race can also play a role. Caucasian women are about twice as likely as African-American women to suffer hip fractures due to osteoporosis. Men get osteoporosis, too, although it's not common among men until after age sixty.

What about Other Risk Factors?
Menopause puts women at risk. During menopause, women stop producing the hormone estrogen, which may change the calcium status and result in rapidly accelerated bone loss. Calcium is one of the primary minerals involved in building and

calcifying, or hardening, bones. Increased calcium in the diet as the single treatment, however, does not seem to be as effective as estrogen-replacement therapy in slowing bone loss after menopause.

Smoking increases risk. The risk for developing osteoporosis is greater if you smoke—regardless of what you smoke. Smoking may negatively affect estrogen levels that place you at an even greater risk of losing bone mass.

Inactivity and too little calcium increase risk. If you are inactive and in general do not get enough calcium in your diet, you are at greater risk for osteoporosis. In particular, weight-bearing activities, such as walking and running, are beneficial to bone health and building bone mass.

Myth

Osteoporosis is a woman's problem.

Truth

Osteoporosis is a woman's problem; one out of every two women over age fifty will suffer a fracture due to osteoporosis. But so will one in eight men. Eating calcium-rich foods and exercising are bone-saving strategies.

How to Prevent Osteoporosis

Ensure you get adequate calcium throughout your lifetime. The process of building bone mass goes on until about age twenty to twenty-five, when bones reach their peak in density. After peaking, new bone tissue continues to be built but at a slower pace than what is breaking down. Eventually, we begin to lose bone (and calcium) at a more rapid pace. Unfortunately, this is an unavoidable consequence of aging.

Adults and children over age two need 1,000 milligrams of calcium daily, according to the National Academy of Sciences. Because the best time to build bone is during the critical growing years (between the ages of nine and eighteen), both boys and girls should consume at least 1,300 milligrams of calcium each day. Choose at least two or three servings of low-fat dairy foods such as milk, yogurt and cheese daily.

To meet the calcium needs of the fetus and the breast-fed infant, pregnant and lactating women should consume at least 1,000 milligrams of calcium per day. Menopausal or postmenopausal women who may be at risk for osteoporosis but who are not undergoing estrogen-replacement therapy may also benefit from 1,200 milligrams of calcium daily. Increase servings of dairy foods to four per day.

Don't forget about vitamin D. Even though you may get enough calcium in your diet, you may not absorb it all. Too little vitamin D (from lack of sunlight or vitamin D-fortified milk products), too much fiber (over 35 grams a day) and too much alcohol can cause calcium absorption problems. To combat these risks effectively, regularly choose vitamin D-fortified milk, avoid fiber supplements (get your fiber from food instead) and be moderate in your consumption of alcohol.

BOTTOM LINE: Eat enough calcium and vitamin D. Besides dairy foods (milk, yogurt and cheese), select canned salmon or sardines with edible bones, dried beans and peas or tofu processed with calcium sulfate. Try dark green vegetables, such as broccoli, kale and collards, and grain products, such as lime-processed tortillas and fortified ready-to-eat cereals. Drink calcium-fortified juices, or check with your doctor about taking a calcium supplement.

Twelve Tips for Wellness

Here are some simple ways to reduce your risk for many of the major illnesses common today. Although there are no guarantees, following these twelve easy tips will start you on the path to wellness.

1. *If you smoke, stop.* Whether you smoke cigarettes, cigars or pipes, smoking more than any other habit has been clearly linked to disease.

2. *Get regular checkups.* Encourage your doctor to monitor blood pressure and blood cholesterol. For women nearing or beginning menopause, consider estrogen-replacement therapy.

3. *Eat well.* That means consuming a diet low in fat that includes fruits, vegetables, grains and calcium-rich foods such as milk and yogurt. Choose small amounts of lean meats, fish and poultry.

4. *Maintain a healthy weight.* Aim for a weight that is achievable and realistic.

5. *Limit sun exposure, and wear sunscreen.* Even if you don't expect to be in the sun for any length of time, protecting your skin is important.

6. *Exercise regularly.* Any physical activity counts. Start with something you know, such as walking or swimming, gardening or housework. If you haven't been active recently, check with your physician before you begin.

7. *Drink plenty of fluids.* Each day, drink at least eight cups of liquid including water, but don't count caffeine-containing teas or coffees because these tend to have the opposite effect.

8. *Limit alcohol.* Drink only moderate amounts of alcohol; experts suggest no more than two drinks daily for men and one drink daily for women.

9. *Consume salt and sodium in moderation.* Limit salt-cured, nitrite-cured and smoked foods such as hot dogs, sausages and pickles. Skimp on salty snacks, too.

10. *Read food labels and menus carefully.* Reading helps you make informed food choices. Select more healthy options whenever possible.

11. *Manage stress and emotional upsets.* Develop a network of supportive friends and family to talk over your life stresses. Exercise regularly to keep your mind and body recharged. And get enough sleep, aiming for at least six to eight hours each night.

12. *Plan your wellness strategy with your doctor.* If you have an illness, ask your doctor and family to help you accomplish your goals.

Mind-Body Connection

All ancient healing practices involve some link between thoughts and emotions and their effects on the physical body. As intricately connected as the brain and body are, it makes sense that each can have an effect on the health of the other.

As many of you know, when you become stressed or angry or do not get enough sleep, you tax your immune system and often end up sick in bed. Over time, these continual stresses add up and can lead to chronic disease. Conversely, you may have heard or read about the powers the mind can have on healing sickness, such as cancer for example, even when conventional therapies are employed, because of faith, positive thinking, hope or even a sense of humor.

In conventional medicine, the mind-body connection is generally ignored. We rely instead on things outside of us, such as medications and surgery, to cure ailments. On the other hand, alternative or complementary medicine places great emphasis on using the inside, our thoughts and emotions, as an integral part of healing and wellness.

Experts say you don't need a practitioner to make the mind-body connection work for you. Practitioners in many of the complementary medical fields act merely as guides, to teach you techniques that may be helpful in tapping into your own mind-body connection. Ultimately, it is you who must do much of the mind-body work on your own.

By way of introduction to the mind-body connection, let's take a look at many of the complementary therapies that may make it easier for you to connect your brain, your physical body and good health—more tools for wellness.

An Alphabetical Guide to Complementary Medicine

You've probably heard the words *alternative* and *complementary* before but perhaps not as they refer to medicine or wellness. Whether you've taken advantage of any of the unconventional medical therapies available, they're here, and apparently to stay.

Many of the therapies listed here began thousands of years ago, in a host of cultures spanning the globe from Europe to China and India to Egypt. The treatments use herbs, needles or body manipulation as a means to heal ailments. Before you venture out to try them, read on for details about what they are, how they work and whom to trust.

The Office of Alternative Medicine, established in the United States about ten years ago, has collected volumes of available research data on alternative medical practices and has developed a report to the National Institutes of Health. This documented research will be useful in helping to establish recommendations and guidelines for scientific testing for safety and effectiveness of these therapies.

If you have any doubts about blending these therapies with your current medications or treatment plan or are unsure of their safety or effectiveness, check with your doctor. Your own wellness is counting on you.

Acupuncture

Part of traditional Chinese medicine, acupuncture is an ancient art and science of healing. The word *acupuncture* comes from two Latin words: *acus*, meaning "needles," and *punctura*, meaning "pricking."

And like its definition, Chinese acupuncture involves the insertion of needles into specific points on your body. Based on a belief that energy flows between body organs along channels, or meridians, healing occurs when the flow of energy in the entire body is balanced. The energy is called *chi*, or *qi* (pronounced CHEE). Chi changes with your mental, physical and spiritual well-being and is made up of two opposing forces called *yin* (the shady side of the mountain) and *yang* (the sunny side).

Worldwide scientific evidence exists to support the idea that acupuncture is a successful treatment for headaches, low back pain, angina, dementia and arthritis and for relief of many other ailments or imbalances. Today, Western practitioners often use acupuncture out of the traditional context. Instead of using it to regain balance, acupuncture has become a treatment for acute or chronic pain and for behavior modification to treat addictions to food, alcohol, smoking and drugs.

Qualified acupuncturists should meet the requirements of the state in which you live, and you should be able to trust them. For more information, contact the American Academy of Medical Acupuncture, 5820 Wilshire Boulevard, Suite 500, Los Angeles, CA 90036; (800) 521-2262.

Aromatherapy

Aromatherapy, or scent therapy, first developed by ancient Egyptians, is the use of "essential oils" to increase relaxation, improve mood and enhance circulation. Essential oils are the concentrated forms of natural oils extracted from petals, leaves, roots, resin, bark, rinds, stalks, stems and seeds of various plants. Large volumes of plant parts are processed to extract very small volumes of essential oils.

Once extracted, essential oils are applied externally, inhaled or used in compresses or lotions. We find them in soaps, candles, perfumes, potpourri, lotions, bath salts, massage oils, antiseptic solutions, sprays, and shampoos and other hair care products. Because essential oils are somewhat fragile, store them in a cool place in dark, airtight glass containers to protect them. For more information, contact the National Association for Holistic Aromatherapy, P.O. Box 17622, Boulder, CO 80308; (888) 275-6242.

Ayurveda

One of the oldest forms of medical practice, Ayurveda (pronounced I-YUR-VAYDA) originated in ancient India. It is based on the concept that energy, called *prana,* keeps the mind and body alive. Each of us is made up of five elements: air, water, earth, fire and space. These five elements are organized into three constitutional states called *doshas* that govern our physical, mental and emotional processes. These doshas are *vata,* representing space and air; *pitta,* for fire and water; and *kapha,* encompassing water and earth. Each of us is a combination of all three doshas, but usually one of them dominates.

Ayurvedic practitioners observe, ask questions about your lifestyle, spirituality and physical health, touch you and take pulses at different places to determine the diagnosis and assess the status of your doshas, depending upon which elements are out of balance. You are then further categorized based on dietary changes needed to rebalance your doshas.

Most Ayurvedic remedies are diet based, using foods, herbs and spices to regain balance by strengthening or weakening the doshas. In addition, other remedies and behavioral changes, such as minerals, gems, yoga postures and breathing, meditation, detoxification processes, or hydrotherapy and massages, may be advised to reestablish the elements.

Research studies examining the effects of Ayurvedic techniques on specific disorders show positive results in reducing the risk of coronary heart disease by lowering blood cholesterol and in achieving better blood glucose control in diabetic patients. Look for practitioners with a Bachelor of Ayurvedic Medicine and Surgery (BAMS), which is a medical school degree of five and a half years from India. For more information, contact The Ayurvedic Institute, 11311 Menaul NE, Suite A, Albuquerque, NM 87112; (505) 291-9698.

Bodywork

Bodywork is a catchall term for many different techniques that treat ailments and promote relaxation through proper movement, posture, exercise, massage and other body manipulations. Interestingly, many bodywork techniques were developed by people in other professions who were seeking relief from their own ailments. Some common techniques include Feldenkrais work, Shiatsu, Rolfing and massage.

Feldenkrais work, developed by a physicist with a knee injury, is a system of movements, floor exercises and bodywork to retrain your nervous system to work around damaged or blocked areas. It is sometimes recommended in place of physical therapy.

Shiatsu, a traditional healing method from Japan, uses a form of acupressure, finger pressure on specific body sites to increase circulation and improve energy flow. The technique involves locating acupoints, sites on your body specific to certain tissues. Pressure is applied to these points for two to ten minutes until a pulse is felt, then the pressure is released slowly. Acupressure techniques can be used in physical therapy and in various types of bodywork and massage.

Rolfing, developed by Ida Rolf, a biochemist with a desire to cure her own spine curvature, is a more vigorous and sometimes painful bodywork technique aimed at restructuring muscles and improving posture. Rolfing works on releasing tension and chronic pain in deep tissues, thus allowing your misaligned body to return to a more aligned state.

Massage is a system of manipulation of soft tissues to relieve sore muscles and promote relaxation. It is used to reduce tension, improve circulation, aid in healing injured soft tissues, control pain and promote overall well-being. Massage can stretch tissue, increase your range of motion and reduce certain kinds of swelling.

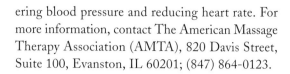

There are more than a hundred different massage therapy methods born out of many cultures, all with one universal element: touch. Studies have shown we all respond positively to touch. There is documented scientific evidence that healing occurs faster and our length of hospital stay is decreased when a caring touch, as in massage, is employed. Research has demonstrated that massage can be effective in reducing stress, lowering blood pressure and reducing heart rate. For more information, contact The American Massage Therapy Association (AMTA), 820 Davis Street, Suite 100, Evanston, IL 60201; (847) 864-0123.

Chiropractic

Chiropractic manipulation, or adjustment of bones, joints, spine, muscles and ligaments, is used to improve posture and reduce pain, particularly low back pain. Chiropractors may use X rays to diagnose problems and to develop treatment plans, but no drugs or medications are prescribed. Chiropractic therapy focuses mainly on mechanical problems, such as spinal alignment and adjustment, and today it is less likely to be sought for curing disease, such as cancer or diabetes, in place of other therapies where medical expertise is required.

Seek a Licensed Doctor of Chiropractic (D.C.) who has passed the National Board of Chiropractic Examiners exam. For more information, contact the American Chiropractic Association, 1701 Clarendon Boulevard, Arlington, VA 22209; (800) 986-4636.

Herbal Medicine

Herbs come from plant materials, mainly leaves, stems, flowers, twigs, roots, seeds, bark, fruit and saps of a variety of different plants. We typically think of herbs as substances that impart flavor to our foods, but some of these herbs have medicine-like qualities.

Many modern medicines, in fact, are derived from plants discovered long ago to have medical properties. An example is digitalis (digoxin), a drug derived from the foxglove plant, now a common treatment for congestive heart failure. Though herbs may be predecessors to modern medicines, they are not regulated by the Food and Drug Administration (FDA) as are conventional over-the-counter and prescription medicines, so purity may be suspect and testing may be minimal.

Herbs and Their Uses

Herb Name	Common Uses
Aloe (*Aloe barbadensis*)	Relieves minor burns, skin infections, irritations. Improves digestion.
Cayenne (*Capsicum annuum*)	Stimulates heart and improves circulation. Improves digestion.
Echinacea (*Echinacea angustifolia*)	Boosts immune system. Aids bladder infections.
Feverfew (*Tanacetum parthenium*)	Helps with migraine headaches.
Garlic (*Allium sativum*)	Relieves colds, coughs. Helps to alleviate high blood pressure. Reduces blood cholesterol and lipids.
Ginger (*Zingiber officinale*)	Relieves motion sickness. Alleviates menstrual cramps. Soothes minor burns.
Ginkgo (*Ginkgo biloba*)	Improves vascular disease by dilating blood vessels. Treats asthma.
Ginseng, Asian (*Panax ginseng*)	Boosts immune system. Reduces stress, fatigue.
Ginseng, Siberian (*Eleutherococcus senticosus*)	Helps with depression. Reduces fatigue. Relieves colds and flu. Reduces inflammation.
Green tea	Acts as an anticarcinogen.
Kava (*Piper methysticum*)	Relieves anxiety, insomnia, stress.
Licorice (*Glycyrrhiza glabra*)	Reduces inflammation. Aids in fighting viral infections. Improves digestion.
Peppermint (*Mentha piperita*)	Relieves stomach pain, nausea.
Psyllium (*Plantago psyllium*)	Relieves constipation, diarrhea, Helps reduce blood cholesterol.
St. John's wort (*Hypericum perforatum*)	Heals cuts, scrapes, wounds. Helps with depression.
Valerian (*Valeriana officinalis*)	Relieves insomnia, anxiety, nervousness, intestinal pain.

You can buy herbal remedies in the form of capsules, tablets, powders or concentrated liquids (called tinctures or extracts), or they can be prepared using fresh or dried ingredients or can be steeped or infused as in making a tea. Experts suggest you purchase prepared herbal medicines from reliable sources because those grown or concocted yourself may be inconsistent or may contain natural variations that can be toxic.

Because some herbs can be toxic or carcinogenic or can cause allergic reactions, they should be used with care and caution. Trained professionals in the fields of botany, Ayurvedic medicine, naturopathy and traditional Chinese medicine can be helpful in selecting the herbs, the form and potency that are appropriate for you and your ailment.

Herbal medicines are usually milder and may act more slowly than conventional medicines. However, certain herbs, such as borage, chaparral, coltsfoot, comfrey, Ma Huang (ephedra), germanium and yohimbe should not be used because they are potentially harmful, causing liver disease, rises in blood pressure and kidney damage. If you're pregnant or lactating, you may want to skip herbal medicines entirely. Some herbs may interact with your medications. Check with your doctor. See page 43 for some common medical herbs and their uses.

Myth

If you want to be a vegetarian, you have to eat certain foods in combination with other foods to get enough protein.

Truth

That used to be the party line. In the past, if you were vegetarian, you were schooled on how to form a complete protein by combining foods that had certain amino acids with foods containing complementary amino acids, such as combining rice with beans. Newer research shows that as long as you eat a variety of foods from the grain, vegetable, nut and legume groups, you will more than likely get plenty of protein. The amino acids you get from these various foods form a "pool" in your body from which complete proteins can be made.

Most vegetarians tend to eat some animal foods, such as milk products or fish. Animal foods are complete proteins and can therefore supplement the missing amino acids in the plant foods you eat.

Homeopathy

The basis for homeopathy is to use natural remedies to strengthen your body's "life energy" and eliminate symptoms of illness based on a principle of "like cures like." If you have a specific illness, a homeopathic doctor will give you a small amount of a remedy that will cause symptoms similar to your present illness to jolt your immune system into action.

Homeopathic remedies are extracted from natural substances, such as herbs, animal products and minerals. These extractions are "potentized," or taken through a series of dilutions and rapid shakings to achieve the correct potency, or strength. The final remedy is made into a tablet that is taken by mouth. Homeopathic remedies are manufactured by drug companies and are regulated by the FDA.

Because everyone responds differently to homeopathic cures, some amount of trial and error, or monitoring of symptoms and progress, by the administering homeopath is required. Symptoms often worsen first or move throughout the body from one organ or tissue to another before the cure is effective. Choose a practitioner who has a Diplomate in Homeotherapeutics (DHt). For more information, contact The National Center for Homeopathy, 801 North Fairfax Street, Suite 306, Alexandria, VA 22314; (703) 548-7790.

Laughter

We've included laughter in this section as, well, comic relief. Seriously though, studies have shown that laughter, particularly the kind that makes your whole body shake, can promote better blood circulation and lower blood pressure and release endorphins, the chemicals in the brain that relieve pain and have a calming effect. Keeping your spirits up and having a smile on your face make it easier to deal with the stresses and strains of the world around you. Laughing to promote health is easy to overlook, yet it is so simple to do.

Meditation

Quiet forms of contemplation, mindfulness or meditation have been recognized worldwide for their effectiveness at establishing a sense of peacefulness, inner calm and relaxation. Developed in Eastern cultures, most techniques require closing your eyes and focusing on a single thought, word, image or sound and allowing other thoughts to float away.

Traditionally used as a spiritual exercise, meditative forms have been helpful for people with chronic pain, post-traumatic stress disorder, panic attacks, high blood pressure and respiratory problems, such as asthma and emphysema, because meditation slows heart rate and regulates breathing. For more information, contact the Insight Meditation Society, 1230 Pleasant Street, Barre, MA 01005; (978) 355-4378.

Naturopathy

Naturopathy originates from the traditions of early European health spas. Emphasizing preventive care, naturopathy takes advantage of your body's own natural healing powers. It avoids many of the traditions of conventional medicine, such as drugs and surgery, and teaches healthy lifestyle habits. Naturopathic treatments vary by practitioner and encompass many elements, such as massage, physical activity, herbal remedies, natural foods, acupuncture and hydrotherapy (internal and external water treatments).

Potential Benefits of Phytochemicals

PHYTOCHEMICAL	BENEFIT	FOOD SOURCES
Allyl sulfides	Lowers risk of stomach and colon cancers	Chives, garlic, leeks, onions, shallots
Alpha-linolenic acid and Vitamin E	Reduces inflammation from exercise-related muscle damage and lowers risk of heart disease	Vegetable oils, margarine
Beta-carotene and Vitamin A	Lowers risk of lung, stomach and prostate cancers. Acts as antioxidant to reduce cancer risk	Apricots, broccoli, cantaloupe, carrots, papaya, peaches, spinach, sweet potatoes, winter squash
Flavonoids	Acts as antioxidant to reduce cancer risk	Citrus fruits, berries, tomatoes, radishes
Genistein and isoflavones	Lowers buildup of fatty plaques in arteries	Soy foods; e.g., tempeh, tofu, soybeans, soy milk
Indoles, Iso-thiocyanates and Sulphoraphanes	Lowers risk of breast, lung and stomach cancers	Broccoli, Brussels sprouts, cabbage, cauliflower, mustard greens, rutabaga, turnips
Lycopene	Lowers risk of prostate and stomach cancers	Tomatoes
Monoterpenes	Lowers risk of breast, skin, liver, lung, stomach and pancreatic cancers	Caraway seed, cherries, dill weed, lemongrass, spearmint
Vitamin C	Lowers risk of esophageal, larynx, pancreatic, stomach, rectal, breast and cervical cancers	Citrus fruits, broccoli, green bell peppers, tomatoes, strawberries

Naturopathy is one of the smaller therapies in terms of the number of practitioners, and it is more widely practiced on the West Coast. For more information, contact the American Association of Naturopathic Physicians, 601 Valley Street, Suite 105, Seattle, WA 98109; (877) 969-2267.

Osteopathy

Osteopathic manipulative therapy (OMT), a system of healing the whole body, originally focused on manipulation of muscles, ligaments, joints and bones, postural positions and exercises, and it now incorporates the use of drugs and surgery to diagnose and treat all ailments. Today, there is little difference between the schooling of conventional medical doctors (M.D.s) and Doctors of Osteopathic Medicine (D.O.s).

Osteopathy has been effective for treating back and neck pain, headaches and temporomandibular joint syndrome (TMJ). Osteopaths tend to be less vigorous than chiropractors in their assessments and manipulations, and they generally have a better understanding of internal body physiology because of their medical training.

Craniosacral therapy, a form of OMT that focuses on correcting stresses to the brain and spinal cord, may be of some benefit to potentially chronic conditions such as earaches, migraine headaches, sleep disorders and asthma in children and adults. In addition, craniosacral therapy can be effective as a means to help process and heal from emotional traumas and post-traumatic stress disorder.

Seek practitioners who have a D.O. degree and training. For more information, contact the American Osteopathic Association, 142 East Ontario Street, Chicago, IL 60611; (800) 621-1773, ext. 8252.

Phytochemicals

Phytochemicals (literally, "plant chemicals") is an umbrella term for many different substances found in plant foods. Found primarily in fruits and vegetables, phytochemicals show promising disease-fighting benefits, according to scientific research. Scientists have identified nearly three thousand different phytochemicals and believe there are thousands more to uncover. You can get an assortment of phytochemicals—all of which may lower your risk for disease—by eating the whole food and a variety of foods, particularly fruits, vegetables and soy foods. On page 45, you'll find a list of some phytochemicals and their potential benefits.

Yoga

Yoga is an ancient practice and philosophy first developed and practiced in India. The word *yoga* is derived from the ancient Sanskrit word *yuj*, meaning "union." Yoga is based on balancing the mind, body and spirit, using exercises, ethical beliefs and dietary restrictions.

Many different types of yoga are practiced worldwide. Western versions of yoga typically practiced in the United States include both body positions and movements, called *postures*, and breathing exercises, in addition to dietary practices. The postures, called *asanas*, are used to stretch and strengthen muscles; the breathing exercises, called *pranayama*, help with relaxation and stress relief. Yoga experts advise that you start slowly with basic breathing techniques and simple postures before moving on to the more advanced exercises that could cause injury if done incorrectly. For more information, contact The American Yoga Association, P.O. Box 19986, Sarasota, FL 34276; (941) 927-4977.

As you can see, there is a wide variety of complementary therapies from different parts of the world that focus on different principles. All are available to you as you make the connection between your mind and body and wellness. Be sure to check with your doctor if you have any questions about your conventional medication or treatment plan or one of these complementary therapies. Here's to wellness!

REFERENCES

"Alternative Medicine." *Prevention,* February 1998.

Alternative Medicine: Expanding Medical Horizons. A Report to the National Institutes of Health on Alternative Medical Systems and Practices in the United States. Washington, D.C.: U.S. Government Printing Office, 1995.

American Cancer Society. *Cancer Facts and Figures 1997.* Atlanta: American Cancer Society, 1997.

American Council on Science and Health. "High Blood Pressure: A Silent Killer, Hypertension." New York, June 1989.

Balch, James F., and Phyllis Balch. *Prescription for Nutritional Healing.* New York: Avery Publishing Group, 1997.

Collinge, William. *The American Holistic Health Association Complete Guide to Alternative Medicine.* New York: Warner Books, 1996.

"Complementary Medicine: Finding a Balance." *Journal of American Dietetic Association,* December 1997.

Eckel, Robert H. "Obesity and Heart Disease." *Circulation,* 96: 1997.

General Mills Dietary Intake Study 1990–1992. Minneapolis: General Mills, 1992.

Larson, David E., ed. *Mayo Clinic Family Health Book.* 2d ed. New York: William Morrow and Company, 1996.

Levinson, David, and Laura Gaccione. *Health and Illness: A Cross-Cultural Encyclopedia.* Santa Barbara, Calif.: ABC-CLIO, 1997.

Mills, Simon, and Steven T. Finando. *Alternatives in Healing.* New York: New American Library, 1989.

Murray, Michael. *The Healing Power of Herbs.* Rocklin, Calif.: Prima Publishing, 1995.

National Academy of Sciences. *Dietary Reference Intakes for Calcium,* 1997.

National Dairy Council. *Calcium: A Summary of Current Research for the Health Professional.* Rosemont, Illinois: National Dairy Council, 1987.

———. "Diet and Cancer Prevention," *Dairy Council Digest,* January–February, 1991.

National Heart, Lung and Blood Institute. *Report of the Expert Panel on Detection, Evaluation and Treatment High Blood Cholesterol in Adults.* NIH Publication No. 88-2925. Washington, D.C.: U.S. Government Printing Office, 1988.

National Research Council. *Diet and Health: Implications for Reducing Chronic Disease Risk.* Washington, D.C.: National Academy Press, 1989.

———. *Recommended Dietary Allowances.* 10th ed. Washington, D.C.: National Academy Press, 1989.

Nattiv, Aurelia. "Osteoporosis: Its Prevention, Recognition and Management." *Family Practice Recertification* 20, no. 2 (February 1998).

"Position of the American Dietetic Association: Health Implications of Dietary Fiber." *Journal of American Dietetic Association,* December 1993.

"Position of the American Dietetic Association and the Canadian Dietetic Association: Nutrition for Physical Fitness and Athletic Performance for Adults." *Journal of American Dietetic Association,* June 1993.

Time-Life Books. *The Alternative Advisor.* Alexandria, Va.: Time–Life Books, 1997.

Tyler, Varro E. *Herbs of Choice.* New York: Pharmaceutical Products Press, 1994.

———. *The Honest Herbal.* New York: Pharmaceutical Products Press, 1993.

U.S. Department of Agriculture, and U.S. Department of Health and Human Services. *Nutrition and Your Health: Dietary Guidelines for Americans.* Home and Garden Bulletin No. 232. Washington, D.C.: U.S. Government Printing Office, 1995.

U.S. Department of Health and Human Services. *Healthy People 2000, National Health Promotion and Disease Prevention Objectives.* DHHS Publication No. (PHS) 91-50212. Washington, D.C.: U.S. Government Printing Office, 1990.

———. *The Surgeon General's Report on Nutrition and Health.* Washington, D.C.: U.S. Government Printing Office, 1988.

———. National Heart, Lung and Blood Institute; and National Institutes of Health. *The Right Moves.* Bethesda, Maryland: U.S. Department of Health and Human Services, 1990.

Warshaw, Hope. *The Restaurant Companion.* Chicago: Surrey Books, 1995.

Weil, Andrew. *Spontaneous Healing.* New York: Fawcett Columbine, 1995.

World Cancer Research Fund, and American Institute for Cancer Research. *Food, Nutrition and the Prevention of Cancer: A Global Perspective.* Washington, D.C.: American Institute for Cancer Research, 1997.

Ziegler, E. E., and L. J. Filer, eds. *Present Knowledge in Nutrition.* 7th ed. Washington, D.C.: International Life Sciences Institute Press, 1996.

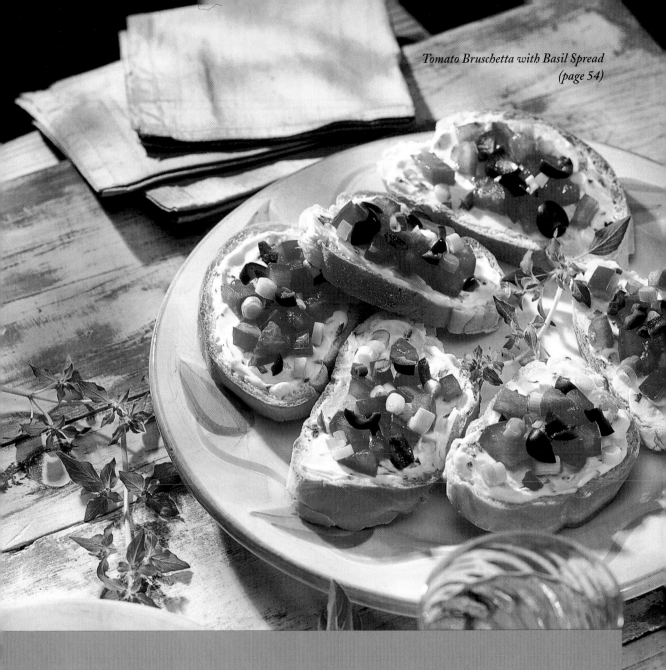

Tomato Bruschetta with Basil Spread
(page 54)

APPETIZERS, SNACKS AND SMOOTHIES

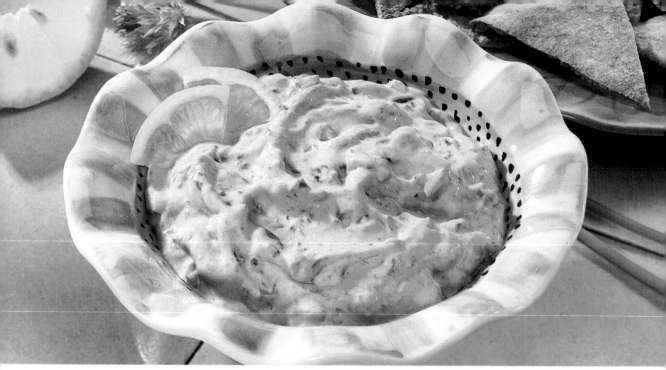

Sun-Dried Tomato Dip with Baked Pita Chips (page 61)

Sun-Dried Tomato Dip

LO CAL / LO FAT / LO CHOL / LO SODIUM

PREP: 20 MIN; CHILL: 2 HR

ABOUT 1½ CUPS DIP

8   sun-dried tomato halves (not oil-packed)

¼   cup chopped fresh parsley

1   tablespoon chopped fresh or 1 teaspoon freeze-dried chives

1   tablespoon olive or vegetable oil

2   teaspoons lemon juice

1   teaspoon red wine vinegar

½   teaspoon salt

½   teaspoon pepper

1   clove garlic, finely chopped

¾   cup plain fat-free yogurt

¾   cup reduced-fat sour cream

Place tomato halves in 1 inch water in 1-quart saucepan. Heat to boiling; reduce heat to medium. Simmer uncovered about 5 minutes or until water has evaporated.

Place tomatoes and remaining ingredients except yogurt and sour cream in blender or food processor. Cover and blend on medium speed until smooth.

Pour tomato mixture into medium glass or plastic bowl. Stir in yogurt and sour cream. Cover and refrigerate about 2 hours or until chilled.

1 Tablespoon: Calories 20 (Calories from Fat 10); Fat 1g (Saturated 0g); Cholesterol 5mg; Sodium 75mg; Carbohydrate 2g (Dietary Fiber 0g); Protein 1g
% Daily Value: Vitamin A 2%; Vitamin C 0%; Calcium 2%; Iron 0%
Diet Exchanges: free food

Almost Guacamole

LO CAL / LO FAT / LO CHOL / LO SODIUM

PREP: 10 MIN; CHILL: 1 HR

ABOUT 2 CUPS DIP

Lime and lemon juice, which are naturally acidic, help preserve the bright green color of this dip. And you can eat all you want—this dip does not have the high fat content of regular guacamole.

1	can (15 ounces) asparagus cuts, drained
1	large tomato, seeded and chopped (1 cup)
1	medium onion, chopped (1/2 cup)
1	clove garlic, finely chopped
2	tablespoons finely chopped fresh cilantro
2	tablespoons reduced-fat mayonnaise or salad dressing
1	tablespoon lime or lemon juice
3 to 6	drops red pepper sauce
	Dash of pepper
	Baked Tortilla Chips (page 62) or reduced-fat tortilla chips, if desired

Place asparagus in blender or food processor. Cover and blend on medium speed until smooth.

Mix asparagus and remaining ingredients except Baked Tortilla Chips. Cover and refrigerate at least 1 hour to blend flavors. Serve with tortilla chips.

1 Tablespoon: Calories 5 (Calories from Fat 0); Fat 0g (Saturated 0g); Cholesterol 0mg; Sodium 50mg; Carbohydrate 1g (Dietary Fiber 0g); Protein 0g
% Daily Value: Vitamin A 0%; Vitamin C 6%; Calcium 0%; Iron 0%
Diet Exchanges: free food

Easy Tuna Spread

LO CAL / LO FAT / LO CHOL / LO SODIUM

PREP: 10 MIN; CHILL: 2 HR

ABOUT 2 CUPS SPREAD

Try spreading this on a toasted bagel half and topping with sliced tomatoes and alfalfa spouts for a quick afternoon snack or a light lunch.

1	cup fat-free ricotta cheese
2	tablespoons chopped fresh or 2 teaspoons dried basil leaves
2	tablespoons lemon juice
2	tablespoons reduced-fat sour cream
1	can (12 ounces) white tuna in water, drained

Place all ingredients in blender or food processor. Cover and blend on medium speed until smooth.

Line 2-cup metal bowl or mold with plastic wrap. Place mixture in bowl. Cover and refrigerate about 2 hours or until set. Carefully unmold onto serving plate.

1 Tablespoon: Calories 20 (Calories from Fat 0); Fat 0g (Saturated 0g); Cholesterol 5mg; Sodium 40mg; Carbohydrate 1g (Dietary Fiber 0g); Protein 4g
% Daily Value: Vitamin A 0%; Vitamin C 0%; Calcium 2%; Iron 0%
Diet Exchanges: free food

Mushroom Pita Pizzas

LO CAL / LO FAT / LO CHOL

PREP: 10 MIN; BAKE: 10 MIN

8 SERVINGS (4 WEDGES EACH)

Choose sliced shiitake mushrooms to give these pizzas a slightly "earthy" flavor.

- 2 pita breads (6 inches in diameter)
- 2 cups sliced mushrooms (6 ounces)
- 1 small red onion, thinly sliced
- 1/4 cup chopped green bell pepper
- 2 tablespoons chopped fresh or 2 teaspoons dried basil leaves
- 1 cup finely shredded reduced-fat mozzarella cheese (4 ounces)
- 1 tablespoon grated Parmesan cheese

Heat oven to 425°. Split each pita bread around edge with knife to make 2 rounds. Place rounds, cut sides up, on ungreased cookie sheet.

Top rounds with mushrooms, onion and bell pepper. Sprinkle with basil and cheeses. Bake 8 to 10 minutes or until cheese is melted. Cut each round into 8 wedges.

1 Serving: Calories 80 (Calories from Fat 20); Fat 2g (Saturated 1g); Cholesterol 0mg; Sodium 190mg; Carbohydrate 14g (Dietary Fiber 1g); Protein 3g
% Daily Value: Vitamin A 6%; Vitamin C 2%; Calcium 10%; Iron 4%
Diet Exchanges: 1 starch

Three-Cheese Pizza Snacks

LO CAL / LO FAT / LO CHOL / LO SODIUM

PREP: 15 MIN; BAKE: 11 MIN

8 SERVINGS (1 SNACK EACH)

For a heartier snack idea, use toasted French bread slices or bagel halves instead of the crackers.

- 1/4 cup fat-free ricotta cheese
- 1/4 teaspoon Italian seasoning
- 1 clove garlic, finely chopped
- 8 crispy rye crackers (any flavor)
- 2 tablespoons shredded reduced-fat mozzarella cheese
- 1 1/2 tablespoons shredded Parmesan cheese
- 1 medium roma (plum) tomato, thinly sliced and slices cut in half
- **Dash of pepper**

Heat oven to 375°. Mix ricotta cheese, Italian seasoning and garlic; spread on crackers. Sprinkle with mozzarella and Parmesan cheeses. Place 2 tomato slice halves on each cracker. Sprinkle with pepper.

Place crackers on ungreased cookie sheet. Bake 9 to 11 minutes or until cheese is melted and begins to turn golden brown.

1 Serving: Calories 60 (Calories from Fat 10); Fat 1g (Saturated 1g); Cholesterol 2mg; Sodium 95mg; Carbohydrate 10g (Dietary Fiber 0g); Protein 3g
% Daily Value: Vitamin A 2%; Vitamin C 2%; Calcium 4%; Iron 4%
Diet Exchanges: 1/2 starch

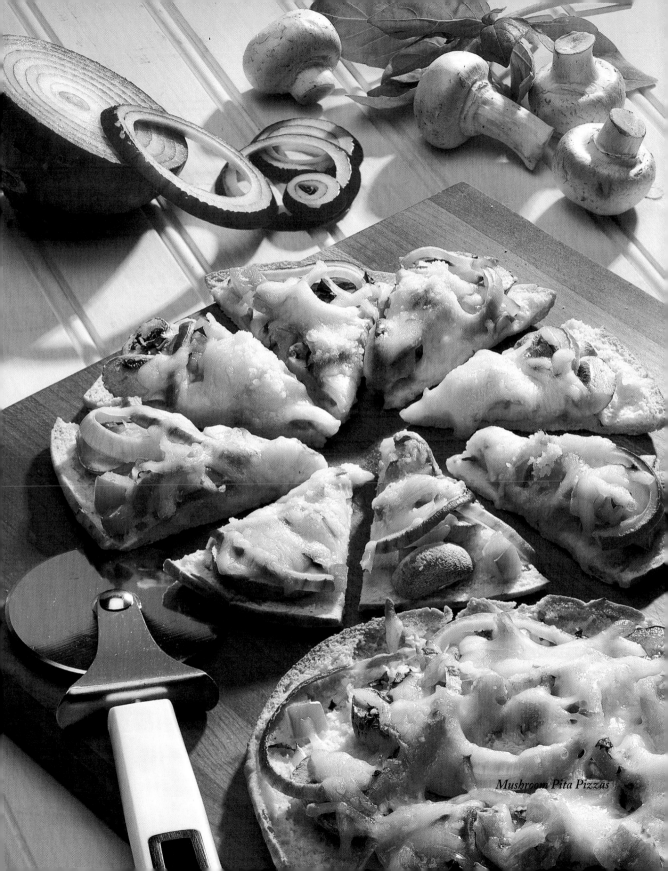

Mushroom Pita Pizzas

Gorgonzola and Caramelized Onion Appetizer

LO CAL / LO CHOL

PREP: 10 MIN; COOK: 25 MIN; BROIL: 3 MIN

4 SERVINGS (2 SLICES EACH)

Using Gorgonzola cheese here will help you cut down on fat, but not on flavor. Gorgonzola has a strong and slightly pungent flavor, so you need only a small amount to make a big flavor impact.

- 2 tablespoons margarine
- 2 medium onions, sliced and separated into rings
- 1 tablespoon packed brown sugar
- 1/2 teaspoon balsamic or red wine vinegar
- 8 slices baguette, 1/2 inch thick
- 2 tablespoons crumbled Gorgonzola cheese

Melt margarine in 10-inch nonstick skillet over medium heat. Cook onions, brown sugar and vinegar in margarine about 25 minutes, stirring frequently, until onions are golden brown.

Set oven control to broil. Place baguette slices on cookie sheet. Broil with tops 2 to 3 inches from heat 1 to 2 minutes or until lightly toasted. Spoon caramelized onions evenly onto each slice. Sprinkle with cheese. Broil about 1 minute or until cheese is melted.

1 Serving: Calories 145 (Calories from Fat 45); Fat 5g (Saturated 2g); Cholesterol 5mg; Sodium 310mg; Carbohydrate 23g (Dietary Fiber 2g); Protein 4g
% Daily Value: Vitamin A 8%; Vitamin C 2%; Calcium 6%; Iron 6%
Diet Exchanges: 1 1/2 starch, 1 fat

Tomato Bruschetta with Basil Spread

LO CAL / LO CHOL

PREP: 15 MIN; BROIL: 3 MIN

6 SERVINGS (2 SLICES EACH)

This appealing appetizer takes the classic bruschetta to new heights. Instead of a toasted bread brushed with olive oil and garnished with a simple topping or two, these savory treats are spread with reduced-fat cream cheese and topped with chopped tomato, green onion and ripe olives. Throw in a simple bean soup, and you might just want to make this dinner (photo, page 49)!

- 12 slices French bread, 1/2 inch thick
- 1/2 package (8-ounce size) reduced-fat cream cheese (Neufchâtel), softened
- 1 tablespoon chopped fresh or 1 teaspoon dried basil or oregano leaves
- 1 small tomato, chopped (1/2 cup)
- 1 medium green onion, sliced (2 tablespoons)
- 1 tablespoon chopped ripe olives

Set oven control to broil. Place bread slices on cookie sheet. Broil with tops 3 to 4 inches from heat 1 to 2 minutes or until lightly toasted.

Mix cream cheese and basil; spread on untoasted sides of bread slices. Broil about 1 minute or until cheese mixture is melted. Top with tomato, onion and olives.

1 Serving: Calories 180 (Calories from Fat 55); Fat 6g (Saturated 3g); Cholesterol 15mg; Sodium 380mg; Carbohydrate 27g (Dietary Fiber 2g); Protein 6g
% Daily Value: Vitamin A 6%; Vitamin C 6%; Calcium 6%; Iron 8%
Diet Exchanges: 2 starch, 1 fat

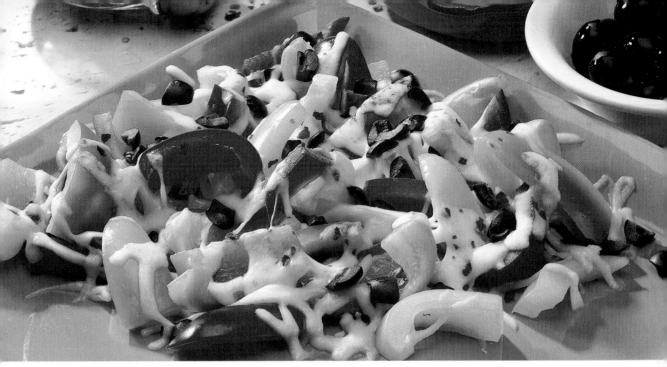

Bell Pepper Nachos

Bell Pepper Nachos

LO CAL / LO FAT / LO CHOL / LO SODIUM

PREP: 10 MIN; BROIL: 3 MIN

6 SERVINGS

Adding a tablespoon of chopped jalapeño chilies will bring some heat to this colorful appetizer without adding calories.

$1/2$	green bell pepper, seeded and cut into 6 strips
$1/2$	red bell pepper, seeded and cut into 6 strips
$1/2$	yellow bell pepper, seeded and cut into 6 strips
$3/4$	cup shredded reduced-fat Monterey Jack cheese (3 ounces)
2	tablespoons chopped ripe olives
$1/4$	teaspoon crushed red pepper

Cut bell pepper strips crosswise in half. Arrange close together in ungreased broilerproof pie pan, $9 \times 1^{1}/_{4}$ inches, or ovenproof serving dish. Sprinkle with cheese, olives and red pepper.

Set oven control to broil. Broil peppers with tops 3 to 4 inches from heat about 3 minutes or until cheese is melted.

1 Serving: Calories 60 (Calories from Fat 25); Fat 3g (Saturated 2g); Cholesterol 10mg; Sodium 135mg; Carbohydrate 3g (Dietary Fiber 0g); Protein 5g
% Daily Value: Vitamin A 10%; Vitamin C 38%; Calcium 12%; Iron 2%
Diet Exchanges: $1/2$ lean meat, 1 vegetable

Phyllo Egg Rolls

LO CAL / LO FAT / LO CHOL

PREP: 35 MIN; BAKE: 20 MIN

18 SERVINGS (1 EGG ROLL EACH)

To prevent phyllo sheets from becoming dry and brittle, keep them in their wrapping until you have prepared the turkey filling.

1	pound ground turkey breast
4	cups coleslaw mix
3	tablespoons reduced-sodium soy sauce
1	teaspoon grated gingerroot
½	teaspoon five-spice powder
1	small onion, chopped (¼ cup)
2	cloves garlic, finely chopped
18	frozen (thawed) phyllo sheets (16 × 12 inches)
	Cooking spray

Heat oven to 350°. Cook turkey in 10-inch non-stick skillet over medium-high heat, stirring occasionally, until no longer pink; drain. Stir in remaining ingredients except phyllo sheets and cooking spray. Cook 2 to 3 minutes, stirring occasionally, until coleslaw mix is wilted; remove from heat.

Unroll phyllo sheets; cover sheets with waxed paper, then with damp towel to prevent them from drying out. Place 1 phyllo sheet on cutting board; spray with cooking spray. Repeat with 2 more phyllo sheets to make stack of 3 sheets. Cut stack of phyllo sheets crosswise into thirds to make 3 rectangles, about 12 × 5 inches.

Spray cookie sheet with cooking spray. Place ¼ cup turkey mixture on short end of each rectangle; roll up, folding in edges of phyllo. Place roll, seam side down, on cookie sheet. Repeat with remaining phyllo and turkey mixture. Spray rolls with cooking spray. Bake 15 to 20 minutes or until light golden brown. Serve warm.

1 Serving: Calories 95 (Calories from Fat 10); Fat 1g (Saturated 0g); Cholesterol 15mg; Sodium 190mg; Carbohydrate 15g (Dietary Fiber 1g); Protein 8g
% Daily Value: Vitamin A 0%; Vitamin C 4%; Calcium 2%; Iron 6%
Diet Exchanges: 1 starch

Caramelized Onion Tartlets

LO CAL / LO FAT / LO CHOL / LO SODIUM

PREP: 1½ HR; BAKE: 8 MIN

20 SERVINGS (2 TARTLETS EACH)

Chopping an onion is easy if you first cut the onion in half from the top to the root. Place each half cut side down, and cut into lengthwise slices. Finally, cut the slices crosswise into desired piece size.

Phyllo Tartlets (right)

9   large onions, chopped (9 cups)

1¼   cups beef broth

¼   teaspoon pepper

2   slices turkey bacon, cooked and chopped

1½   cups grated Parmesan cheese

Prepare Phyllo Tartlets. Cook remaining ingredients except cheese in 10-inch nonstick skillet over medium heat 20 minutes, stirring occasionally; reduce heat to medium-low. Cook uncovered about 50 minutes, stirring occasionally, until all liquid is absorbed and onions are consistency of marmalade.

Heat oven to 400°. Fill each tartlet with 2 teaspoons onion mixture. Place on ungreased cookie sheet. Sprinkle tartlets with cheese. Bake 6 to 8 minutes or until cheese is light brown. Serve hot.

Phyllo Tartlets

¼   cup apple juice

2   tablespoons margarine

4   frozen (thawed) phyllo sheets (13 × 9 inches)

Heat oven to 400°. Heat apple juice and margarine in 6-inch nonstick skillet over low heat, stirring occasionally, until margarine is melted.

Brush one phyllo sheet at a time with apple juice mixture. (Keep remaining phyllo sheets covered with waxed paper or a damp towel to prevent them from drying out.) Fold each sheet crosswise into thirds, overlapping; cut lengthwise in half, then cut crosswise to make 10 pieces.

Place pieces in ungreased small muffin cups, 1¾ × 1 inch, making pleats as necessary to fit into cups. Bake 5 to 7 minutes or until golden brown. Remove from pan. Cool on wire rack.

1 Serving: Calories 50 (Calories from Fat 20); Fat 2g (Saturated 0g); Cholesterol 0mg; Sodium 130mg; Carbohydrate 8g (Dietary Fiber 2g); Protein 2g
% Daily Value: Vitamin A 0%; Vitamin C 2%; Calcium 2%; Iron 0%
Diet Exchanges: 2 vegetable

Cheesy Ranch Potato Skins

LO CAL / LO FAT / LO CHOL / LO SODIUM

PREP: 10 MIN; BROIL: 5½ MIN

4 SERVINGS (2 POTATO SKINS EACH)

To enjoy these crispy skins in just minutes, start with leftover baked potatoes or bake the potatoes in your microwave oven. Then set up a "potato bar," let your guests choose the toppings they like best and pop the potato skins into the oven to heat.

2	medium unpeeled baking potatoes, baked*
	Butter-flavored cooking spray
	Garlic powder
¼	cup finely chopped cooked chicken or turkey
¼	cup shredded reduced-fat Cheddar cheese
2	tablespoons imitation bacon-flavor bits
	Reduced-calorie ranch dressing, if desired

Cut potatoes lengthwise into fourths. Carefully scoop out pulp, leaving ¼-inch shells. Cover and refrigerate potato pulp for another use.

Set oven control to broil. Place potato shells, skin sides down, on rack in broiler pan. Spray with butter-flavored cooking spray. Sprinkle with garlic powder. Broil with tops 4 to 5 inches from heat about 5 minutes or until crisp and brown.

Sprinkle chicken and cheese over potato shells. Broil about 30 seconds or until cheese is melted. Sprinkle with bacon bits. Serve hot with ranch dressing.

Tex-Mex Potato Skins: Substitute fat-free refried beans for the chicken. Omit bacon-flavor bits. Sprinkle each potato skin with 1 tablespoon chopped green bell pepper and 1 tablespoon sliced green onion. Serve hot with reduced-fat sour cream and salsa.

*To "bake" potatoes in microwave oven, pierce potatoes with fork. Arrange potatoes about 1 inch apart in circle on microwavable paper towel. Microwave uncovered on High 8 to 10 minutes or until tender. To bake potatoes in conventional oven, pierce potatoes with fork. Bake in 375° oven 1 to 1½ hours or until tender. Let potatoes stand until cool enough to handle.

1 Serving: Calories 105 (Calories from Fat 20); Fat 2g (Saturated 1g); Cholesterol 10mg; Sodium 120mg; Carbohydrate 17g (Dietary Fiber 2g); Protein 7g
% Daily Value: Vitamin A 0%; Vitamin C 6%; Calcium 4%; Iron 6%
Diet Exchanges: 1 starch, ½ lean meat

Chicken Pot Stickers

LO CAL / LO FAT / LO CHOL

PREP: 1 HR; COOK: 40 MIN

16 SERVINGS (3 POT STICKERS EACH)

Look for round wonton skins in the produce section of your supermarket.

1½   pounds ground chicken

1   small red bell pepper, finely chopped
     (½ cup)

3   medium green onions, chopped
     (3 tablespoons)

½   cup shredded green cabbage

2   tablespoons fat-free cholesterol-free egg
     product or 1 egg white

2   teaspoons chopped gingerroot

1   teaspoon sesame or vegetable oil

¼   teaspoon white pepper

1   package (10 ounces) round wonton skins

2   cups chicken broth

4   teaspoons reduced-sodium soy sauce

Mix all ingredients except wonton skins, broth and soy sauce. Brush each wonton skin with water. Place 1 scant tablespoon chicken mixture on center of wonton skin. Pinch 5 pleats on one side of wonton circle. Fold circle in half over chicken mixture, pressing pleated edge to unpleated edge. Repeat with remaining wonton skins and chicken mixture.

Spray 12-inch nonstick skillet with cooking spray; heat over medium heat. Cook 12 pot stickers at a time in skillet about 3 minutes or until light brown; turn. Stir in ½ cup of the broth and 1 teaspoon of the soy sauce. Cover and cook 5 minutes. Uncover and cook 1 minute longer or until liquid has evaporated. Repeat with remaining pot stickers, broth and soy sauce.

1 Serving: Calories 115 (Calories from Fat 25); Fat 3g (Saturated 1g); Cholesterol 35mg; Sodium 220mg; Carbohydrate 11g (Dietary Fiber 0g); Protein 11g
% Daily Value: Vitamin A 4%; Vitamin C 8%; Calcium 0%; Iron 6%
Diet Exchanges: ½ starch, 1 lean meat

Stuffed Mushrooms

LO CAL / LO FAT / LO CHOL / LO SODIUM

PREP: 15 MIN; BAKE: 10 MIN

6 SERVINGS (2 MUSHROOMS EACH)

½   pound ground chicken

1   small onion, chopped (¼ cup)

1   clove garlic, finely chopped

2   tablespoons chopped fresh cilantro

3   tablespoons fat-free cholesterol-free egg
     product or 1 egg white

1   tablespoon Dijon mustard

1½   teaspoons finely chopped gingerroot

2   teaspoons reduced-sodium soy sauce

12   large white mushrooms (about 2½ inches
      in diameter), stems removed

Heat oven to 450°. Spray cookie sheet with cooking spray. Mix all ingredients except mushrooms. Fill mushroom caps with chicken mixture. Place mushrooms, filled sides up, on cookie sheet.

Bake 7 to 10 minutes or until tops are light brown and chicken is no longer pink. Serve hot.

1 Serving: Calories 70 (Calories from Fat 20); Fat 2g (Saturated 0g); Cholesterol 20mg; Sodium 130mg; Carbohydrate 4g (Dietary Fiber 0g); Protein 10g
% Daily Value: Vitamin A 0%; Vitamin C 0%; Calcium 0%; Iron 2%
Diet Exchanges: 1 lean meat

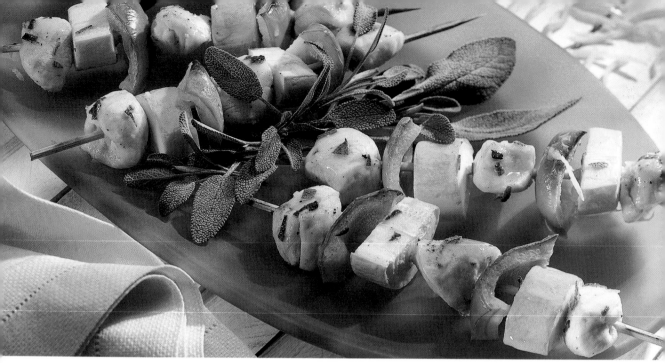

Maple-Glazed Chicken Kabobs

Maple-Glazed Chicken Kabobs

LO CAL / LO FAT / LO CHOL / LO SODIUM

PREP: 25 MIN; MARINATE: 4 HR; BROIL: 6 MIN

8 SERVINGS (1 KABOB EACH)

1/2   pound skinless, boneless chicken breast halves

3   tablespoons reduced-calorie maple-flavored syrup

2   tablespoons lemon juice

1   tablespoon margarine, melted

1 1/2   teaspoons chopped fresh or 1/2 teaspoon ground sage leaves

1   teaspoon grated lemon peel

1/4   teaspoon pepper

1   medium bell pepper, cut into 16 pieces

1   medium yellow summer squash, cut lengthwise in half, then cut crosswise into 16 pieces

Remove fat from chicken. Cut chicken into 24 pieces. Mix remaining ingredients except bell pepper and squash in large glass or plastic bowl. Stir in chicken, bell pepper and squash. Cover and refrigerate at least 4 hours but no longer than 24 hours.

Set oven control to broil. Thread chicken, bell pepper and squash alternately on each of eight 8-inch skewers.* Place on rack in broiler pan. Broil with tops 4 inches from heat 2 to 3 minutes; turn. Broil 2 to 3 minutes longer or until chicken is no longer pink in center.

*If using bamboo skewers, soak in water at least 30 minutes before using to prevent burning.

1 Serving: Calories 55 (Calories from Fat 20); Fat 2g (Saturated 1g); Cholesterol 15mg; Sodium 45mg; Carbohydrate 3g (Dietary Fiber 1g); Protein 7g
% Daily Value: Vitamin A 4%; Vitamin C 14%; Calcium 0%; Iron 2%
Diet Exchanges: 1 lean meat

Hot and Peppery Cocktail Shrimp

LO CAL / LO FAT / LO SODIUM

PREP: 20 MIN; CHILL: 4 HR; BAKE: 12 MIN

12 SERVINGS (5 SHRIMP EACH)

A little sesame oil goes a long way, but its strong and pungent flavor is perfect for these spicy shrimp. You could also serve this as a main dish. Just add a side of steamed or stir-fried veggies and hot cooked rice for a delicious dinner for six.

1½	pounds uncooked peeled deveined medium shrimp (about 60)
2	medium green onions, chopped (2 tablespoons)
2	cloves garlic, finely chopped
2	teaspoons grated lime peel
¼	cup lime juice
1	tablespoon reduced-sodium soy sauce
¼	teaspoons pepper
⅛	teaspoon crushed red pepper
2	teaspoons sesame oil

Mix all ingredients except oil in large glass or plastic bowl. Cover and refrigerate for 4 hours but no longer than 24 hours.

Heat oven to 400°. Spray rectangular pan, 13 × 9 × 2 inches, with cooking spray. Arrange shrimp in single layer in pan. Bake 10 to 12 minutes or until shrimp are pink and firm. Drizzle with oil. Serve hot.

1 Serving: Calories 50 (Calories from Fat 10); Fat 1g (Saturated 0g); Cholesterol 80mg; Sodium 140mg; Carbohydrate 1g (Dietary Fiber 0g); Protein 9g
% Daily Value: Vitamin A 2%; Vitamin C 2%; Calcium 2%; Iron 8%
Diet Exchanges: 1 very lean meat

Baked Pita Chips

LO CAL / LO FAT / LO CHOL

PREP: 5 MIN; BAKE: 9 MIN

8 SERVINGS (8 CHIPS EACH)

These pita chips are great for dunking into a bowl of hearty Spicy Chicken Chili (page 87), or to serve with your favorite dips (photo, page 50).

4	whole wheat pita breads (6 inches in diameter)

Heat oven to 400°. Split each pita bread around each edge with knife to make 2 rounds. Cut each round into 8 wedges. Place in single layer on 2 ungreased cookie sheets.

Bake about 9 minutes or until crisp and light brown; cool. Store in airtight container at room temperature.

1 Serving: Calories 85 (Calories from Fat 10); Fat 1g (Saturated 0g); Cholesterol 0mg; Sodium 170mg; Carbohydrate 18g (Dietary Fiber 2g); Protein 3g
% Daily Value: Vitamin A 0%; Vitamin C 0%; Calcium 0%; Iron 4%
Diet Exchanges: 1 starch

Baked Tortilla Chips

LO CAL / LO FAT / LO CHOL / LO SODIUM

PREP: 5 MIN; BAKE: 6 MIN

8 SERVINGS (8 CHIPS EACH)

Craving something sweet? Create a simple and delicious low-fat treat by spraying the tortillas lightly with butter-flavored cooking spray and sprinkling them with brown sugar and ground cinnamon before cutting into wedges.

8   corn tortillas (5 or 6 inches in diameter)

Heat oven to 450°. Spray 2 cookie sheets with cooking spray. Cut each tortilla into 8 wedges. Place in single layer on cookie sheets.

Bake about 6 minutes or until crisp but not brown; cool. Store in airtight container at room temperature.

1 Serving: Calories 50 (Calories from Fat 10); Fat 1g (Saturated 0g); Cholesterol 0mg; Sodium 35mg; Carbohydrate 10g (Dietary Fiber 1g); Protein 1g
% Daily Value: Vitamin A 0%; Vitamin C 0%; Calcium 4%; Iron 2%
Diet Exchanges: 1/2 starch

Spicy Popcorn

LO CAL / LO FAT / LO CHOL / LO SODIUM

PREP: 5 MIN; COOK: 3 MIN

10 SERVINGS (1 CUP EACH)

Ground turmeric, a popular spice used in East Indian cooking, is what gives this flavorful snack its bright yellow color (photo, page 64).

1   **tablespoon water**

4   **teaspoons margarine**

1   **teaspoon ground cinnamon**

1   **teaspoon ground turmeric**

1/2   **teaspoon salt**

1/4   **teaspoon white pepper**

1/8   **teaspoon ground red pepper (cayenne)**

10   **cups hot-air-popped popcorn**

Heat water and margarine in 6-inch nonstick skillet over low heat about 3 minutes or until margarine is melted. Stir in remaining ingredients except popcorn.

Drizzle over popcorn; toss. Serve immediately.

1 Serving: Calories 45 (Calories from Fat 20); Fat 2g (Saturated 0g); Cholesterol 0mg; Sodium 135mg; Carbohydrate 7g (Dietary Fiber 1g); Protein 1g
% Daily Value: Vitamin A 2%; Vitamin C 0%; Calcium 0%; Iron 2%
Diet Exchanges: 1/2 starch

Southwestern Popcorn Snack

LO CAL / LO CHOL / LO SODIUM

PREP: 10 MIN

8 SERVINGS (1 CUP EACH)

If your popcorn has lost some of its crispness, spread it in a single layer in a jelly roll pan and heat in a 325° oven for 5 to 10 minutes (photo, page 64).

6	cups hot-air-popped popcorn
2	cups Cheerios® cereal
2	tablespoons margarine
$\frac{1}{2}$	teaspoon chili powder
$\frac{1}{4}$	teaspoon ground cumin
$\frac{1}{4}$	teaspoon garlic powder
2	tablespoons grated Parmesan cheese

Mix popcorn and cereal. Heat margarine, chili powder, cumin and garlic powder in 6-inch nonstick skillet over low heat, stirring occasionally, until margarine is melted.

Drizzle over popcorn mixture; toss. Immediately sprinkle with cheese; toss. Serve warm.

1 Serving: Calories 85 (Calories from Fat 35); Fat 4g (Saturated 1g); Cholesterol 0mg; Sodium 120mg; Carbohydrate 11g (Dietary Fiber 1g); Protein 2g
% Daily Value: Vitamin A 10%; Vitamin C 2%; Calcium 2%; Iron 12%
Diet Exchanges: $\frac{1}{2}$ starch, 1 fat

Honey-Spice Pretzels

LO CAL / LO FAT / LO CHOL

PREP: 10 MIN; BAKE: 8 MIN

4 SERVINGS (1 CUP EACH)

Honey, chili powder and fat-free pretzels team up for a healthy yet spunky snack that you can nibble by the handful without feeling guilty.

4	cups fat-free pretzel sticks
3	tablespoons honey
2	teaspoons margarine, melted
1	teaspoon onion powder
1	teaspoon chili powder

Heat oven to 350°. Line cookie sheet with aluminum foil; spray with cooking spray. Place pretzels in large bowl. Mix remaining ingredients; drizzle over pretzels, stirring to coat.

Spread pretzels evenly on cookie sheet. Bake 8 minutes, stirring once. Cool on sheet. Loosen pretzels from foil. Store in airtight container at room temperature.

1 Serving: Calories 225 (Calories from Fat 20); Fat 2g (Saturated 1g); Cholesterol 0mg; Sodium 800mg; Carbohydrate 50g (Dietary Fiber 29g); Protein 4g
% Daily Value: Vitamin A 4%; Vitamin C 0%; Calcium 2%; Iron 12%
Diet Exchanges: 3 starch

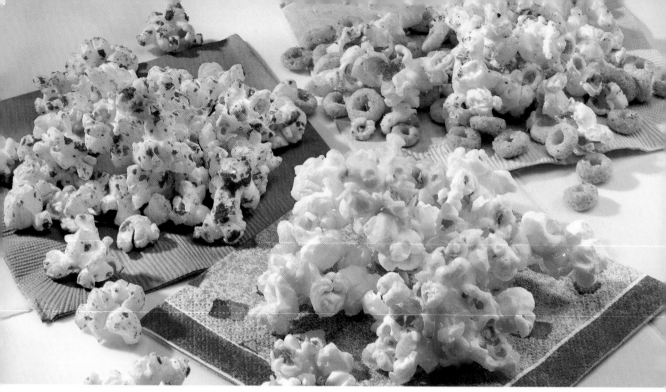

Caramelized-Sugar Popcorn, Southwestern Popcorn Snack (page 63), Spicy Popcorn (page 62)

Caramelized-Sugar Popcorn

LO CAL / LO FAT / LO CHOL / LO SODIUM

PREP: 10 MIN; COOK: 5 MIN

10 SERVINGS (1 CUP EACH)

If you don't have a hot-air popcorn popper, purchase popped popcorn at the supermarket. Just be sure to select a "light" type, and if the purchased popcorn is already salted, omit the salt in this recipe.

  $^1/_4$ teaspoon salt

  10 cups hot-air-popped popcorn

  $^1/_2$ cup sugar

  2 teaspoons margarine

Sprinkle salt over popcorn in large bowl; set aside.

Place sugar in Dutch oven. Heat over medium heat, shaking Dutch oven occasionally (do not stir), until sugar starts to melt. Reduce heat to low. Add margarine, stirring constantly, until sugar is completely melted and golden.

Remove from heat. Immediately add popcorn, stirring to coat. Quickly transfer to large bowl; cool.

1 Serving: Calories 75 (Calories from Fat 10); Fat 1g (Saturated 0g); Cholesterol 0mg; Sodium 70mg; Carbohydrate 16g (Dietary Fiber 1g); Protein 1g
% Daily Value: Vitamin A 2%; Vitamin C 0%; Calcium 0%; Iron 2%
Diet Exchanges: 1 starch

Wake-Up Shake

LO CAL / LO FAT / LO CHOL / LO SODIUM / HI FIB

PREP: 5 MIN

2 SERVINGS

A teaspoon of wheat germ stirred into each serving will increase the nutritional content of this shake and help get you going in the morning!

> 1 cup vanilla low-fat yogurt
>
> 1/2 cup frozen berries (such as raspberries or blueberries)
>
> 1/4 cup orange juice
>
> 1 medium banana, cut into chunks

Place all ingredients in blender. Cover and blend on high speed about 30 seconds or until smooth. Serve immediately.

1 Serving: Calories 215 (Calories from Fat 10); Fat 1g (Saturated 1g); Cholesterol 2mg; Sodium 55mg; Carbohydrate 49g (Dietary Fiber 4g); Protein 6g
% Daily Value: Vitamin A 10%; Vitamin C 46%; Calcium 18%; Iron 8%
Diet Exchanges: 3 fruit, 1/2 skim milk

Orange-Papaya Cooler

LO CAL / LO FAT / LO CHOL / LO SODIUM

PREP: 5 MIN

1 SERVING

Oranges, papayas and many other fruits are a super source of vitamin C. This healthy vitamin is thought to be protective against certain types of cancer. Be sure to have at least two or three servings of fruits daily.

> Juice of 1 large orange (1/2 cup)
> or 1/2 cup unsweetened orange juice
>
> 1/2 cup papaya or pear juice
>
> 1 tablespoon lemon juice
>
> Ice cubes or crushed ice

Pour fruit juices over ice. Stir before serving.

1 Serving: Calories 100 (Calories from Fat 0); Fat 1g (Saturated 0g); Cholesterol 0mg; Sodium 5mg; Carbohydrate 24g (Dietary Fiber 2g); Protein 1g
% Daily Value: Vitamin A 2%; Vitamin C 82%; Calcium 2%; Iron 4%
Diet Exchanges: 1 1/2 fruit

Strawberry-Yogurt Smoothie

LO CAL / LO FAT / LO CHOL / LO SODIUM

PREP: 5 MIN

4 SERVINGS

Although variations of this popular drink are endless, the basic smoothie recipe is quite simple—a blending of fruit, yogurt and milk.

- 1 pint (2 cups) strawberries
- 1 cup skim milk
- 1⅓ cups strawberry low-fat yogurt

Reserve 4 strawberries for garnish, if desired. Place remaining strawberries, the milk and yogurt in blender. Cover and blend on high speed about 30 seconds or until smooth. Garnish with reserved strawberries.

1 Serving: Calories 125 (Calories from Fat 10); Fat 1g (Saturated 1g); Cholesterol 5mg; Sodium 80mg; Carbohydrate 24g (Dietary Fiber 1g); Protein 6g
% Daily Value: Vitamin A 4%; Vitamin C 70%; Calcium 20%; Iron 2%
Diet Exchanges: 1½ fruit, ½ skim milk

Mixed-Berry Smoothie

LO CAL / LO FAT / LO CHOL / LO SODIUM / HI FIB

PREP: 10 MIN

3 SERVINGS

If you can't find frozen mixed berries at your supermarket, substitute 1½ cups each of frozen unsweetened strawberries and unsweetened red raspberries.

- 1 cup strawberry or raspberry low-fat yogurt
- 1 cup skim milk
- 1 tablespoon powdered sugar
- 1 bag (14 to 16 ounces) frozen mixed berries (strawberries, blackberries, blueberries and raspberries), slightly thawed

Place yogurt, milk and powdered sugar in blender or food processor. Cover and blend on high speed about 30 seconds or until smooth.

Add half the berries. Cover and blend on high speed 1 minute. Add remaining berries. Cover and blend on high speed about 1 minute or until smooth, adding a small amount of additional milk if necessary. Serve immediately.

1 Serving: Calories 175 (Calories from Fat 20); Fat 2g (Saturated 1g); Cholesterol 5mg; Sodium 90mg; Carbohydrate 38g (Dietary Fiber 6g); Protein 7g
% Daily Value: Vitamin A 6%; Vitamin C 74%; Calcium 24%; Iron 4%
Diet Exchanges: 1 starch, 1 fruit, ½ skim milk

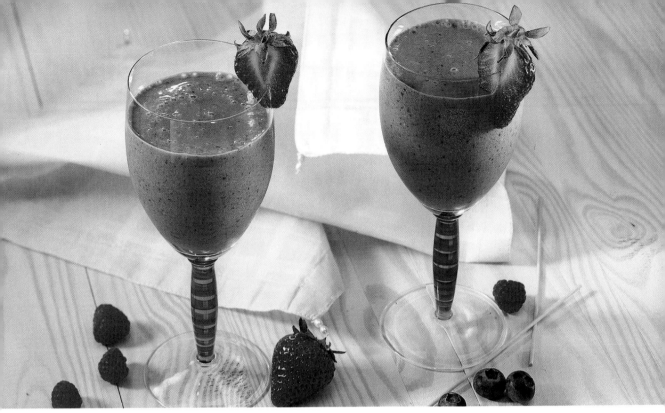

Mixed-Berry Smoothie

Banana-Peach Shake

LO CAL / LO FAT / LO CHOL / LO SODIUM

PREP: 5 MIN; FREEZE: 2 HOURS

3 SERVINGS

If you like your shakes extra-thick use vanilla fat-free frozen yogurt in place of the milk. You can also freeze the bananas ahead of time so you won't have to wait to make your shake.

1 cup mashed ripe bananas (2 medium)

¹⁄₂ cup skim milk

1 cup peach nectar

Spoon mashed bananas into ice-cube trays. Freeze about 2 hours or until frozen; transfer frozen banana cubes to freezer bags to store, if desired.

Place frozen bananas, milk and peach nectar in blender. Cover and blend on high speed about 30 seconds or until smooth. Serve immediately over ice cubes.

1 Serving: Calories 150 (Calories from Fat 10); Fat 1g (Saturated 0g); Cholesterol 0mg; Sodium 30mg; Carbohydrate 35g (Dietary Fiber 2g); Protein 2g
% Daily Value: Vitamin A 4%; Vitamin C 22%; Calcium 6%; Iron 2%
Diet Exchanges: 2 fruit

Pineapple-Orange Colada

LO CAL / LO CHOL / LO SODIUM

PREP: 5 MIN

4 SERVINGS

For an extra boost of potassium, add a sliced banana to this thick and creamy drink.

1½ cups fresh pineapple chunks
    or 1 can (20 ounces) pineapple
    chunks in juice, drained

½ cup frozen piña colada concentrate or
    pineapple juice

2 cups orange sherbet

   Sliced pineapple, if desired

   Fresh mint, if desired

Place all ingredients except sliced pineapple and mint in blender. Cover and blend on high speed about 30 seconds until smooth. Garnish with sliced pineapple and mint.

1 Serving: Calories 210 (Calories from Fat 35); Fat 4g (Saturated 3g); Cholesterol 5mg; Sodium 60mg; Carbohydrate 44g (Dietary Fiber 1g); Protein 1g
% Daily Value: Vitamin A 2%; Vitamin C 24%; Calcium 6%; Iron 2%
Diet Exchanges: 3 fruit, ½ fat

Fresh Fruit Frappé

LO CAL / LO FAT / LO CHOL / LO SODIUM

PREP: 15 MIN

4 SERVINGS

A frappé is simply a slushy drink made by blending fruit, fruit juice and ice.

1 cup cut-up cantaloupe or honeydew melon

1 cup cut-up pineapple

1 cup cut-up mango

1 cup strawberry halves

1 cup orange juice

2 tablespoons sugar

   Crushed ice

   Halved strawberries, if desired

Mix all ingredients except ice and halved strawberries. Fill blender one-half full with fruit mixture; add crushed ice to fill to top. Cover and blend on high speed about 30 seconds until smooth. Repeat with remaining fruit mixture. Garnish with halved strawberries. Serve immediately.

1 Serving: Calories 125 (Calories from Fat 10); Fat 1g (Saturated 0g); Cholesterol 0mg; Sodium 5mg; Carbohydrate 30g (Dietary Fiber 2g); Protein 1g
% Daily Value: Vitamin A 28%; Vitamin C 100%; Calcium 2%; Iron 4%
Diet Exchanges: 2 fruit

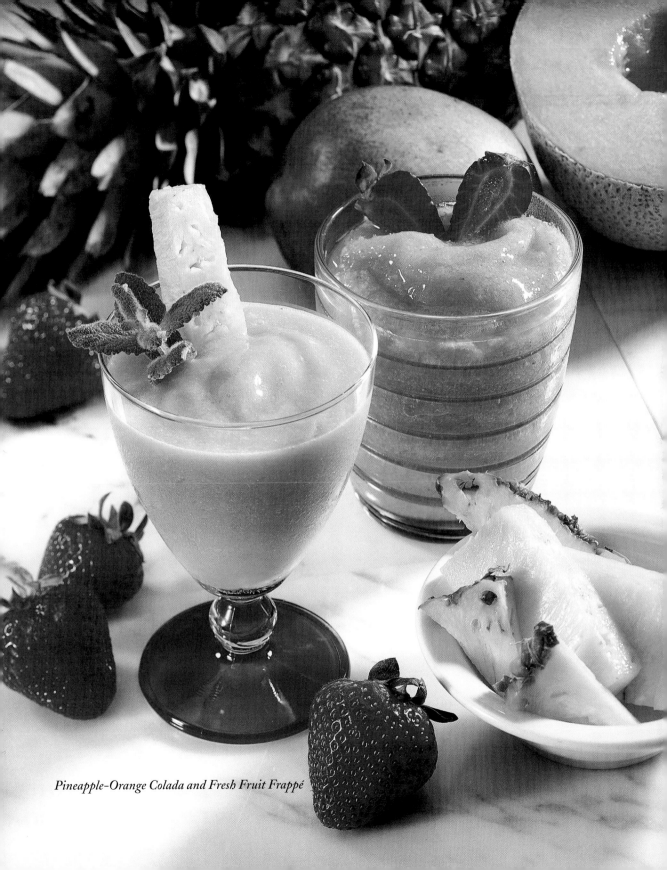

Pineapple–Orange Colada and Fresh Fruit Frappé

Strawberry-Lime Slush

LO CAL / LO FAT / LO CHOL / LO SODIUM / HI FIB

PREP: 10 MIN

4 SERVINGS

If you want a sweeter drink, frozen limeade concentrate that's been thawed can be used in place of the lime juice.

2   pints (4 cups) fresh strawberries
    or 4 cups frozen (thawed) strawberries

1½ cups crushed ice

¼   cup powdered sugar

2   tablespoons lime juice

Reserve 4 strawberries for garnish if desired. Place crushed ice and 1 pint of the strawberries in blender or food processor. Cover and blend on high speed until mixture is almost smooth. Pour into 1-quart (or larger) pitcher.

Place remaining 1 pint strawberries, the powdered sugar and lime juice in blender or food processor. Cover and blend on high speed until almost smooth. Add mixture to pitcher; stir. Serve in 4 tall glasses. Garnish sides of glasses with reserved strawberries. Serve immediately.

1 Serving: Calories 95 (Calories from Fat 10); Fat 1g (Saturated 0g); Cholesterol 0mg; Sodium 5mg; Carbohydrate 23g (Dietary Fiber 3g); Protein 1g
% Daily Value: Vitamin A 0%; Vitamin C 100%; Calcium 2%; Iron 2%
Diet Exchanges: 1½ fruit

Peachy Raspberry Sodas

LO CAL / LO FAT / LO CHOL / LO SODIUM

PREP: 10 MIN

4 SERVINGS

Sugar-free lemon-lime carbonated beverage is a lively and lemony substitute for the ginger ale.

1   cup peach nectar

1   pint (2 cups) raspberry sherbet

1½ cups chilled sugar-free ginger ale

Pour ¼ cup peach nectar into each of 4 short, wide glasses. Place 1 scoop (about ½ cup) sherbet in each glass. Fill with ginger ale.

1 Serving: Calories 175 (Calories from Fat 20); Fat 2g (Saturated 1g); Cholesterol 5mg; Sodium 60mg; Carbohydrate 39g (Dietary Fiber 1g); Protein 1g
% Daily Value: Vitamin A 2%; Vitamin C 12%; Calcium 6%; Iron 2%
Diet Exchanges: 2½ fruit, ½ fat

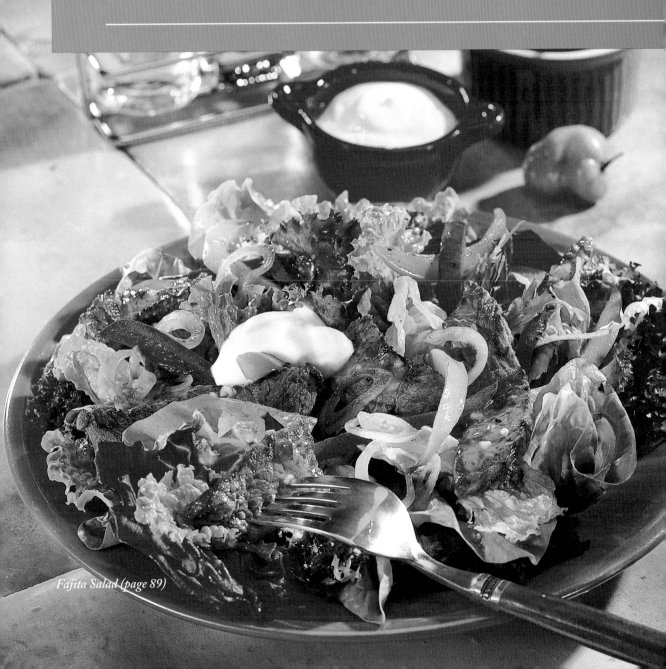

SANDWICHES, SOUPS AND SIZEABLE SALADS

Fajita Salad (page 89)

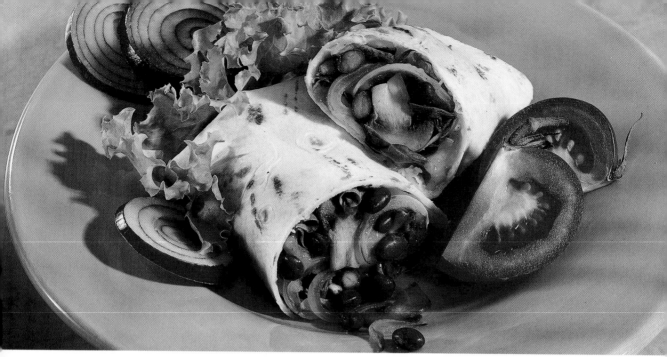

Bean and Veggie Wrap

Bean and Veggie Wrap

LO CAL / LO FAT / LO CHOL / HI FIB

PREP: 10 MIN; COOK: 6 MIN

4 SERVINGS

Prewashed spinach sold in your supermarket makes this black bean wrap super easy and nutritionally rich.

- 4 fat-free flour tortillas (6 to 8 inches in diameter)
- 2 cups sliced mushrooms (5 ounces)
- 1 medium onion, cut lengthwise in half, then cut crosswise into thin slices
- 1 can (15 ounces) black beans, rinsed and drained
- 4 cups fresh spinach leaves
- 1/2 cup shredded reduced-fat Cheddar cheese (2 ounces)

Heat tortillas as directed on package. While tortillas are heating, spray 10-inch nonstick skillet with cooking spray; heat over medium heat. Cook mushrooms and onion in skillet about 4 minutes, stirring frequently, until onion is crisp-tender. Stir in beans; heat through. Stir in spinach; remove from heat.

Divide bean mixture among tortillas. Sprinkle with cheese. Fold one end of each tortilla up about 1 inch over filling; fold right and left sides over folded end, overlapping. Fold remaining end down.

1 Serving: Calories 275 (Calories from Fat 20); Fat 2g (Saturated 1g); Cholesterol 5mg; Sodium 860mg; Carbohydrate 57g (Dietary Fiber 10g); Protein 18g
% Daily Value: Vitamin A 26%; Vitamin C 10%; Calcium 16%; Iron 12%
Diet Exchanges: 3 starch, 1/2 very lean meat, 2 vegetable

Quick Chicken Barbecue Sandwiches

LO CAL / LO FAT / LO CHOL

PREP: 5 MIN; COOK: 5 MIN

6 SERVINGS

Are you wrap happy? Then fill fat-free flour tortillas with this barbecue mixture for a simple and delicious Chicken Barbecue Wrap.

1 cup barbecue sauce

3 packages (2.5 ounces each) sliced smoked chicken, cut into 1-inch strips (3 cups)

6 hamburger buns, split

Mix barbecue sauce and chicken in 2-quart saucepan. Heat to boiling; reduce heat to low. Cover and simmer about 5 minutes or until hot. Fill buns with chicken mixture.

1 Serving: Calories 195 (Calories from Fat 45); Fat 5g (Saturated 2g); Cholesterol 20mg; Sodium 600mg; Carbohydrate 27g (Dietary Fiber 1g); Protein 11g
% Daily Value: Vitamin A 4%; Vitamin C 2%; Calcium 6%; Iron 10%
Diet Exchanges: 1 starch, 1 lean meat, 2 vegetable

Turkey Sloppy Joes

LO CAL / LO FAT

PREP: 5 MIN; COOK: 15 MIN

6 SERVINGS

If you prefer the flavor of beef, use diet-lean or extra-lean ground beef in place of the ground turkey breast. Multigrain or whole wheat buns would also be a delicious and fiber-rich alternative to regular hamburger buns.

1 pound ground turkey breast

1 medium onion, chopped ($\frac{1}{2}$ cup)

1 can ($10\frac{3}{4}$ ounces) reduced-fat condensed tomato soup

2 teaspoons Worcestershire sauce

3 drops red pepper sauce

6 hamburger buns, split

Cook turkey and onion in 2-quart saucepan over medium-high heat, stirring occasionally, until turkey is no longer pink; drain.

Stir in remaining ingredients except buns. Cook, stirring occasionally, until hot. Fill buns with turkey mixture.

1 Serving: Calories 240 (Calories from Fat 35); Fat 4g (Saturated 2g); Cholesterol 50mg; Sodium 482mg; Carbohydrate 31g (Dietary Fiber 2g); Protein 22g
% Daily Value: Vitamin A 2%; Vitamin C 84%; Calcium 6%; Iron 12%
Diet Exchanges: 2 starch, 2 very lean meat

Turkey Fajita Pitas

LOW CALORIE

PREP: 10 MIN

4 SERVINGS

Turn these pitas into quick and easy vegetarian sandwiches by substituting fat-free refried beans for the turkey.

- ¼ cup thick-and-chunky salsa
- 4 pita breads (6 inches in diameter), cut in half to form pockets
- 1 pound deli-style sliced fat-free turkey
- 1 small red bell pepper, cut into ¼-inch strips
- ¼ cup finely chopped red onion
- ½ cup shredded reduced-fat Monterey Jack cheese (2 ounces)

Spoon salsa into pita bread halves. Top with turkey, bell pepper, onion and cheese.

1 Serving: Calories 330 (Calories from Fat 65); Fat 7g (Saturated 3g); Cholesterol 60mg; Sodium 1810mg; Carbohydrate 39g (Dietary Fiber 2g); Protein 30g
% Daily Value: Vitamin A 16%; Vitamin C 32%; Calcium 20%; Iron 14%
Diet Exchanges: 2 starch, 3 lean meat, 1 vegetable

Cranberry-Turkey Wrap

LOW CALORIE

PREP: 15 MIN

4 SERVINGS

You don't have to wait until you have Thanksgiving leftovers to make this wrap! Substitute cooked chicken for the turkey and strawberry spreadable fruit for the cranberry sauce. For a fresh summer sandwich bursting with flavor, top each tortilla with 2 tablespoons of sliced strawberries before rolling up into a wrap.

- 4 fat-free flour tortillas (6 to 8 inches in diameter)
- ½ tub (8-ounce size) reduced-fat cream cheese (Neufchâtel) (½ cup)
- ¼ cup jellied cranberry sauce or strawberry spreadable fruit
- 2 teaspoons mustard
- 1½ cups chopped cooked turkey or chicken
- ½ cup shredded reduced-fat mozzarella cheese (2 ounces)
- ½ cup alfalfa sprouts, if desired

Spread each tortilla with 2 tablespoons cream cheese, 1 tablespoon cranberry sauce and ½ teaspoon mustard. Sprinkle with turkey, mozzarella cheese and sprouts.

Fold one end of each tortilla up about 1 inch over filling; fold right and left sides over folded end, overlapping. Fold remaining end down.

1 Serving: Calories 305 (Calories from Fat 80); Fat 9g (Saturated 5g); Cholesterol 60mg; Sodium 600mg; Carbohydrate 33g (Dietary Fiber 1g); Protein 24g
% Daily Value: Vitamin A 8%; Vitamin C 0%; Calcium 14%; Iron 4%
Diet Exchanges: 2 starch, 2 lean meat, ½ vegetable

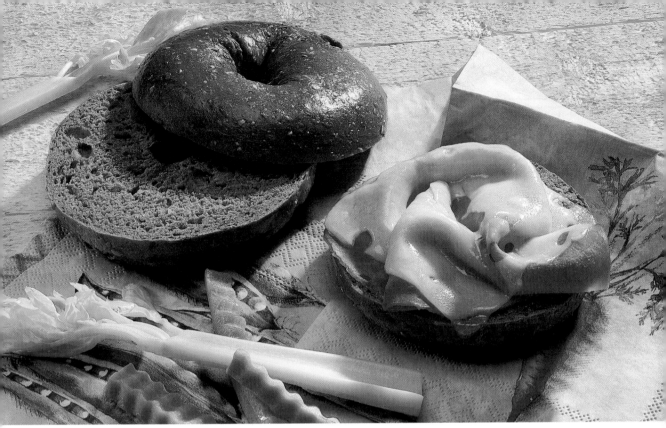

Honey Ham Bagel Sandwiches

Honey Ham Bagel Sandwiches

LOW CALORIE

PREP: 5 MIN; BAKE: 5 MIN

4 SERVINGS

Make your own fat-free spread for these sandwiches by mixing equal parts of honey and mustard.

2 pumpernickel bagels, split and toasted

4 teaspoons honey mustard

4 slices (1 ounce each) fully cooked honey ham

4 thin slices ($^1/_2$ ounce each) Swiss cheese

Heat oven to 400°. Spread each bagel half with 1 teaspoon mustard. Top each with one slice of ham and cheese. Place on cookie sheet. Bake 3 to 5 minutes or until cheese is melted.

1 Serving: Calories 185 (Calories from Fat 65); Fat 7g (Saturated 4g); Cholesterol 30mg; Sodium 620mg; Carbohydrate 18g (Dietary Fiber 1g); Protein 13g
% Daily Value: Vitamin A 2%; Vitamin C 0%; Calcium 14%; Iron 6%
Diet Exchanges: 1 starch, 2 lean meat

Three-Bean and Barley Soup

LO FAT / LO CHOL / HI FIB

PREP: 10 MIN; COOK: 20 MIN

5 SERVINGS

Mixing grains, such as barley, with beans builds complete proteins. Grains or beans alone don't contain all the protein building blocks our bodies need. But when they are added together, we get all the benefits!

- 1 tablespoon olive or vegetable oil
- 2 small onions, cut in half and thinly sliced
- 2 cloves garlic, finely chopped
- 1 teaspoon ground cumin
- 1 can (15 to 16 ounces) garbanzo beans, undrained
- 1 can (15 to 16 ounces) lima beans, drained
- 1 can (15 ounces) black beans, rinsed and drained
- 1 can (14$\frac{1}{2}$ ounces) Italian-style stewed tomatoes, undrained
- $\frac{1}{2}$ cup uncooked quick-cooking barley
- $\frac{1}{2}$ teaspoon salt
- 3 cups water
- 2 tablespoons chopped fresh parsley

Heat oil in Dutch oven over medium-high heat. Cook onions, garlic and cumin in oil 4 to 5 minutes, stirring occasionally, until onions are tender.

Stir in remaining ingredients except parsley. Heat to boiling; reduce heat to low. Cover and simmer about 10 minutes or until lima beans are tender. Stir in parsley.

1 Serving: Calories 370 (Calories from Fat 55); Fat 6g (Saturated 1g); Cholesterol 0mg; Sodium 970mg; Carbohydrate 77g (Dietary Fiber 19g); Protein 21g
% Daily Value: Vitamin A 4%; Vitamin C 12%; Calcium 14%; Iron 38%
Diet Exchanges: 4 starch, 3 vegetable

Minestrone Soup

LO CAL / LO FAT / LO CHOL / HI FIB

PREP: 20 MIN; COOK: 20 MIN

6 SERVINGS

Use freshly grated Parmesan cheese to get the full benefit of the rich, sharp and nutty flavor of this cheese.

1	can (28 ounces) whole tomatoes, undrained
1	can (15 to 16 ounces) great northern beans, undrained
1	can (8 ounces) kidney beans, undrained
1	can (about 8 ounces) whole kernel corn, undrained
2	medium stalks celery, thinly sliced (1 cup)
1	small zucchini, sliced (1 cup)
1	medium onion, chopped ($^1/_2$ cup)
1	cup shredded cabbage
$^1/_2$	cup uncooked elbow macaroni or broken spaghetti
$1^1/_4$	cups water
2	teaspoons vegetable bouillon granules
1	teaspoon Italian seasoning
1	clove garlic, crushed
	Grated Parmesan cheese

Heat all ingredients except cheese to boiling in Dutch oven, breaking up tomatoes; reduce heat to low. Cover and simmer about 15 minutes, stirring occasionally, until macaroni is tender. Serve with cheese.

1 Serving: Calories 250 (Calories from Fat 25); Fat 3g (Saturated 1g); Cholesterol 5mg; Sodium 900mg; Carbohydrate 47g (Dietary Fiber 9g); Protein 15g
% Daily Value: Vitamin A 10%; Vitamin C 24%; Calcium 18%; Iron 26%
Diet Exchanges: 2 starch, 3 vegetable

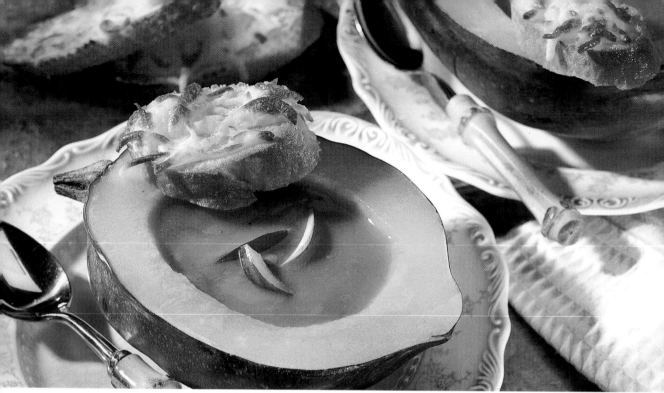

Winter Squash and Lentil Bisque

Vegetable and Tortellini Soup

LO CAL / LO FAT

PREP: 5 MIN; COOK: 10 MIN

6 SERVINGS

For a vegetarian version of this soup, substitute cheese-filled tortellini for the beef-filled.

- 4 cups water
- 1 package (1.4 ounces) vegetable soup and recipe mix
- 1 package (9 ounces) refrigerated cheese-filled tortellini
- 1 package (10 ounces) frozen chopped spinach, thawed and squeezed to drain

  Grated Parmesan cheese, if desired

Mix water and soup mix in 3-quart saucepan. Heat to boiling, stirring occasionally; reduce heat to low.

Stir in tortellini and spinach. Simmer uncovered about 5 minutes, stirring occasionally, until tortellini is tender. Sprinkle each serving with cheese.

1 Serving: Calories 105 (Calories from Fat 25); Fat 3g (Saturated 1g); Cholesterol 40mg; Sodium 710mg; Carbohydrate 15g (Dietary Fiber 2g); Protein 7g
% Daily Value: Vitamin A 32%; Vitamin C 4%; Calcium 8%; Iron 8%
Diet Exchanges: 1 starch, 1 very lean meat

Winter Squash and Lentil Bisque

LO CAL / LO FAT / LO CHOL / HI FIB

PREP: 20 MIN; COOK: 55 MIN; BROIL: 2 MIN

6 SERVINGS

Create a sensation by serving this soup in edible squash bowls. Cut butternut or acorn squash in half, remove seeds and fibers and cook the squash halves before filling.

2	medium butternut or acorn squash, cooked and chopped
2	medium green apples, chopped (2 cups)
1	medium red onion, chopped
½	cup unsweetened applesauce
1	cup apple juice
¼	teaspoon ground nutmeg
⅛	teaspoon ground red pepper (cayenne)
1	can (14½ ounces) ready-to-serve vegetable broth
½	cup dried lentils (4 ounces), sorted and rinsed
¾	cup shredded reduced-fat mozzarella cheese (3 ounces)
6	slices French bread, ¼ inch thick
	Additional chopped red onion, if desired

Heat squash, apples, onion, applesauce, apple juice, nutmeg, red pepper and 1 cup of the broth to boiling in 3-quart saucepan, stirring occasionally; reduce heat to low. Cover and simmer 20 minutes.

Place squash mixture in blender or food processor. Cover and blend on medium speed until smooth; return mixture to saucepan. Stir in lentils and remaining broth. Heat to boiling; reduce heat. Cover and simmer 25 to 30 minutes, stirring occasionally, until lentils are tender.

Set oven control to broil. Sprinkle cheese on bread slices. Place on rack in broiler pan. Broil bread with tops 3 inches from heat about 2 minutes or until cheese is bubbly. Top each serving of soup with a slice of cheese bread and onion.

1 Serving: Calories 220 (Calories from Fat 35); Fat 4g (Saturated 2g); Cholesterol 10mg; Sodium 490mg; Carbohydrate 43g (Dietary Fiber 8g); Protein 11g
% Daily Value: Vitamin A 50%; Vitamin C 12%; Calcium 16%; Iron 14%
Diet Exchanges: 1 starch, 2 vegetable, 1 fruit, 1 fat

Tomato and Red Lentil Soup

LO CAL / LO FAT / LO CHOL / HI FIB

PREP: 15 MIN; COOK: 35 MIN

6 SERVINGS

Although most supermarkets carry at least one variety of lentils, red lentils may be slightly harder to find. They usually can be purchased in Middle Eastern or East Indian markets. If you have trouble finding red lentils, the familiar grayish-green lentils can be used instead.

1 tablespoon margarine

1 medium onion, chopped ($^{1}/_{2}$ cup)

2 medium carrots, sliced (1 cup)

2 medium stalks celery, sliced (1 cup)

1 small red bell pepper, chopped ($^{1}/_{2}$ cup)

2 cans (14$^{1}/_{2}$ ounces each) ready-to-serve vegetable broth

1 can (28 ounces) crushed tomatoes with puree, undrained

1 cup dried red lentils (8 ounces), sorted and rinsed*

1 tablespoon chopped fresh or 1 teaspoon dried thyme leaves

1 tablespoon chopped fresh or 1 teaspoon dried dill weed

$^{1}/_{2}$ teaspoon pepper

Melt margarine in Dutch oven over medium-high heat. Cook onion, carrots, celery and bell pepper in margarine 5 minutes, stirring occasionally.

Stir in remaining ingredients. Heat to boiling; reduce heat to low. Cover and simmer 25 to 30 minutes, stirring occasionally, until lentils are tender. Garnish with additional fresh dill weed if desired.

*Rinse red lentils just before adding to soup, or they will stick together.

1 Serving: Calories 145 (Calories from Fat 25); Fat 3g (Saturated 1g); Cholesterol 0mg; Sodium 820mg; Carbohydrate 30g (Dietary Fiber 10g); Protein 10g
% Daily Value: Vitamin A 58%; Vitamin C 40%; Calcium 8%; Iron 22%
Diet Exchanges: 2 starch

Chicken Meatball-Tomato Minestrone

LO CAL / HI FIB

PREP: 15 MIN; COOK: 40 MIN

8 SERVINGS

Acini de pepe is tiny pasta that's shaped like peppercorns. Other small pastas, such as anellini or coralli, would also be well suited to this soup.

1	large onion, chopped (1 cup)
2	medium carrots, chopped (1 cup)
2	medium stalks celery, chopped (1 cup)
3	cloves garlic, finely chopped
1	can (46 ounces) tomato juice (5³/₄ cups)
3¹/₄	cups chicken broth
9	cups chopped Chinese (napa) cabbage
	Chicken Meatballs (right)
1	cup uncooked acini de pepe (dot shape) pasta (8 ounces)
1¹/₂	cups chopped fresh parsley

Heat onion, carrots, celery, garlic, tomato juice and 2 cups of the broth to boiling in Dutch oven; reduce heat. Simmer uncovered 15 minutes. Stir in cabbage. Simmer uncovered 5 minutes.

While mixture is simmering, prepare Chicken Meatballs. Stir meatballs and pasta into soup mixture. Simmer uncovered about 15 minutes or until pasta is tender and meatballs are no longer pink in centers.

Place parsley and remaining 1¹/₄ cups broth in blender. Cover and blend on medium speed until pureed; stir into soup.

Chicken Meatballs

1¹/₂	pounds ground chicken
5	medium green onions, chopped (¹/₃ cup)
1	cup soft whole wheat or white bread crumbs
¹/₃	cup chicken broth
¹/₄	cup fat-free cholesterol-free egg product or 2 egg whites
¹/₄	teaspoon pepper

Mix all ingredients. Shape by rounded tablespoonfuls into 24 balls. Spray 12-inch nonstick skillet with cooking spray; heat over medium heat. Cook meatballs in skillet about 5 minutes or until light brown on all sides (they will not be cooked through).

1 Serving: Calories 345 (Calories from Fat 65); Fat 7g (Saturated 2g); Cholesterol 55mg; Sodium 1260mg; Carbohydrate 47g (Dietary Fiber 6g); Protein 29g
% Daily Value: Vitamin A 50%; Vitamin C 60%; Calcium 16%; Iron 28%
Diet Exchanges: 3 starch, 2 lean meat

Mediterranean Fish Stew

LO CAL / LO FAT / HI FIB

PREP: 40 MIN; COOK: 20 MIN

6 SERVINGS

Red snapper and other fish are outstanding sources of omega-3 fatty acids, a type of polyunsaturated fat that may help to reduce the risk of heart disease. Try to serve fish at two meals each week.

- 3   pounds clams in shells
- 1/3   cup white vinegar
- 1   cup chicken broth
- 1/2   cup white wine or chicken broth
- 1   tablespoon tomato paste
- 2   teaspoons chopped fresh or 1/2 teaspoon dried oregano leaves
- 1   teaspoon fennel seed
- 1/8   teaspoon saffron, if desired
- 1/8   teaspoon ground red pepper (cayenne)
- 2   large tomatoes, chopped (2 cups)
- 1   large onion, chopped (1 cup)
- 1   pound red snapper or whitefish fillets, cut into 2-inch pieces
- 3   cups cooked brown rice
- 2   tablespoons chopped fresh parsley
- 2   teaspoons grated lemon peel
- 1   clove garlic, finely chopped

Discard any broken-shell or open (dead) clams. Place remaining clams in large container. Cover with 6 cups water and the vinegar. Let stand 30 minutes; drain. Scrub clams in cold water.

Cook broth, wine, tomato paste, oregano, fennel seed, saffron, red pepper, tomatoes and onion in Dutch oven over medium heat about 10 minutes, stirring occasionally, until onion is tender.

Stir in clams and fish. Cover and cook 5 minutes. Stir in rice. Cover and cook about 3 minutes, removing clams as they open, until all clams have opened. (Discard any unopened clams.) Mix remaining ingredients; sprinkle over stew.

1 Serving: Calories 220 (Calories from Fat 25); Fat 3g (Saturated 1g); Cholesterol 45mg; Sodium 280mg; Carbohydrate 30g (Dietary Fiber 3g); Protein 21g
% Daily Value: Vitamin A 8%; Vitamin C 16%; Calcium 4%; Iron 34%
Diet Exchanges: 2 starch, 2 very lean meat

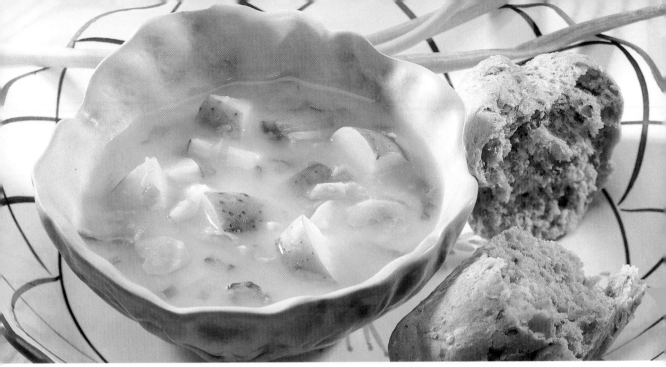

New England Clam Chowder

New England Clam Chowder

LO CAL / LO FAT

PREP: 10 MIN; COOK: 20 MIN

4 SERVINGS

Turning this chowder into a tasty and nourishing meal is easy—serve it with a loaf of rustic bread and, for dessert, Baked Maple Apples (page 407).

2 slices bacon, cut into ¹/₂-inch pieces

2 medium green onions, sliced
(2 tablespoons)

2 cans (6¹/₂ ounces each) minced clams,
drained and liquid reserved

2 medium potatoes, diced (2 cups)

Dash of pepper

2 cups skim milk

Cook bacon and onion in 2-quart saucepan over medium-high heat, stirring frequently, until bacon is crisp.

Add enough water, if necessary, to reserved clam liquid to measure 1 cup. Stir clams, clam liquid, potatoes and pepper into onion mixture. Heat to boiling; reduce heat to medium. Cover and cook about 15 minutes or until potatoes are tender.

Stir in milk. Heat, stirring occasionally, just until hot (do not boil).

1 Serving: Calories 185 (Calories from Fat 30); Fat 3g (Saturated 1g); Cholesterol 35mg; Sodium 170mg; Carbohydrate 25g (Dietary Fiber 2g); Protein 17g
% Daily Value: Vitamin A 14%; Vitamin C 10%; Calcium 20%; Iron 70%
Diet Exchanges: ¹/₂ starch, 1 lean meat, 1 skim milk

Chunky Ham and Veggie Soup

LO CAL / LO FAT

PREP: 5 MIN; COOK: 15 MIN

6 SERVINGS

Leftovers? Freeze individual portions of soup in air-tight plastic containers. Simply reheat in the microwave for a quick and nutritious dinner prepared in minutes.

- 2 cups cubed fully cooked ham
- 3/4 teaspoon dried thyme leaves
- 1/4 teaspoon pepper
- 1 bag (16 ounces) frozen green beans, potatoes, onions and red peppers
- 2 cans (14 1/2 ounces each) ready-to-serve chicken broth

  Reduced-fat sour cream, if desired

Mix all ingredients except sour cream in 2-quart saucepan. Heat to boiling; reduce heat. Simmer uncovered 6 to 8 minutes, stirring occasionally, until vegetables are tender. Top each serving with sour cream.

1 Serving: Calories 125 (Calories from Fat 45); Fat 5g (Saturated 2g); Cholesterol 25mg; Sodium 1300mg; Carbohydrate 7g (Dietary Fiber 1g); Protein 14g
% Daily Value: Vitamin A 8%; Vitamin C 28%; Calcium 2%; Iron 8%
Diet Exchanges: 2 lean meat, 1 vegetable

Ham 'n' Corn Chowder

LO CAL / LO FAT / LO CHOL / HI FIB

PREP: 5 MIN; COOK: 15 MIN

4 SERVINGS

Corn adds a sweet flavor plus offers the benefits of complex carbohydrates, fiber, and vitamins A and B.

- 1/2 cup chopped fully cooked ham
- 1 1/2 cups skim milk
- 1 bag (16 ounces) frozen whole kernel corn
- 1 can (10 3/4 ounces) condensed cream of celery soup
- 2 medium green onions, sliced (2 tablespoons)

Mix ham, milk, corn and soup in 3-quart saucepan. Heat to boiling, stirring occasionally; reduce heat to low. Simmer uncovered 10 minutes, stirring occasionally. Sprinkle with onions.

1 Serving: Calories 215 (Calories from Fat 55); Fat 6g (Saturated 2g); Cholesterol 15mg; Sodium 860mg; Carbohydrate 32g (Dietary Fiber 3g); Protein 11g
% Daily Value: Vitamin A 10%; Vitamin C 6%; Calcium 16%; Iron 6%
Diet Exchanges: 1 starch, 2 vegetable, 1/2 skim milk, 1 fat

Black Bean Chili

LO CAL / LO FAT / LO CHOL / HI FIB

PREP: 15 MIN; COOK: 50 MIN

6 SERVINGS

Garnish this hearty chili with chopped red bell peppers and crushed Baked Tortilla Chips (page 62).

- 1 large onion, chopped (1 cup)
- 2 cups water
- 2 cups apple juice
- 1 tablespoon chopped fresh or 1 teaspoon dried oregano leaves
- 2 tablespoons tomato paste
- 1 teaspoon ground cumin
- $\frac{1}{8}$ teaspoon ground red pepper (cayenne)
- 2 cans (4 ounces each) chopped mild green chilies, drained
- 3 cans (15 ounces each) black beans, rinsed and drained
- 1 medium red bell pepper, chopped (1 cup)
- 3 tablespoons chopped fresh cilantro
- 1 cup shredded reduced-fat Cheddar cheese (4 ounces)
- 1 cup plain fat-free yogurt

Heat onion, water, apple juice, oregano, tomato paste, cumin, red pepper and chilies to boiling in Dutch oven; reduce heat to low. Cover and simmer 30 minutes.

Stir in beans, bell pepper and cilantro. Cover and simmer about 15 minutes or until beans are hot. Serve with cheese and yogurt.

1 Serving: Calories 300 (Calories from Fat 25); Fat 3g (Saturated 1g); Cholesterol 5mg; Sodium 810mg; Carbohydrate 58g (Dietary Fiber 11g); Protein 21g
% Daily Value: Vitamin A 16%; Vitamin C 52%; Calcium 28%; Iron 26%
Diet Exchanges: 3 starch, 1 very lean meat, 2 vegetable

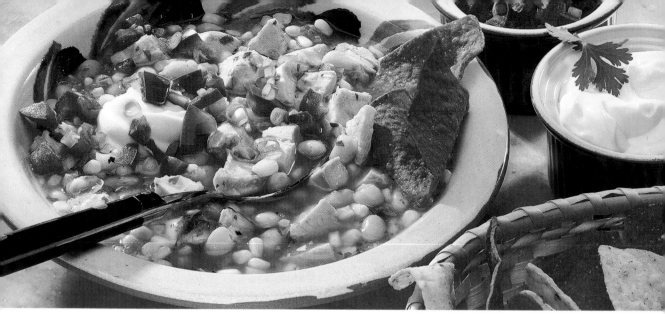

Chili Verde with Fresh Tomato Salsa

Chili Verde with Fresh Tomato Salsa

LO CAL / LO FAT / HI FIB

PREP: 10 MIN; COOK: 25 MIN

4 SERVINGS

Salsa verde is a green salsa made up of tomatillos, green chilies and cilantro.

- 2 cups chopped cooked chicken breast
- 1 can (15 to 16 ounces) cannellini or great northern beans, rinsed and drained
- 1 can (14½ ounces) ready-to-serve chicken broth
- 1 cup green salsa (salsa verde)
- 1 package (9 ounces) frozen shoepeg white corn, thawed
- ¼ cup chopped fresh cilantro

  Fresh Tomato Salsa (right)
  or 1 cup thick-and-chunky salsa

  Reduced-fat sour cream, if desired

Mix all ingredients except cilantro and Fresh Tomato Salsa in 3-quart saucepan. Heat to boiling; reduce heat to low. Cover and simmer 20 minutes. Stir in cilantro. Serve chili with Fresh Tomato Salsa and sour cream.

Fresh Tomato Salsa

- 1 large tomato, chopped (1 cup)
- 2 medium green onions, sliced (2 tablespoons)
- 1 jalapeño chili, seeded and finely chopped
- ¼ teaspoon grated lime peel
- 2 tablespoons lime juice

Mix all ingredients.

1 Serving: Calories 290 (Calories from Fat 45); Fat 5g (Saturated 1g); Cholesterol 60mg; Sodium 810mg; Carbohydrate 37g (Dietary Fiber 8g); Protein 33g
% Daily Value: Vitamin A 18%; Vitamin C 32%; Calcium 12%; Iron 26%
Diet Exchanges: 2 starch, 3 lean meat

Spicy Chicken Chili

LO CAL / LO FAT / HI FIB

PREP: 5 MIN; COOK: 15 MIN

4 SERVINGS

For added heat and flavor, use Southwestern salsa-style diced tomatoes with green chilies or Southwestern-style diced tomatoes with chili spices.

- 1 pound skinless, boneless chicken breast halves
- 1 can (14$\frac{1}{2}$ ounces) salsa-style chunky tomatoes, undrained
- 1 can (15 ounces) spicy chili beans, undrained
- $\frac{1}{2}$ cup shredded reduced-fat Cheddar cheese (2 ounces)

Remove fat from chicken. Cut chicken into $\frac{3}{4}$-inch pieces. Spray 12-inch nonstick skillet with cooking spray; heat over medium-high heat. Cook chicken in skillet 3 to 5 minutes, stirring frequently, until light brown.

Stir in tomatoes and beans; reduce heat to medium-low. Cook uncovered 8 to 10 minutes, stirring frequently, until chicken is no longer pink in center. Sprinkle each serving with 2 tablespoons cheese.

1 Serving: Calories 245 (Calories from Fat 45); Fat 5g (Saturated 2g); Cholesterol 70mg; Sodium 1070mg; Carbohydrate 21g (Dietary Fiber 5g); Protein 34g
% Daily Value: Vitamin A 12%; Vitamin C 20%; Calcium 12%; Iron 18%
Diet Exchanges: 1 starch, 1 very lean meat, 2 lean meat, 1 vegetable

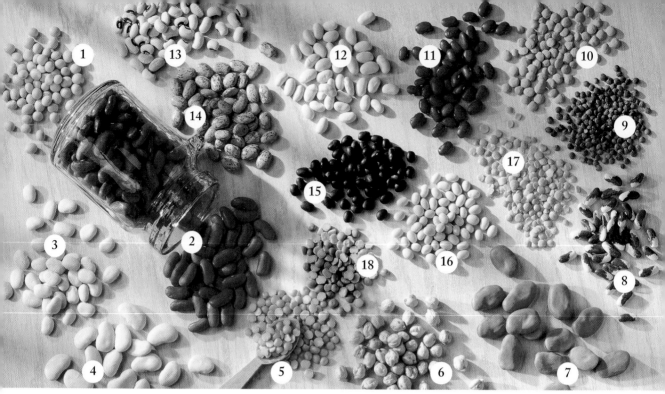

Know Your Beans: 1) soybeans; 2) red kidney beans; 3) lima beans; 4) butter beans; 5) yellow split peas; 6) garbanzo beans; 7) fava beans; 8) appaloosa beans; 9) green lentils; 10) lentils; 11) small red beans (small reds); 12) great northern beans; 13) black-eyed peas; 14) pinto beans; 15) black turtle beans; 16) navy beans; 17) red lentils; 18) green split peas

Caesar Tortellini

LO CAL / LO FAT

PREP: 20 MIN

4 SERVINGS

For a nutrient-packed salad, add chopped vegetables such as broccoli, cauliflower, celery and carrots.

1　package (9 ounces) refrigerated cheese-filled tortellini

1　bag (7¹/₂ ounces) complete fat-free Caesar salad mix

1　medium tomato, chopped (³/₄ cup)

¹/₄　cup imitation bacon-flavor bits

¹/₄　teaspoon freshly ground pepper

Cook and drain tortellini as directed on package. Rinse with cold water; drain.

Toss tortellini, all ingredients in salad mix and remaining ingredients. Serve immediately.

1 Serving: Calories 130 (Calories from Fat 45); Fat 5g (Saturated 2g); Cholesterol 55mg; Sodium 160mg; Carbohydrate 15g (Dietary Fiber 2g); Protein 8g
% Daily Value: Vitamin A 6%; Vitamin C 10%; Calcium 6%; Iron 10%
Diet Exchanges: 1 starch, 1 lean meat

Northern Italian White Bean Salad

LO CAL / LO CHOL / HI FIB

PREP: 15 MIN; CHILL: 2 HR

6 SERVINGS

Cannellini beans are large white kidney beans origi-nally from South America. They have been adopted by Italy and are a delicious part of their cuisine.

- 1 large tomato, seeded and coarsely chopped (1 cup)
- 1 small red bell pepper, chopped ($^1/_2$ cup)
- $^1/_2$ cup chopped red onion
- $^1/_4$ cup chopped fresh parsley
- $^1/_4$ cup olive or vegetable oil
- 2 tablespoons chopped fresh or 2 teaspoons dried basil leaves
- 2 tablespoons red wine vinegar
- $^1/_2$ teaspoon salt
- $^1/_8$ teaspoon pepper
- 2 cans (19 ounces each) cannellini beans, rinsed and drained
- 12 leaves red leaf lettuce

Carefully mix all ingredients except lettuce in glass or plastic bowl. Cover and refrigerate at least 2 hours to blend flavors. Serve on lettuce.

1 Serving: Calories 245 (Calories from Fat 90); Fat 10g (Saturated 2g); Cholesterol 0mg; Sodium 210mg; Car-bohydrate 35g (Dietary Fiber 9g); Protein 13g
% Daily Value: Vitamin A 4%; Vitamin C 36%; Calcium 12%; Iron 28%
Diet Exchanges: 2 starch, 1 vegetable, 1 fat

Fajita Salad

LO CAL / LO FAT

PREP: 15 MIN; COOK: 7 MIN

4 SERVINGS

For a colorful presentation, use a variety of sweet bell peppers, such as red, yellow, orange and green (photo, page 71).

- $^3/_4$ pound lean beef boneless sirloin steak
- 2 teaspoons vegetable oil
- 2 medium bell peppers, cut into strips
- 1 small onion, thinly sliced
- 4 cups bite-size pieces salad greens
- $^1/_3$ cup fat-free Italian dressing
- $^1/_4$ cup plain fat-free yogurt

Remove fat from beef. Cut beef with grain into 2-inch strips; cut strips across grain into $^1/_8$-inch slices.

Heat oil in 10-inch nonstick skillet over medium-high heat. Cook beef in oil about 3 minutes, stirring occasionally, until brown. Remove beef from skillet.

Cook bell peppers and onion in skillet about 3 min-utes, stirring occasionally, until bell peppers are crisp-tender. Stir in beef. Place salad greens on serving platter. Top with beef mixture. Pour dressing over salad. Top with yogurt.

1 Serving: Calories 150 (Calories from Fat 45); Fat 5g (Saturated 1g); Cholesterol 45mg; Sodium 240mg; Car-bohydrate 8g (Dietary Fiber 1g); Protein 19g
% Daily Value: Vitamin A 10%; Vitamin C 30%; Calcium 4%; Iron 12%
Diet Exchanges: $2^1/_2$ lean meat

Raspberry-Chicken Salad

LO CAL / LO FAT / HI FIB

PREP: 10 MIN

4 SERVINGS

Round up those raspberries! Not only do raspberries add a delectable sweetness to this salad, they also bump up the fiber.

Raspberry Dressing (right)

6 cups bite-size pieces mixed salad greens (such as Bibb, iceberg, romaine or spinach)

2 cups cut-up cooked chicken breast

1 cup fresh raspberries

1/3 cup thinly sliced celery

Freshly ground pepper, if desired

Prepare Raspberry Dressing. Toss salad greens, chicken, raspberries and celery. Serve with dressing and pepper.

Raspberry Dressing

1 cup plain fat-free yogurt

1/2 cup fresh raspberries*

1 tablespoon raspberry or red wine vinegar

2 teaspoons sugar

Place all ingredients in blender. Cover and blend on high speed about 15 seconds or until smooth.

*Frozen loose-pack unsweetened raspberries can be substituted for the fresh raspberries in the dressing.

1 Serving: Calories 170 (Calories from Fat 35); Fat 4g (Saturated 1g); Cholesterol 60mg; Sodium 110mg; Carbohydrate 14g (Dietary Fiber 4g); Protein 25g
% Daily Value: Vitamin A 6%; Vitamin C 30%; Calcium 16%; Iron 8%
Diet Exchanges: 3 lean meat, 1 fruit

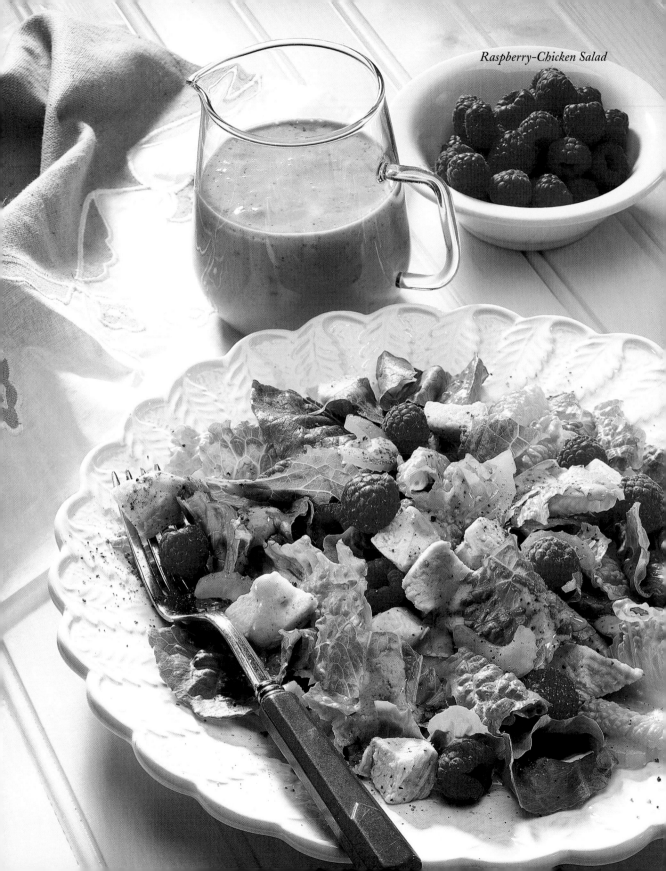

Raspberry-Chicken Salad

Chicken-Pesto Salad

Pesto will keep up to five days if stored tightly covered in the refrigerator. Make a double batch, and toss half of it with hot cooked pasta for an easy weeknight meal.

Pesto (right)

2 cups cut-up cooked chicken or turkey

1 medium tomato, chopped ($^3/_4$ cup)

1 medium green onion, sliced (1 tablespoon)

1 can (8 ounces) sliced water chestnuts, drained

4 cups shredded Bibb lettuce

2 tablespoons crumbled feta cheese

Prepare Pesto. Mix chicken, tomato, onion and water chestnuts. Serve on lettuce. Spoon Pesto over salad. Sprinkle with cheese.

Pesto

2 tablespoons olive or vegetable oil

1 tablespoon plain fat-free yogurt

1 tablespoon lemon juice

$^1/_4$ cup grated Parmesan cheese

1 tablespoon pine nuts

2 cloves garlic

$^3/_4$ cup firmly packed fresh basil leaves

Place all ingredients in blender or food processor. Cover and blend on medium speed about 2 minutes, stopping occasionally to scrape sides, until almost smooth.

1 Serving: Calories 275 (Calories from Fat 145); Fat 16g (Saturated 5g); Cholesterol 70mg; Sodium 220mg; Carbohydrate 11g (Dietary Fiber 2g); Protein 24g
% Daily Value: Vitamin A 8%; Vitamin C 22%; Calcium 14%; Iron 10%
Diet Exchanges: 3 lean meat, 2 vegetable, 1 fat

Penne-Turkey Salad

LO CAL / HI FIB

PREP: 20 MIN; CHILL: 4 HR

6 SERVINGS

Toss in chopped tomatoes and sliced carrots for extra vitamins A and C.

1½ cups uncooked penne pasta (4½ ounces)

1   package (10 ounces) frozen green peas

2   cups cut-up cooked turkey

¾   cup reduced-fat mayonnaise or salad dressing

½   cup shredded reduced-fat Cheddar cheese (2 ounces)

⅓   cup sweet pickle relish

5   medium green onions, sliced (⅓ cup)

1   medium stalk celery, sliced (½ cup)

3   cups bite-size pieces lettuce

Cook and drain pasta as directed on package—except omit salt and add frozen peas to cooking water before draining pasta. Rinse with cold water; drain.

Mix pasta, peas and remaining ingredients except lettuce in large glass or plastic bowl. Cover and refrigerate about 4 hours or until chilled. Serve on lettuce.

1 Serving: Calories 335 (Calories from Fat 100); Fat 11g (Saturated 3g); Cholesterol 40mg; Sodium 500mg; Carbohydrate 41g (Dietary Fiber 4g); Protein 22g
% Daily Value: Vitamin A 6%; Vitamin C 14%; Calcium 8%; Iron 16%
Diet Exchanges: 2 starch, 2 lean meat, 2 vegetable

Turkey Salad with Fruit

LO CAL / LO FAT

PREP: 15 MIN; CHILL: 2 HR

6 SERVINGS

Fill up on fiber by serving this salad with slices of crusty whole wheat bread.

3   cups cut-up cooked turkey

¾   cup sliced green grapes

2   medium stalks celery, sliced (1 cup)

2   medium green onions, thinly sliced (2 tablespoons)

1   can (11 ounces) mandarin orange segments, drained

1   can (8 ounces) sliced water chestnuts, drained

1   cup peach or lemon low-fat yogurt

2   tablespoons reduced-sodium soy sauce
    Mixed salad greens

Mix turkey, grapes, celery, onions, orange segments and water chestnuts in large glass or plastic bowl. Mix yogurt and soy sauce. Pour over turkey mixture; toss. Cover and refrigerate at least 2 hours to blend flavors. Serve on salad greens.

1 Serving: Calories 220 (Calories from Fat 55); Fat 6g (Saturated 2g); Cholesterol 60mg; Sodium 270mg; Carbohydrate 21g (Dietary Fiber 2g); Protein 22g
% Daily Value: Vitamin A 8%; Vitamin C 34%; Calcium 8%; Iron 10%
Diet Exchanges: 2½ lean meat, 1½ fruit

Salmon Salad with Cucumber Noodles

LO CAL / LO FAT / HI FIB

PREP: 10 MIN; CHILL: 1 HR

6 SERVINGS

Although English cucumbers may be a bit more expensive, they are virtually seedless and will save you from removing the seeds, which can tend to be bitter in regular cucumbers. If stored whole and unwashed in a plastic bag, cucumbers will keep up to 10 days in the refrigerator.

Cucumber-Yogurt Sauce (right)

2   English cucumbers

1   pound grilled salmon or tuna, cut into
    3-inch pieces (3 cups)

3   cups cooked cut green beans

2   cups cherry tomatoes, cut in half

2   medium green onions, chopped
    (2 tablespoons)

Prepare Cucumber-Yogurt Sauce. Peel cucumbers; cut into thin strips, 8 × ¼ inches, using vegetable peeler. Divide cucumbers, salmon, green beans and tomatoes among 6 plates. Sprinkle with onions. Serve with sauce.

Cucumber-Yogurt Sauce

¾   cup plain fat-free yogurt

½   cup chopped peeled cucumber

2   tablespoons chopped fresh chives

2   tablespoons reduced-fat sour cream

2   teaspoons Dijon mustard

½   teaspoon salt

¼   teaspoon pepper

Mix all ingredients. Cover and refrigerate 1 hour to blend flavors.

1 Serving: Calories 165 (Calories from Fat 45); Fat 5g (Saturated 2g); Cholesterol 50mg; Sodium 310mg; Carbohydrate 14g (Dietary Fiber 4g); Protein 20g
% Daily Value: Vitamin A 12%; Vitamin C 38%; Calcium 12%; Iron 10%
Diet Exchanges: 2 lean meat, 3 vegetable

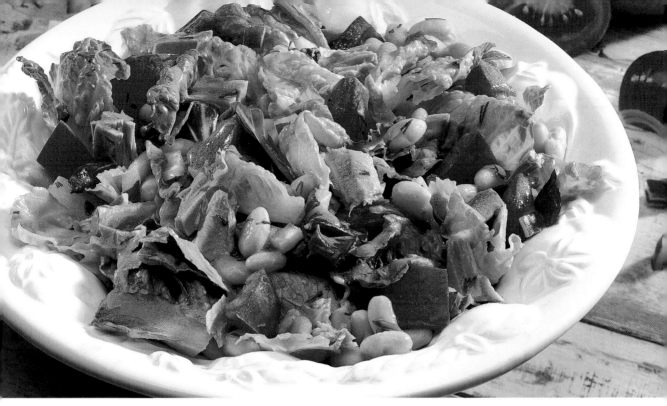

Tuscan Tuna Salad

Tuscan Tuna Salad

LO CAL / LO CHOL / HI FIB

PREP: 10 MIN

4 SERVINGS

Water-packed tuna has two advantages over oil-packed: a fresher flavor and fewer calories.

$1/2$ package (10-ounce size) Italian blend lettuce pieces (4 cups)

1 large tomato, coarsely chopped (1 cup)

1 can (15 to 16 ounces) great northern beans, rinsed and drained

1 can (6 ounces) tuna in water, drained

3 tablespoons chopped red onion

2 tablespoons olive or vegetable oil

1 tablespoon balsamic or red wine vinegar

1 tablespoon Dijon mustard

$1/2$ teaspoon dried dill weed

1 teaspoon chopped fresh or $1/4$ teaspoon dried dill weed

Gently toss lettuce, tomato, beans and tuna in large bowl. Mix remaining ingredients; toss with tuna mixture just until coated. Serve immediately.

1 Serving: Calories 220 (Calories from Fat 70); Fat 8g (Saturated 2g); Cholesterol 10mg; Sodium 200mg; Carbohydrate 24g (Dietary Fiber 6g); Protein 19g
% Daily Value: Vitamin A 4%; Vitamin C 18%; Calcium 8%; Iron 22%
Diet Exchanges: 1 starch, 1 medium-fat meat, 2 vegetable

California Club Pasta Salad

LO CAL / LO FAT / LO CHOL / HI FIB

PREP: 20 MIN

6 SERVINGS

A Mixed-Berry Smoothie (page 66) turns this cool pasta salad into a healthy and delicious meal.

3	cups uncooked medium pasta shells ($7^1/_2$ ounces)
$^3/_4$	cup fat-free ranch dressing
1	medium tomato, chopped ($^3/_4$ cup)
$^1/_4$	pound deli-style sliced fat-free ham, cut into $^1/_2$-inch strips
$^1/_4$	pound deli-style sliced fat-free turkey, cut into $^1/_2$-inch strips
2	medium green onions, sliced (2 tablespoons)
1	bag (10 ounces) washed fresh spinach
$^1/_4$	cup imitation bacon-flavor bits

Cook and drain pasta as directed on package. Rinse with cold water; drain.

Toss pasta, dressing, tomato, ham, turkey and onions. Place spinach on serving platter. Top with pasta mixture. Sprinkle with bacon bits.

1 Serving: Calories 230 (Calories from Fat 20); Fat 2g (Saturated 0g); Cholesterol 15mg; Sodium 840mg; Carbohydrate 42g (Dietary Fiber 3g); Protein 14g
% Daily Value: Vitamin A 40%; Vitamin C 30%; Calcium 8%; Iron 18%
Diet Exchanges: 2 starch, 1 very lean meat, 2 vegetable

Bacon-Spinach Salad

LO CAL / LO FAT

PREP: 10 MIN; COOK: 10 MIN

4 SERVINGS

This salad is best when served immediately, before it has a chance to become soggy.

4	slices bacon, diced
$^1/_4$	cup white vinegar
4	teaspoons sugar
$^1/_4$	teaspoon salt
$^1/_8$	teaspoon pepper
1	cup chopped cooked chicken
1	cup sliced mushrooms
1	bag (10 ounces) washed fresh spinach
3	medium green onions, chopped (3 tablespoons)

Cook bacon in 12-inch nonstick skillet over low heat, stirring occasionally, until crisp. Stir in vinegar, sugar, salt and pepper. Heat through, stirring constantly, until sugar is dissolved; remove from heat.

Add chicken, mushrooms, spinach and onions to bacon mixture. Toss 1 to 2 minutes or until spinach is wilted.

1 Serving: Calories 130 (Calories from Fat 45); Fat 5g (Saturated 2g); Cholesterol 35mg; Sodium 320mg; Carbohydrate 9g (Dietary Fiber 2g); Protein 14g
% Daily Value: Vitamin A 42%; Vitamin C 28%; Calcium 6%; Iron 12%
Diet Exchanges: $1^1/_2$ lean meat, 2 vegetable

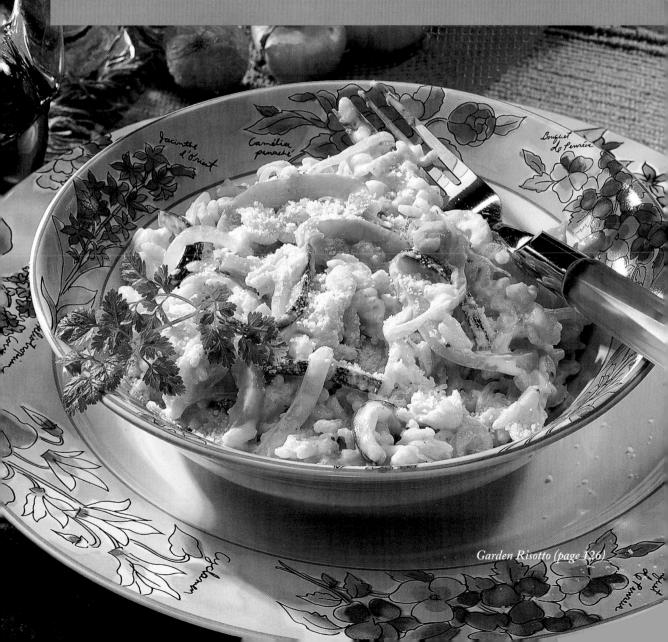

PASTA, RICE AND GRAINS

Garden Risotto (page 126)

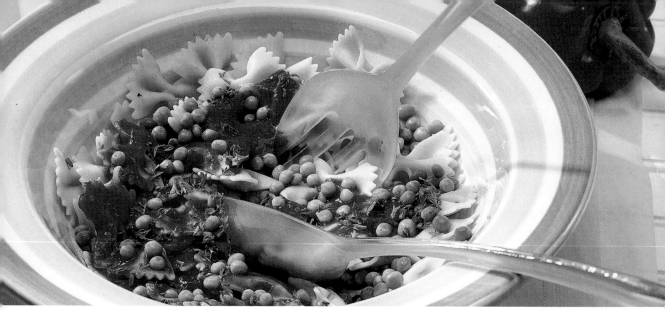

Red Pepper Bows with Peas

Red Pepper Bows with Peas

LO CAL / LO FAT / LO CHOL / HI FIB

PREP: 10 MIN; COOK: 20 MIN

4 SERVINGS

Peppers are more easily cut from the flesh side, so keep the skin side down on your cutting board. And on the nutrition front, bell peppers are an excellent source of vitamin C.

Red Pepper Sauce (right)

2 cups uncooked farfalle (bow-tie) pasta (6 ounces)

1 cup cooked green peas

2 tablespoons chopped fresh parsley

Prepare Red Pepper Sauce. Cook and drain pasta as directed on package—except omit salt. Mix pasta, sauce, peas and parsley.

Red Pepper Sauce

2 medium red bell peppers, chopped (2 cups)

½ cup chicken broth

1 tablespoon chopped fresh or 1 teaspoon dried oregano leaves

¼ teaspoon salt

¼ teaspoon pepper

1 tablespoon tomato paste

1 tablespoon balsamic vinegar

1 teaspoon honey

Cover and cook bell peppers, broth, oregano, salt and pepper in 2-quart saucepan over medium-low heat 20 minutes, stirring occasionally, until bell peppers are tender. Stir in remaining ingredients; remove from heat. Place mixture in blender. Cover and blend on medium speed until smooth.

1 Serving: Calories 210 (Calories from Fat 10); Fat 1g (Saturated 0g); Cholesterol 0mg; Sodium 350mg; Carbohydrate 46g (Dietary Fiber 5g); Protein 9g
% Daily Value: Vitamin A 38%; Vitamin C 100%; Calcium 2%; Iron 16%
Diet Exchanges: 2 starch, 2 vegetable

Lemon-Chive Fettuccine

LO CAL / LO FAT

PREP: 20 MIN

4 SERVINGS

Try adding slices of grilled chicken breast or grilled shrimp to this zesty-tasting pasta for a hearty main dish. Also, when grating the lemon peel, grate only the yellow portion; the white part, or pith, is bitter.

6	ounces uncooked fettuccine
1/3	cup reduced-fat sour cream
3	tablespoons chopped fresh or 1 tablespoon freeze-dried chives
1	tablespoon grated lemon peel
2	tablespoons lemon juice
1	teaspoon margarine, softened
1/2	teaspoon salt
1/4	teaspoon white pepper

Cook and drain fettuccine as directed on package—except omit salt. Mix remaining ingredients; toss with fettuccine.

1 Serving: Calories 185 (Calories from Fat 35); Fat 4g (Saturated 2g); Cholesterol 45mg; Sodium 340mg; Carbohydrate 31g (Dietary Fiber 1g); Protein 7g
% Daily Value: Vitamin A 6%; Vitamin C 2%; Calcium 4%; Iron 10%
Diet Exchanges: 2 starch, 1/2 fat

Ravioli with Tomato-Alfredo Sauce

LOW CALORIE

PREP: 10 MIN; COOK: 10 MIN

6 SERVINGS

This healthy, can't-miss recipe lets you re-create a rich, restaurant-style pasta dish at home without all of the fat and calories. If you can't find fat-free half-and-half in your area, refrigerated fat-free nondairy creamer makes an excellent substitute.

2   packages (9 ounces each) refrigerated dried tomato- or cheese-filled ravioli

1   package (8 ounces) sliced mushrooms (3 cups)

1   large onion, coarsely chopped (1 cup)

1   jar (24 to 28 ounces) fat-free spaghetti sauce

1/2   cup fat-free half-and-half or refrigerated fat-free nondairy creamer

1/4   cup grated Parmesan cheese

1/4   cup chopped fresh parsley

Cook and drain ravioli as directed on package; keep warm.

Spray same saucepan with cooking spray; heat over medium heat. Cook mushrooms and onion in saucepan about 5 minutes, stirring frequently, until onion is crisp-tender.

Stir in spaghetti sauce and half-and-half. Heat to boiling; reduce heat. Stir in ravioli, cheese and parsley.

1 Serving: Calories 225 (Calories from Fat 65); Fat 7g (Saturated 4g); Cholesterol 85mg; Sodium 1100mg; Carbohydrate 30g (Dietary Fiber 2g); Protein 12g
% Daily Value: Vitamin A 12%; Vitamin C 10%; Calcium 20%; Iron 10%
Diet Exchanges: 2 starch, 1 fat

Fettuccine with Creamy Tomato Sauce

LO CAL / LO FAT

PREP: 10 MIN; COOK: 10 MIN

6 SERVINGS

Dried chives are labeled "freeze-dried chives," which refers to the drying method that was used, not where they are found in the supermarket.

- 1   package (16 ounces) fettuccine
- 1   small onion, chopped ($\frac{1}{4}$ cup)
- 2   cloves garlic, finely chopped
- 1   can (14$\frac{1}{2}$ ounces) whole tomatoes, undrained
- $\frac{2}{3}$ cup reduced-fat ricotta cheese
- 1   tablespoon chopped fresh or 1 teaspoon dried basil leaves
- 1   tablespoon chopped fresh or 1 teaspoon freeze-dried chives
- 2   teaspoons sugar
- $\frac{1}{8}$ teaspoon pepper

Cook and drain fettuccine as directed on package—except omit salt. While fettuccine is cooking, spray 3-quart saucepan with cooking spray; heat over medium-high heat. Cook onion and garlic in saucepan, stirring occasionally, until onion is crisp-tender. Stir in remaining ingredients, breaking up tomatoes.

Heat to boiling; reduce heat. Simmer uncovered about 5 minutes, stirring occasionally, until mixture thickens slightly. Add fettuccine; toss with tomato sauce.

1 Serving: Calories 310 (Calories from Fat 45); Fat 5g (Saturated 2g); Cholesterol 75mg; Sodium 150mg; Carbohydrate 56g (Dietary Fiber 3g); Protein 13g
% Daily Value: Vitamin A 8%; Vitamin C 8%; Calcium 12%; Iron 20%
Diet Exchanges: 3 starch, 2 vegetable, $\frac{1}{2}$ fat

Pasta with Tomato-Lentil Sauce

LO CAL / LO FAT / LO CHOL / HI FIB

PREP: 15 MIN; COOK: 45 MIN

6 SERVINGS

Lentils are truly ancient, known to have been eaten in southwestern Asia around 7000 B.C. There are literally hundreds of types of lentils, or "pulses," but the most common type is grayish green in color and widely available in most supermarkets.

1	large onion, chopped (1 cup)
1	medium stalk celery, chopped (1/2 cup)
1	medium carrot, chopped (1/2 cup)
1/2	cup chicken broth
2	cloves garlic, finely chopped
1/2	cup dried lentils (4 ounces), sorted and rinsed
1	tablespoon chopped fresh or 1 teaspoon dried basil leaves
1 1/2	teaspoons chopped fresh or 1/2 teaspoon dried thyme leaves
1	bay leaf
1	can (8 ounces) tomato sauce
4	cups uncooked spiral macaroni (12 ounces)
1	package (10 ounces) frozen chopped spinach, thawed and squeezed to drain
2	tablespoons grated Parmesan cheese

Cook onion, celery, carrot, broth and garlic in 2-quart saucepan over medium heat about 10 minutes or until liquid has evaporated. Stir in remaining ingredients except macaroni, spinach and cheese. Heat to boiling; reduce heat. Cover and simmer 25 to 30 minutes, stirring occasionally, until lentils are tender.

While mixture is simmering, cook and drain macaroni as directed on package—except omit salt.

Stir spinach into lentil mixture. Cook about 3 minutes, stirring frequently, until spinach is hot. Remove bay leaf. Serve lentil mixture over macaroni, sprinkle with cheese.

1 Serving: Calories 286 (Calories from Fat 20); Fat 2g (Saturated 1g); Cholesterol 0mg; Sodium 390mg; Carbohydrate 61g (Dietary Fiber 8g); Protein 14g
% Daily Value: Vitamin A 44%; Vitamin C 10%; Calcium 10%; Iron 26%
Diet Exchanges: 4 starch

Roasted Red Pepper Mostaccioli

LO CAL / LO FAT / LO CHOL

PREP: 5 MIN; COOK: 20 MIN

6 SERVINGS

Mostaccioli is a short, tubular pasta measuring about 2 inches long. Both ends are cut at a slant, and the surface can be smooth or grooved. Penne, rigatoni or ziti can be substituted for mostaccioli.

3 cups uncooked mostaccioli pasta (9 ounces)

1 can (14$\frac{1}{2}$ ounces) Italian-style stewed tomatoes, undrained

1 jar (7 ounces) roasted red bell peppers, drained

1 tablespoon olive or vegetable oil

1 clove garlic, finely chopped

2 teaspoons chopped fresh or $\frac{1}{2}$ teaspoon dried oregano leaves

2 teaspoons capers

Freshly ground pepper, if desired

Cook and drain pasta as directed on package—except omit salt. While pasta is cooking, place tomatoes and bell peppers in blender or food processor. Cover and blend on high speed until smooth.

Heat oil in 1-quart nonstick saucepan over medium heat. Cook garlic in oil, stirring occasionally, until golden. Stir in tomato mixture, oregano and capers. Simmer uncovered 15 minutes, stirring occasionally. Serve over pasta with pepper.

1 Serving: Calories 205 (Calories from Fat 25); Fat 3g (Saturated 0g); Cholesterol 0mg; Sodium 220mg; Carbohydrate 40g (Dietary Fiber 2g); Protein 6g
% Daily Value: Vitamin A 12%; Vitamin C 40%; Calcium 2%; Iron 12%
Diet Exchanges: 2 starch, 2 vegetable

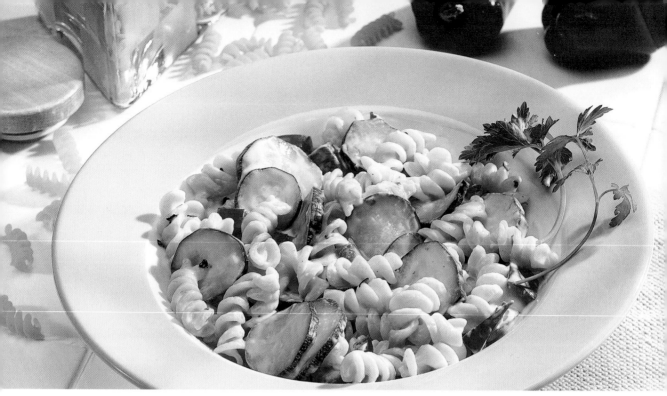

Rotini and Vegetables with Blue Cheese Sauce

Rotini and Vegetables with Blue Cheese Sauce

LO CAL / HI FIBER

PREP: 10 MIN; COOK: 20 MIN

6 SERVINGS

Corkscrew-shaped rotini has lots of ridges to trap all of the scrumptious blue cheese sauce.

2²/₃   cups uncooked rotini pasta (8 ounces)

3   medium zucchini, thinly sliced (4 cups)

1   medium red bell pepper, chopped (1 cup)

1   cup skim milk

2   tablespoons all-purpose flour

1   teaspoon salt

1   teaspoon dried basil leaves

1¹/₂   cups reduced-fat sour cream

1   ounce finely crumbled blue cheese or Gorgonzola

Cook pasta as directed on package, adding zucchini and bell pepper for the last 3 minutes of cooking.

While pasta and vegetables are cooking, mix milk, flour, salt, and basil in 1-quart saucepan. Heat to boiling over medium heat, stirring constantly. Boil and stir 1 minute. Stir in sour cream; heat through.

Drain pasta and vegetables; stir in cheese. Pour sour cream sauce over pasta and vegetables; toss.

1 Serving: Calories 275 (Calories from Fat 55); Fat 6g (Saturated 4g); Cholesterol 25mg; Sodium 540mg; Carbohydrate 45g (Dietary Fiber 3g); Protein 13g
% Daily Value: Vitamin A 28%; Vitamin C 36%; Calcium 18%; Iron 12%
Diet Exchanges: 2 starch, 3 vegetable, 1 fat

Portabella Stroganoff

LO CAL / LO FAT / LO CHOL / HI FIB

PREP: 10 MIN; COOK: 10 MIN

4 SERVINGS

Portabella mushrooms have a texture similar to beef and make a great substitute in this stroganoff.

4	cups uncooked cholesterol-free noodles (8 ounces)
1	tablespoon margarine
³/₄	pound fresh portabella mushrooms, cut into 2 × ¹/₂-inch strips
1	medium onion, chopped (¹/₂ cup)
1	clove garlic, finely chopped
³/₄	cup beef broth
2	tablespoons ketchup
¹/₂	cup reduced-fat sour cream
	Freshly ground pepper
	Chopped fresh parsley, if desired

Cook and drain noodles as directed on package—except omit salt. While noodles are cooking, melt margarine in 12-inch nonstick skillet over medium heat. Cook mushrooms, onion and garlic in margarine, stirring occasionally, until mushrooms are brown and tender.

Stir broth and ketchup into mushroom mixture. Cook 5 minutes, stirring occasionally. Stir in sour cream. Serve over noodles. Sprinkle with pepper and parsley.

1 Serving: Calories 215 (Calories from Fat 25); Fat 3g (Saturated 0g); Cholesterol 0mg; Sodium 280mg; Carbohydrate 40g (Dietary Fiber 3g); Protein 10g
% Daily Value: Vitamin A 10%; Vitamin C 4%; Calcium 10%; Iron 16%
Diet Exchanges: 2 starch, 2 vegetable

Asian Noodle Salad

LO CAL / LO FAT

PREP: 15 MIN; CHILL: 2 HR

4 SERVINGS

If you can't find Chinese-style egg noodles, you can substitute thin spaghetti or vermicelli.

6	ounces uncooked Chinese-style egg noodles
1	cup chopped cooked chicken breast
2	tablespoons chopped fresh cilantro
2	tablespoons frozen (thawed) apple juice concentrate
1	tablespoon balsamic vinegar
1	tablespoon reduced-sodium soy sauce
2	teaspoons finely chopped gingerroot
¹/₂	teaspoon sesame oil
5	medium green onions, chopped (¹/₃ cup)
1	clove garlic, finely chopped

Cook and drain noodles as directed on package—except omit salt. Toss noodles and remaining ingredients. Cover and refrigerate about 2 hours or until chilled.

1 Serving: Calories 230 (Calories from Fat 35); Fat 4g (Saturated 1g); Cholesterol 65mg; Sodium 170mg; Carbohydrate 33g (Dietary Fiber 1g); Protein 16g
% Daily Value: Vitamin A 0%; Vitamin C 4%; Calcium 2%; Iron 14%
Diet Exchanges: 2 starch, 1¹/₂ lean meat

Creamy Vegetable Macaroni and Cheese

LO FAT / LO CHOL / HI FIB

PREP: 10 MIN; COOK: 20 MIN

4 SERVINGS

If the youngsters at your house are a little wary of vegetables, cook the vegetables and macaroni for this recipe in separate saucepans. Then add the vegetables only to the servings for the adults.

1 package (7 ounces) elbow macaroni (2 cups)

1 bag (16 ounces) frozen cauliflower, carrots and snow pea pods, thawed, or 1 bag (16 ounces) frozen carrots, green beans and cauliflower, thawed

2 cups fat-free half-and-half or evaporated skimmed milk

$1/4$ cup all-purpose flour

$3/4$ teaspoon dried marjoram leaves

$3/4$ teaspoons ground mustard (dry)

$1/2$ teaspoon salt

$1/4$ teaspoon pepper

1 package (8 ounces) shredded reduced-fat Cheddar cheese (2 cups)

Cook macaroni as directed on package—except add vegetables with pasta.

While macaroni and vegetables are cooking, beat half-and-half, flour, marjoram, mustard, salt and pepper in $1^1/2$-quart saucepan with wire whisk. Heat to boiling over medium heat, stirring constantly. Boil and stir 1 minute; remove from heat. Stir in cheese until melted.

Drain macaroni and vegetables. Pour sauce over macaroni and vegetables; toss.

1 Serving: Calories 375 (Calories from Fat 45); Fat 5g (Saturated 3g); Cholesterol 15mg; Sodium 450mg; Carbohydrate 59g (Dietary Fiber 5g); Protein 29g
% Daily Value: Vitamin A 46%; Vitamin C 30%; Calcium 46%; Iron 18%
Diet Exchanges: 2 starch, 1 vegetable, 1 skim milk, 1 fat

Spicy Confetti Noodles

LO CAL / LO FAT / LO CHOL

PREP: 20 MIN; COOK: 5 MIN

4 SERVINGS

Sesame oil is made by pressing sesame seed, so it has a nutty flavor. It can be found in both light and dark varieties. The dark variety is usually made by pressing toasted sesame seed and has a more intense, distinctive flavor. Look for this oil in the Asian foods section of the supermarket.

3	green onions
2	medium bell peppers
2	medium carrots
2	packages (5 ounces each) Japanese curly noodles or 10 ounces uncooked spaghetti
2	teaspoons sesame oil
1/3	cup water
1/4	cup dry sherry or water
1	tablespoon finely chopped gingerroot
2	tablespoons soy sauce
1	tablespoon chili puree with garlic
1	teaspoon curry powder
1/2	teaspoon chicken bouillon granules
1/4	teaspoon sugar
2	cloves garlic, finely chopped

Cut onions into 2-inch pieces; cut pieces into thin strips. Cut bell peppers into thin strips. Cut carrots into julienne strips.

Cook and drain noodles as directed on package—except omit salt. Toss noodles and sesame oil in large bowl. Stir in onions, bell peppers and carrots.

Mix remaining ingredients in nonstick wok or 12-inch nonstick skillet. Heat to boiling over medium heat, stirring occasionally. Add noodle mixture; toss with sauce. Heat through, stirring constantly.

1 Serving: Calories 85 (Calories from Fat 25); Fat 3g (Saturated 1g); Cholesterol 0mg; Sodium 690mg; Carbohydrate 14g (Dietary Fiber 2g); Protein 2g
% Daily Value: Vitamin A 38%; Vitamin C 22%; Calcium 2%; Iron 4%
Diet Exchanges: 1 starch

Baked Ziti and Bean Casserole

LO CAL / LO FAT / LO CHOL / HI FIB

PREP: 15 MIN; BAKE: 30 MIN

6 SERVINGS

Ziti is a short, tubular pasta with a smooth surface. This type of pasta stands up well to thick or chunky sauces.

1   can (28 ounces) whole tomatoes, drained

1   cup fat-free ricotta cheese

¼   cup chopped red onion

1   tablespoon chopped fresh parsley

1   tablespoon chopped fresh or 1 teaspoon dried thyme leaves

½   teaspoon salt

¼   teaspoon crushed red pepper

4   cups hot cooked ziti or penne pasta

1   can (15 to 16 ounces) great northern beans, rinsed and drained

3   slices reduced-fat mozzarella cheese, about 6½ × 4 inches

Grated Parmesan cheese, if desired

Heat oven to 400°. Spray rectangular baking dish, 11 × 7 × 1½ inches, with cooking spray. Break up tomatoes in large bowl. Stir in ricotta cheese, onion, parsley, thyme, salt and red pepper. Carefully fold in pasta and beans.

Spread pasta mixture in baking dish. Arrange mozzarella cheese on top. Bake uncovered about 30 minutes or until mixture is hot and cheese is golden brown. Sprinkle with Parmesan cheese.

1 Serving: Calories 325 (Calories from Fat 55); Fat 6g (Saturated 4g); Cholesterol 15mg; Sodium 580mg; Carbohydrate 50g (Dietary Fiber 6g); Protein 24g
% Daily Value: Vitamin A 14%; Vitamin C 16%; Calcium 36%; Iron 22%
Diet Exchanges: 3 starch, 2 very lean meat, 1 vegetable

Vegetable Manicotti

LO CAL / LO FAT / LO CHOL / HI FIB

PREP: 25 MIN; BAKE: 45 MIN

4 SERVINGS

Zucchini, or "zukes," are a good source of vitamin C and also contain vitamin A. Look for firm zucchini with bright-colored skin that is free of soft spots.

8	uncooked manicotti shells
1	can (8 ounces) tomato sauce
1	teaspoon olive or vegetable oil
1	small carrot, shredded ($^1/_2$ cup)
1	small zucchini, shredded ($^1/_2$ cup)
$^1/_2$	cup sliced mushrooms
4	medium green onions, sliced ($^1/_4$ cup)
1	clove garlic, finely chopped
1	container (15 ounces) fat-free ricotta cheese
$^1/_4$	cup grated Parmesan cheese
2	tablespoons chopped fresh or 2 teaspoons dried basil leaves
$^1/_4$	cup fat-free cholesterol-free egg product or 2 egg whites
$^1/_2$	cup shredded reduced-fat mozzarella cheese (2 ounces)

Heat oven to 350°. Spray rectangular baking dish, $11 \times 7 \times 1^1/_2$ inches, with cooking spray. Cook and drain manicotti shells as directed on package—except omit salt. Pour $^1/_3$ cup of the tomato sauce into baking dish.

While manicotti is cooking, heat oil in 10-inch nonstick skillet over medium-high heat. Cook carrot, zucchini, mushrooms, onions and garlic in oil, stirring frequently, until vegetables are crisp-tender. Stir in remaining ingredients except mozzarella cheese.

Fill manicotti shells with vegetable mixture; place in baking dish. Pour remaining tomato sauce over manicotti. Sprinkle with mozzarella cheese. Cover and bake 40 to 45 minutes or until hot and bubbly.

1 Serving: Calories 330 (Calories from Fat 55); Fat 6g (Saturated 3g); Cholesterol 10mg; Sodium 640mg; Carbohydrate 42g (Dietary Fiber 3g); Protein 30g
% Daily Value: Vitamin A 36%; Vitamin C 10%; Calcium 40%; Iron 14%
Diet Exchanges: 2 starch, 2 lean meat, 2 vegetable

Mushroom and Spinach Lasagna

LO CAL / LO FAT / LO CHOL / HI FIB

PREP: 25 MIN; BAKE: 1 HR; STAND: 10 MIN

6 SERVINGS

Check out your freezer case for precooked uncut sheets of lasagna noodles or the dried pasta section for precooked lasagna noodles. Use the precooked noodles just as you would traditional cooked noodles.

1   package (8 ounces) lasagna noodles

1¼ cups fat-free ricotta cheese

½   cup fat-free cholesterol-free egg product or 4 egg whites

1   cup chopped mushrooms (4 ounces)

1   large onion, chopped (1 cup)

1   package (10 ounces) frozen chopped spinach, thawed and squeezed to drain

½   teaspoon salt

¼   teaspoon ground nutmeg, if desired

1   jar (14 ounces) spaghetti sauce

3   tablespoons grated Parmesan cheese

Heat oven to 350°. Grease rectangular baking dish, 11 × 7 × 1½ inches. Cook and drain noodles as directed on package—except omit salt.

Mix ½ cup of the ricotta cheese, ¼ cup egg product, the mushrooms and onion. Mix remaining ¾ cup ricotta cheese, ¼ cup egg product, the spinach, salt and nutmeg. Spread ½ cup of the spaghetti sauce in baking dish. Top with 4 noodles, overlapping to fit. Layer with mushroom mixture, 3 noodles, spinach mixture, 3 noodles and remaining spaghetti sauce.

Cover loosely and bake 50 minutes. Sprinkle with Parmesan cheese. Bake uncovered about 10 minutes or until cheese is melted. Let stand 10 minutes before cutting.

1 Serving: Calories 290 (Calories from Fat 35); Fat 4g (Saturated 1g); Cholesterol 2mg; Sodium 670mg; Carbohydrate 50g (Dietary Fiber 4g); Protein 17g
% Daily Value: Vitamin A 34%; Vitamin C 2%; Calcium 20%; Iron 16%
Diet Exchanges: 3 starch, 1 vegetable, 1 very lean meat

Tuna Marinara with Linguine

LO CAL / LO FAT / HI FIB

PREP: 15 MIN; COOK: 20 MIN

6 SERVINGS

Capers are the flower buds of the caper bush. Some capers are not much larger than the end of a cotton swab, and others are twice that size. After the buds are harvested, they are pickled in brine. There isn't a good substitute for capers, so if you can't find them, just leave them out of the recipe.

8	ounces uncooked linguine
³/₄	cup tomato puree
³/₄	cup white wine or apple juice
2	cloves garlic, finely chopped
1	teaspoon olive or vegetable oil
1	can (14¹/₂ ounces) whole tomatoes, undrained
1	pound yellowfin tuna or other lean fish fillets, cut into 1-inch pieces
3	tablespoons chopped fresh or 1 tablespoon dried basil leaves
1	teaspoon grated lemon peel
2	tablespoons lemon juice
2	teaspoons capers
¹/₄	teaspoon pepper

Cook and drain linguine as directed on package—except omit salt. Cook tomato puree, wine, garlic, oil and tomatoes in 2-quart saucepan over medium heat 10 minutes, breaking up tomatoes and stirring occasionally.

Stir in fish. Cover and simmer about 7 minutes or until fish flakes easily with fork. Stir in linguine and remaining ingredients.

1 Serving: Calories 275 (Calories from Fat 45); Fat 5g (Saturated 2g); Cholesterol 30mg; Sodium 290mg; Carbohydrate 37g (Dietary Fiber 3g); Protein 24g
% Daily Value: Vitamin A 54%; Vitamin C 14%; Calcium 4%; Iron 18%
Diet Exchanges: 2 starch, 2 lean meat, 1 vegetable

Spring Chicken Pasta

LO FAT / HI FIB

PREP: 20 MIN; COOK: 10 MIN

6 SERVINGS

Ricotta is a fresh, unaged cheese that is just a bit grainy but smoother than cottage cheese. It is very moist with a slightly sweet flavor and is widely used in both main dishes and desserts.

1½   pounds skinless, boneless chicken breast halves

8   ounces uncooked spaghetti

1   pound asparagus, cut into 2-inch pieces

8   sun-dried tomato halves (not oil-packed), chopped

2   cloves garlic, finely chopped

1   large yellow bell pepper, chopped (1½ cups)

¾   cup chopped red onion

2   cups chicken broth

¾   cup fat-free ricotta cheese

⅓   cup chopped fresh basil leaves

2   tablespoons reduced-fat sour cream

½   teaspoon salt

¼   teaspoon pepper

Remove fat from chicken. Cut chicken into ½-inch strips. Cook and drain spaghetti as directed on package—except omit salt.

While spaghetti is cooking, cook asparagus, tomatoes, garlic, bell pepper, onion and broth in 3-quart saucepan over medium heat 5 minutes. Stir in chicken. Cook 2 to 3 minutes, stirring constantly, until asparagus is crisp-tender and chicken is no longer pink in center.

Stir in spaghetti and remaining ingredients. Toss about 30 seconds or until heated through.

1 Serving: Calories 355 (Calories from Fat 55); Fat 6g (Saturated 2g); Cholesterol 70mg; Sodium 680mg; Carbohydrate 40g (Dietary Fiber 3g); Protein 38g
% Daily Value: Vitamin A 8%; Vitamin C 54%; Calcium 10%; Iron 18%
Diet Exchanges: 2 starch, 4 very lean meat, 2 vegetable

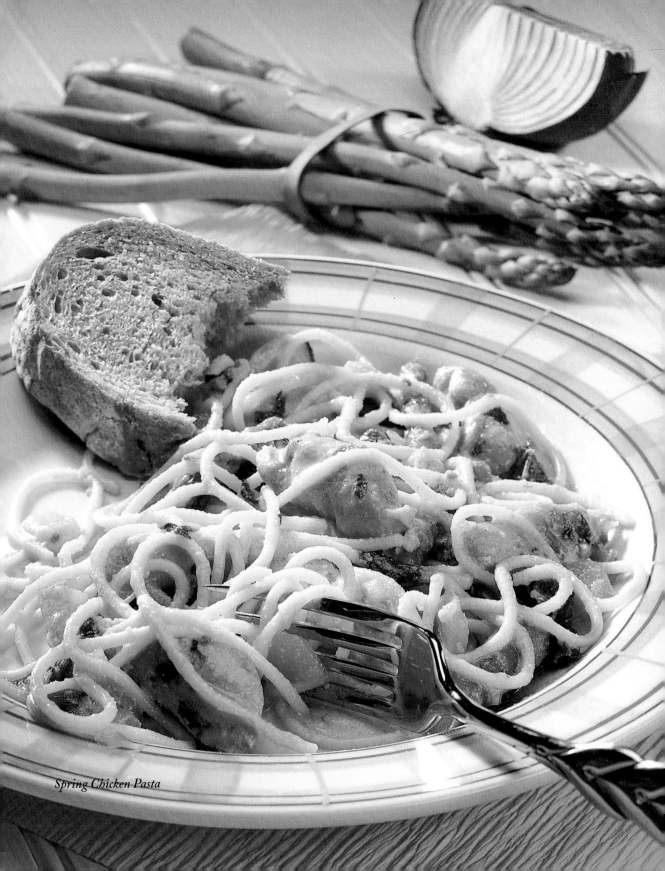

Spring Chicken Pasta

Noodles with Smoked Turkey

LO CAL / HI FIB

PREP: 10 MIN; COOK: 12 MIN

6 SERVINGS

For added zest, dust this sophisticated pasta with a sprinkling of finely shredded Parmesan cheese.

- 10 ounces uncooked yolk-free wide noodles
- 1 package (9 ounces) frozen artichoke hearts, thawed
- 1 small red onion, cut lengthwise in half, then cut crosswise into thin slices
- 1½ cups skim milk
- 3 tablespoons all-purpose flour
- ¾ teaspoon garlic salt
- ½ package (8-ounce size) reduced-fat cream cheese (Neufchâtel)
- 4 ounces sliced fat-free smoked turkey, cut into julienne strips (¾ cup)

  Grated Parmesan cheese, if desired

Cook and drain noodles as directed on package—except add artichokes and onion with noodles.

While noodles and vegetables are cooking, beat milk, flour and garlic salt in 1½-quart saucepan with wire whisk until blended. Heat to boiling over medium heat, stirring constantly. Boil and stir 1 minute. Stir in cream cheese until melted.

Drain noodles and vegetables. Toss noodles, vegetables, turkey and sauce until well coated. Sprinkle with Parmesan cheese.

1 Serving: Calories 285 (Calories from Fat 65); Fat 7g (Saturated 3g); Cholesterol 65mg; Sodium 570mg; Carbohydrate 44g (Dietary Fiber 4g); Protein 15g
% Daily Value: Vitamin A 10%; Vitamin C 4%; Calcium 12%; Iron 16%
Diet Exchanges: 3 starch, 1 lean meat

Shanghai Chicken and Noodles

LO CAL / LO FAT

PREP: 20 MIN; COOK: 10 MIN

6 SERVINGS

Hoisin sauce is a sweet, medium-spicy, thick, reddish-brown sauce made from soybeans, vinegar, chilies, spices and garlic. It is used in cooking and as a condiment. Look for it in the Asian foods section in your supermarket. Sorry, there's no substitute.

1   pound skinless, boneless chicken breast halves

8   ounces uncooked fettuccine

1   bag (16 ounces) chopped vegetables for stir-fry or chop suey (about 5 cups)

1   cup sliced mushrooms (3 ounces)

1/4   cup hoisin sauce

Remove fat from chicken. Cut chicken into 1/4-inch slices. Cook and drain fettuccine as directed on package—except omit salt.

While fettuccine is cooking, spray nonstick wok or 12-inch nonstick skillet with cooking spray; heat over medium-high heat. Add chicken; stir-fry 3 to 4 minutes or until brown and no longer pink in center. Add vegetables and mushrooms; stir-fry about 3 minutes or until vegetables are crisp-tender.

Stir in hoisin sauce. Heat to boiling, stirring constantly. Boil and stir 1 minute. Add fettuccine; toss until well coated and heated through.

1 Serving: Calories 250 (Calories from Fat 35); Fat 4g (Saturated 1g); Cholesterol 75mg; Sodium 55mg; Carbohydrate 34g (Dietary Fiber 2g); Protein 22g
% Daily Value: Vitamin A 6%; Vitamin C 16%; Calcium 4%; Iron 16%
Diet Exchanges: 2 starch, 2 very lean meat, 1 vegetable

Mixed Herb Spaghetti and Clam Sauce

LO CAL / LO FAT / HI FIB

PREP: 15 MIN; COOK: 10 MIN

6 SERVINGS

Canned whole baby clams may not be available in your supermarket, so use minced clams instead.

2   large tomatoes, chopped (2 cups)

1   cup tomato juice

$^1\!/_2$ cup dry white wine or tomato juice

2   tablespoons lemon juice

1   teaspoon olive or vegetable oil

$^1\!/_4$ teaspoon salt

$^1\!/_4$ teaspoon pepper

$^1\!/_4$ cup chopped fresh parsley

2   tablespoons chopped fresh or 2 teaspoons dried basil leaves

2   cans (10 ounces each) whole baby clams, drained

6   cups hot cooked spaghetti

Heat tomatoes, tomato juice, wine, lemon juice, oil, salt and pepper to boiling in 4-quart saucepan; reduce heat. Simmer uncovered about 5 minutes or until slightly thickened. Stir in parsley, basil and clams. Serve over spaghetti.

1 Serving: Calories 275 (Calories from Fat 25); Fat 3g (Saturated 0g); Cholesterol 30mg; Sodium 300mg; Carbohydrate 47g (Dietary Fiber 3g); Protein 18g
% Daily Value: Vitamin A 14%; Vitamin C 26%; Calcium 6%; Iron 14%
Diet Exchanges: 3 starch, 1 very lean meat

Creamy Scallops and Pasta

LO CAL / LO FAT / LO CHOL

PREP: 15 MIN; COOK: 10 MIN

6 SERVINGS

Scallops are available in two sizes: sea scallops, which are about 2 inches in diameter, and bay scallops, which average about ¹/₂ inch in diameter. Both should have a mild, sweet odor and be moist looking but not be in liquid or in direct contact with ice. Bay scallops are a little bit sweeter than sea scallops and are creamy white in color or may be tinted light tan or pink.

2	large shallots or 1 small onion, chopped (¹/₄ cup)
1¹/₂	cups chicken broth
1¹/₂	teaspoons chopped fresh or ¹/₂ teaspoon dried thyme leaves
2	tablespoons all-purpose flour
2¹/₃	cups skim milk
2	tablespoons reduced-fat sour cream
¹/₄	teaspoon salt
¹/₄	teaspoon pepper
1	pound bay scallops
4	cups hot cooked medium pasta shells
¹/₄	cup dry bread crumbs
2	tablespoons chopped fresh parsley
1	teaspoon grated lemon peel

Cook shallots, broth and thyme in 12-inch nonstick skillet over medium heat until shallots are tender. Stir in flour. Cook 2 minutes, stirring constantly. Stir in milk, sour cream, salt and pepper. Simmer about 3 minutes, stirring frequently, until slightly thickened. Stir in scallops and pasta. Cook about 2 minutes longer or until scallops are white.

Set oven control to broil. Mix remaining ingredients; sprinkle over scallop mixture. Wrap aluminum foil around handle of skillet if not ovenproof. Broil with top about 4 inches from heat 2 to 3 minutes or until topping is brown.

1 Serving: Calories 245 (Calories from Fat 35); Fat 4g (Saturated 2g); Cholesterol 20mg; Sodium 550mg; Carbohydrate 35g (Dietary Fiber 1g); Protein 18g
% Daily Value: Vitamin A 8%; Vitamin C 2%; Calcium 18%; Iron 16%
Diet Exchanges: 2 starch, 1 lean meat, 1 vegetable

Beef with Bow-Tie Pasta

LO CAL / LO FAT / HI FIB

PREP: 20 MIN; COOK: 10 MIN

6 SERVINGS

Usher in spring with this asparagus-packed pasta dish. Choose asparagus stalks that are straight, firm and crisp with tightly closed tips. All of the stalks should be about the same size and thickness; that way, they will cook evenly.

1/2	cup hot water
1/4	cup sun-dried tomatoes (not oil-packed)
1 1/2	pounds beef boneless sirloin steak
1	pound asparagus, cut into 2-inch pieces (3 cups)
2	medium onions, sliced
1 1/2	cups beef broth
4	cups cooked farfalle (bow-tie) pasta
1	cup tomato puree
3	tablespoons chopped fresh or 1 tablespoon dried basil leaves
3	tablespoons chopped sun-dried tomatoes (not oil-packed)
1/4	teaspoon pepper
2	tablespoons freshly grated Parmesan cheese

Pour hot water over 1/4 cup tomatoes in small bowl. Let stand 15 minutes; drain well. Chop tomatoes.

Remove fat from beef. Cut beef into 2-inch strips; cut strips crosswise into 1/8-inch slices. (Beef is easier to cut if partially frozen, about 1 1/2 hours.)

Spray 12-inch nonstick skillet with cooking spray; heat over medium heat. Cook asparagus, onions and 1 cup of the broth in skillet 5 to 7 minutes, stirring occasionally, until liquid has evaporated; remove mixture from skillet.

Add beef to skillet. Cook over medium heat about 2 minutes, stirring frequently, until beef is no longer pink. Return vegetable mixture to skillet. Stir in remaining 1/2 cup broth and remaining ingredients except cheese. Cook about 2 minutes, stirring frequently, until mixture is hot. Sprinkle with cheese.

1 Serving: Calories 290 (Calories from Fat 45); Fat 5g (Saturated 2g); Cholesterol 55mg; Sodium 530mg; Carbohydrate 36g (Dietary Fiber 3g); Protein 28g
% Daily Value: Vitamin A 8%; Vitamin C 16%; Calcium 6%; Iron 22%
Diet Exchanges: 2 starch, 2 lean meat, 1 vegetable

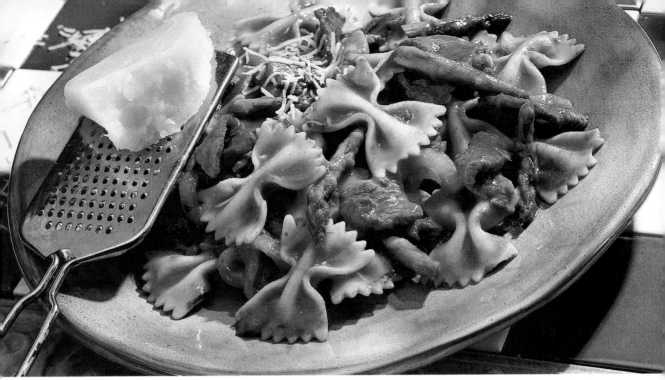

Beef with Bow-Tie Pasta

Onion-Smothered Pasta

LO CAL / LO FAT / LO CHOL / HI FIB

PREP: 5 MIN; COOK: 20 MIN

6 SERVINGS

Onions, like garlic, contain allyl sulfides. These substances may help to reduce the risk of stomach and colon cancers.

3 cups uncooked ziti pasta (10½ ounces)

2 tablespoons olive or vegetable oil

4 medium onions, cut into ¼-inch slices (2 cups)

½ cup beef broth or water

¼ cup dry red wine or beef broth

1 tablespoon chopped fresh or 1 teaspoon dried basil leaves

1 tablespoon chopped fresh or 1 teaspoon dried oregano leaves

1 can (8 ounces) tomato sauce

Cook and drain pasta as directed on package—except omit salt. While pasta is cooking, heat oil in 3-quart nonstick saucepan over medium heat. Cook onions in oil 8 to 10 minutes, stirring occasionally, until tender.

Stir in remaining ingredients; cook until hot. Serve over pasta. Sprinkle with additional oregano if desired.

1 Serving: Calories 295 (Calories from Fat 55); Fat 6g (Saturated 1g); Cholesterol 0mg; Sodium 230mg; Carbohydrate 55g (Dietary Fiber 4g); Protein 9g
% Daily Value: Vitamin A 4%; Vitamin C 8%; Calcium 2%; Iron 16%
Diet Exchanges: 3 starch, 2 vegetable

Cilantro Orzo and Beef

LO CAL / LO FAT / LO CHOL

PREP: 10 MIN; COOK: 15 MIN

6 SERVINGS

Tiny and shaped like grains of rice, orzo is often sold under the name rosamarina. *This mini-pasta is ideal for soups or to use in casseroles or one-dish skillet meals.*

3	cups beef broth
1½	cups uncooked orzo (rosamarina) pasta (9 ounces)
1	can (12 ounces) vacuum-packed whole kernel corn, undrained
1	can (4 ounces) chopped green chilies, undrained
2	teaspoons olive or vegetable oil
½	pound cut-up extra-lean beef for stir-fry
1	medium bell pepper, cut into ¼-inch strips
¼	cup chopped fresh cilantro

Mix broth, pasta, corn and chilies in 2-quart saucepan. Heat to boiling; reduce heat. Cover and simmer about 10 minutes or until pasta is just tender; remove from heat. Let stand about 5 minutes or until almost all liquid is absorbed.

While pasta mixture is cooking, spray 10-inch nonstick skillet with cooking spray. Add oil; heat over medium-high heat. Cook beef and bell pepper in skillet about 5 minutes, stirring occasionally, until beef is brown.

Stir beef mixture into pasta mixture. Stir in cilantro.

1 Serving: Calories 230 (Calories from Fat 35); Fat 4g (Saturated 1g); Cholesterol 20mg; Sodium 700mg; Carbohydrate 36g (Dietary Fiber 2g); Protein 15g
% Daily Value: Vitamin A 2%; Vitamin C 38%; Calcium 2%; Iron 14%
Diet Exchanges: 2½ starch, 1 lean meat

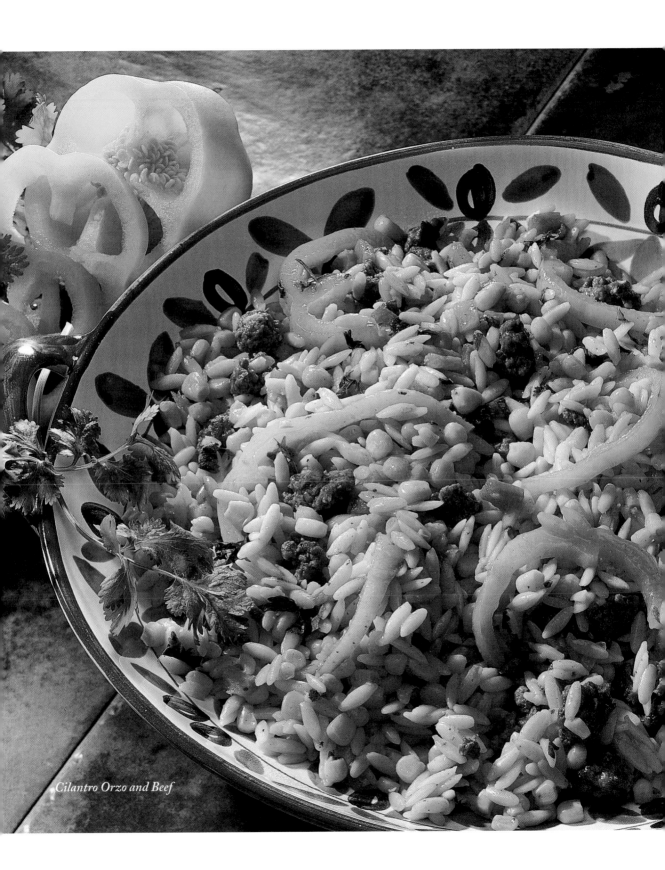

Cilantro Orzo and Beef

Mostaccioli and Beef

LOW CALORIE

PREP: 30 MIN; BAKE: 35 MIN

6 SERVINGS

Romano cheese is usually made from sheep's milk, not cow's milk as is Parmesan cheese. Some of the Romano cheese made in the United States, however, may be made with cow's milk or a combination of sheep and cow's milk. Romano has a drier, sharper flavor than Parmesan.

1½   cups uncooked mostaccioli pasta
     (4½ ounces)

1   pound extra-lean ground beef

1   medium onion, chopped (½ cup)

2   teaspoons chopped fresh or ½ teaspoon
     dried oregano leaves

¼   teaspoon salt

¼   teaspoon ground cinnamon

⅛   teaspoon ground nutmeg

1   can (8 ounces) tomato sauce

1   clove garlic, finely chopped

1   tablespoon margarine

2   tablespoons all-purpose flour
     Dash of ground nutmeg

1½   cups skim milk

¼   cup grated Romano cheese

Heat oven to 350°. Cook and drain pasta as directed on package—except omit salt. Cook beef and onion in 10-inch nonstick skillet over medium heat, stirring occasionally, until beef is brown; drain. Stir in oregano, salt, cinnamon, ⅛ teaspoon nutmeg, the tomato sauce and garlic. Alternate layers of pasta and beef mixture in ungreased 2-quart casserole.

Melt margarine in 1-quart saucepan over low heat. Stir in flour and dash of nutmeg. Cook over low heat, stirring constantly, until smooth and bubbly; remove from heat. Stir in milk. Heat to boiling, stirring constantly. Boil and stir 1 minute. Spoon sauce over pasta and beef mixture. Sprinkle with cheese. Bake uncovered about 35 minutes or until bubbly and cheese is light brown.

1 Serving: Calories 320 (Calories from Fat 110); Fat 12g (Saturated 5g); Cholesterol 50mg; Sodium 480mg; Carbohydrate 32g (Dietary Fiber 2g); Protein 23g
% Daily Value: Vitamin A 10%; Vitamin C 6%; Calcium 14%; Iron 18%
Diet Exchanges: 2 starch, 3 lean meat

Manicotti

LO CAL / HI FIB

PREP: 40 MIN; BAKE: 1½ HR

7 SERVINGS

Filling uncooked manicotti shells makes this recipe very convenient and easy. The liquid from the beef mixture will rehydrate the pasta shells, and they will cook completely as they bake.

1	pound extra-lean ground beef
1	large onion, chopped (1 cup)
2	cloves garlic, finely chopped
1	can (28 ounces) whole tomatoes, undrained
1	package (8 ounces) sliced mushrooms (3 cups)
¼	cup chopped fresh parsley
1	tablespoon chopped fresh or 1 teaspoon dried basil leaves
1	teaspoon fennel seed
¼	teaspoon salt
2	cups fat-free cottage cheese
⅓	cup grated Parmesan cheese
¼	teaspoon ground nutmeg, if desired
¼	teaspoon pepper
2	packages (10 ounces each) frozen chopped spinach, thawed and squeezed to drain
14	uncooked manicotti shells
2	tablespoons grated Parmesan cheese

Heat oven to 350°. Cook beef, onion and garlic in 10-inch nonstick skillet over medium heat, stirring occasionally, until beef is brown; drain. Stir in tomatoes, mushrooms, parsley, basil, fennel seed and salt, breaking up tomatoes. Heat to boiling; reduce heat. Cover and simmer 10 minutes. Spread about one-third of the beef mixture in ungreased rectangular baking dish, 13 × 9 × 2 inches.

Mix cottage cheese, ⅓ cup Parmesan cheese, the nutmeg, pepper and spinach. Fill uncooked manicotti shells with spinach mixture; place shells on beef mixture in baking dish. Pour remaining beef mixture evenly over shells, covering shells completely. Sprinkle with 2 tablespoons Parmesan cheese. Cover and bake about 1½ hours or until manicotti shells are tender.

1 Serving: Calories 345 (Calories from Fat 90); Fat 10g (Saturated 5g); Cholesterol 45mg; Sodium 650mg; Carbohydrate 39g (Dietary Fiber 5g); Protein 30g
% Daily Value: Vitamin A 52%; Vitamin C 24%; Calcium 24%; Iron 26%
Diet Exchanges: 2 starch, 2½ lean meat, 2 vegetable

Pork Lo Mein

LO CAL / LO FAT / LO CHOL / HI FIB

PREP: 20 MIN; COOK: 5 MIN

5 SERVINGS

Fresh gingerroot adds such spunk to foods—it really livens up the flavor! If you don't use gingerroot often but like to keep it on hand, store it tightly wrapped in the freezer. To use, just peel off the thin brown skin and grate the amount you need.

- ½   **pound pork boneless loin**
- ½   **pound snap pea pods, strings removed (2 cups)**
- 1   **cup baby-cut carrots, cut lengthwise into ¼-inch sticks**
- ½   **package (9-ounce size) refrigerated linguine, cut into 2-inch pieces**
- 2   **teaspoons cornstarch**
- 1   **teaspoon sugar**
- 2   **teaspoons cold water**
- ⅓   **cup chicken broth**
- 1   **tablespoon reduced-sodium soy sauce**
- 4   **cloves garlic, finely chopped**
- 2   **teaspoons finely chopped gingerroot**
- ½   **cup thinly sliced red onion**

  Sesame seed, toasted, if desired*

Remove fat from pork. Cut pork with grain into 2 × 1-inch strips; cut strips across grain into ⅛-inch slices.

Heat 2 quarts water to boiling in 3-quart saucepan. Add pea pods, carrots and linguine; heat to boiling. Boil 2 to 3 minutes or until linguine is just tender; drain.

Mix cornstarch, sugar and cold water. Mix broth, soy sauce, garlic and gingerroot; stir in cornstarch mixture.

Spray nonstick wok or 12-inch nonstick skillet with cooking spray; heat over medium-high heat. Add pork and onion; stir-fry about 2 minutes or until pork is no longer pink. Stir broth mixture; stir into pork mixture. Stir in pea pods, carrots and linguine. Cook 2 minutes, stirring occasionally. Sprinkle with sesame seed.

*To toast sesame seed, sprinkle in ungreased skillet. Cook over medium heat about 2 minutes, stirring frequently until browning begins, then stirring constantly until golden brown.

1 Serving: Calories 185 (Calories from Fat 25); Fat 3g (Saturated 1g); Cholesterol 20mg; Sodium 200mg; Carbohydrate 30g (Dietary Fiber 3g); Protein 13g
% Daily Value: Vitamin A 40%; Vitamin C 20%; Calcium 4%; Iron 12%
Diet Exchanges: 2 starch, 1 very lean meat

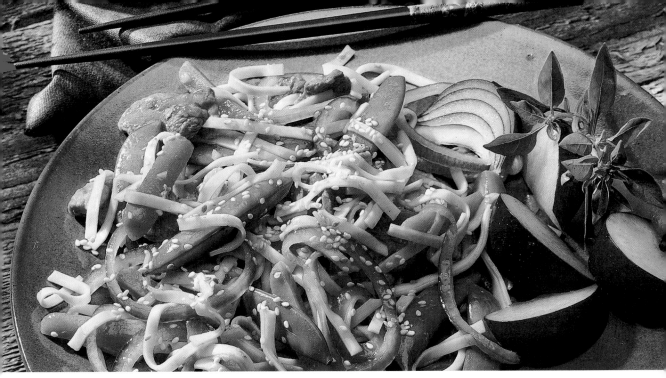

Pork Lo Mein

Bulgur-Shrimp Pilaf

LO CAL / LO FAT / HI FIB

PREP: 10 MIN; COOK: 16 MIN

4 SERVINGS

When red, orange and yellow bell peppers are in season, substitute one or a combination of all three to vary the color combo in this delightful rice dish.

2¹/₂ cups reduced-sodium chicken broth

1¹/₂ cups uncooked bulgur

1 teaspoon lemon pepper

1 medium green or red bell pepper, chopped (1 cup)

2 medium carrots, thinly sliced (1 cup)

1 jar (2¹/₂ ounces) sliced mushrooms, undrained

¹/₂ pound cooked peeled deveined medium shrimp, thawed if frozen

1 teaspoon grated lemon peel

Heat broth to boiling in 2-quart saucepan. Stir in remaining ingredients except shrimp and lemon peel.

Heat to boiling; reduce heat. Cover and simmer 12 minutes (do not lift cover or stir). Stir in shrimp and lemon peel; heat through.

1 Serving: Calories 235 (Calories from Fat 20); Fat 2g (Saturated 1g); Cholesterol 80mg; Sodium 580mg; Carbohydrate 47g (Dietary Fiber 12g); Protein 19g
% Daily Value: Vitamin A 52%; Vitamin C 24%; Calcium 6%; Iron 18%
Diet Exchanges: 2¹/₂ starch, 1¹/₂ lean meat, 1 vegetable

Garden Risotto

LO CAL / LO FAT / LO CHOL

PREP: 15 MIN; COOK: 35 MIN

6 SERVINGS

We've cut 28 grams of fat in this recipe by using fat-free instead of regular half-and-half. Fat-free half-and-half is sold in the dairy case in pints and quarts. It can be used for both cooking and baking (photo, page 97).

1	tablespoon olive or vegetable oil
1	medium onion, thinly sliced
2	medium zucchini, cut into julienne strips
2	medium yellow bell peppers, cut into julienne strips
$1/3$	cup dry white wine or water
2	cups uncooked Arborio rice or regular medium-grain white rice
$3^{1/3}$	cups hot water
4	teaspoons chicken bouillon granules
1	cup fat-free half-and-half
$1/2$	teaspoon pepper
2	tablespoons freshly grated Parmesan cheese, if desired

Heat oil in 12-inch nonstick skillet or Dutch oven over medium-high heat. Cook onion in oil, stirring frequently, until tender. Stir in zucchini and bell peppers. Cook about 2 minutes, stirring frequently, until crisp-tender. Remove from skillet; set aside.

Stir in wine. Cook until liquid has evaporated; reduce heat to medium. Stir in rice. Cook uncovered, stirring frequently, until rice begins to brown.

Mix hot water, bouillon granules, half-and-half and pepper. Pour $1/2$ cup bouillon mixture over rice mixture. Cook uncovered, stirring occasionally, until liquid is absorbed. Repeat with remaining bouillon mixture, $1/2$ cup at a time, until rice is tender. Stir in zucchini and bell peppers. Sprinkle with cheese.

1 Serving: Calories 305 (Calories from Fat 25); Fat 3g (Saturated 1g); Cholesterol 0mg; Sodium 900mg; Carbohydrate 64g (Dietary Fiber 2g); Protein 8g
% Daily Value: Vitamin A 6%; Vitamin C 66%; Calcium 10%; Iron 16%
Diet Exchanges: 3 starch, 3 vegetable

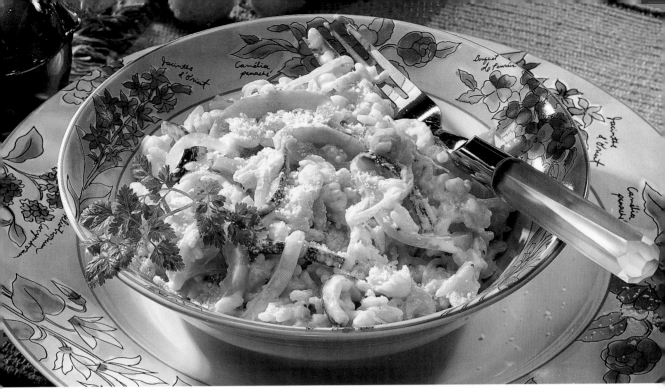

Garden Risotto

Spring Vegetable Risotto

LO CAL / LO FAT / LO CHOL

PREP: 10 MIN; COOK: 25 MIN

4 SERVINGS

¾ cup uncooked Arborio rice or regular medium-grain white rice

2¼ cups chicken broth

½ cup chopped red onion

10 medium spears asparagus, cut into ½-inch pieces (1 cup)

1 medium zucchini, chopped (2 cups)

¼ teaspoon pepper

3 tablespoons chopped fresh parsley

Spray 2-quart saucepan with cooking spray. Cook rice in saucepan over medium-high heat about 5 minutes, stirring occasionally, until rice begins to brown.

Stir in ¾ cup of the broth and the onion; reduce heat to medium. Cook about 15 minutes, stirring occasionally and adding remaining broth, ¾ cup at a time, as liquid is absorbed.

Stir in asparagus, zucchini and pepper. Cook 5 to 6 minutes, stirring occasionally, until all liquid is absorbed and rice is tender. Stir in parsley.

1 Serving: Calories 170 (Calories from Fat 10); Fat 1g (Saturated 0g); Cholesterol 0mg; Sodium 590mg; Carbohydrate 35g (Dietary Fiber 2g); Protein 7g
% Daily Value: Vitamin A 6%; Vitamin C 14%; Calcium 4%; Iron 12%
Diet Exchanges: 2 starch, 1 vegetable

Mushroom and Mozzarella Risotto

LO CAL / LO FAT / LO CHOL

PREP: 10 MIN; COOK: 35 MIN

6 SERVINGS

The meaty texture of mushrooms belies the fact that they are so low in calories and are fat free. Try a variety of fresh or dried wild mushrooms in this creamy risotto.

- 2 cups chopped mushrooms (8 ounces)
- 2 large onions, chopped (2 cups)
- 2 cups uncooked Arborio rice or regular medium-grain white rice
- 2 cups white wine or apple juice
- 5½ to 6 cups vegetable or chicken broth, heated
- ½ cup shredded reduced-fat mozzarella cheese (2 ounces)
- 2 tablespoons grated Parmesan cheese
- 2 tablespoons chopped fresh chives

Spray 3-quart saucepan with cooking spray. Cook mushrooms and onions in saucepan over medium heat about 5 minutes, stirring occasionally, until onions are tender. Stir in rice. Cook 3 minutes, stirring constantly.

Stir in wine and 2 cups of the broth. Heat to boiling; reduce heat to medium. Cook uncovered about 5 minutes, stirring occasionally, until most liquid is absorbed. Stir in 1 cup of the broth. Cook uncovered, stirring occasionally, until most liquid is absorbed. Repeat with remaining broth, 1 cup at a time, until rice is tender and mixture is slightly thickened. Stir in remaining ingredients.

1 Serving: Calories 340 (Calories from Fat 25); Fat 3g (Saturated 2g); Cholesterol 5mg; Sodium 1000mg; Carbohydrate 63g (Dietary Fiber 2g); Protein 10g
% Daily Value: Vitamin A 16%; Vitamin C 4%; Calcium 14%; Iron 16%
Diet Exchanges: 3 starch, 1 vegetable, 1 fruit

Rice Stir-Fry

LO CAL / LO FAT / LO CHOL / HI FIB

PREP: 1 HR; COOK: 10 MIN

4 SERVINGS

Wild rice is actually an aquatic grass native to North America. It is more expensive than other rices because of its limited supply. Nutritionally, it packs a punch, containing fiber, B vitamins, iron, phosphorus, magnesium, calcium and zinc.

- 1/3 cup uncooked regular long grain rice
- 1/3 cup uncooked wild rice
- 3/4 cup thinly sliced red onion
- 2 cloves garlic, finely chopped
- 3/4 cup chicken broth
- 1 small yellow bell pepper, chopped (1/2 cup)
- 1/4 cup raisins
- 1/4 cup chopped dried apricots
- 1/4 teaspoon salt
- 1/4 teaspoon pepper
- 1/4 cup chopped fresh parsley
- 2 tablespoons red wine vinegar
- 1 teaspoon olive or vegetable oil

Cook and drain regular rice as directed on package—except omit salt. Cook and drain wild rice as directed on package—except omit salt.

Cook onion, garlic and broth in 10-inch nonstick skillet over medium-high heat 5 to 6 minutes, stirring occasionally, until liquid has almost evaporated. Stir in regular rice, wild rice, bell pepper, raisins, apricots, salt and pepper. Cook over medium heat about 2 minutes, stirring constantly, until heated through. Stir in parsley, vinegar and oil.

1 Serving: Calories 195 (Calories from Fat 20); Fat 2g (Saturated 1g); Cholesterol 0mg; Sodium 350mg; Carbohydrate 42g (Dietary Fiber 3g); Protein 5g
% Daily Value: Vitamin A 8%; Vitamin C 34%; Calcium 2%; Iron 10%
Diet Exchanges: 2 starch, 2 vegetable

Marinated-Pork Fried Rice

LO CAL / LO FAT

PREP: 15 MIN; MARINATE: 1 HR; COOK: 25 MIN

4 SERVINGS

Using cold cooked rice is the secret to keeping rice kernels separate and fluffy in fried rice. Leftover white rice can be tightly covered and stored in the refrigerator for up to five days.

- 1/2   pound pork tenderloin
- 1/4   cup unsweetened pineapple juice
- 1/2   teaspoon grated gingerroot or 1/4 teaspoon ground ginger
- 1/4   teaspoon red pepper sauce
- 1   clove garlic, finely chopped
- 1   medium onion, chopped (1/2 cup)
- 1   small red bell pepper, cut into thin strips
- 2   tablespoons reduced-sodium soy sauce or fish sauce
- 3   cups cold cooked white rice
-      Chopped fresh chives, if desired
-      Soy sauce, if desired

Remove fat from pork. Cut pork into 1/2-inch cubes. Mix pork, pineapple juice, gingerroot, pepper sauce and garlic in glass or plastic bowl. Cover and refrigerate at least 1 hour but no longer than 12 hours.

Remove pork from marinade; drain. Spray wok or 12-inch nonstick skillet with cooking spray; heat over medium-high heat. Add pork; stir-fry 5 to 10 minutes or until no longer pink. Remove pork from wok.

Add onion and bell pepper to wok; stir-fry about 8 minutes or until onion is tender. Stir in pork, 2 tablespoons soy sauce and the rice. Cook about 10 minutes, stirring constantly, until rice is hot and golden. Sprinkle with chives; serve with soy sauce.

1 Serving: Calories 250 (Calories from Fat 25); Fat 3g (Saturated 1g); Cholesterol 35mg; Sodium 300mg; Carbohydrate 40g (Dietary Fiber 1g); Protein 17g
% Daily Value: Vitamin A 10%; Vitamin C 32%; Calcium 2%; Iron 14%
Diet Exchanges: 2 starch, 1 lean meat, 2 vegetable

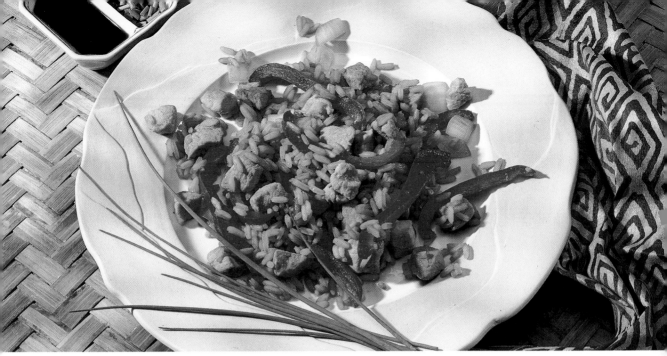

Spanish Pork and Rice

LO CAL / LO FAT

PREP: 10 MIN; COOK: 15 MIN

4 SERVINGS

Using lean pork loin in this main-dish version of Spanish rice helps keep the fat in check.

$1/2$ pound pork boneless center-cut loin

1 medium onion, chopped ($1/2$ cup)

2 cloves garlic, finely chopped

$1^1/2$ cups uncooked instant rice

$1^1/4$ cups reduced-sodium chicken broth

1 teaspoon chili powder

1 can (10 ounces) diced tomatoes and green chilies, undrained

Remove fat from pork. Cut pork into about $1^1/2 \times 1/4$-inch strips. Spray 10-inch nonstick skillet with cooking spray; heat over medium heat.

Cook pork, onion and garlic in skillet about 6 minutes, stirring frequently, until pork is no longer pink. Stir in remaining ingredients. Heat to boiling; remove from heat. Cover and let stand 5 minutes.

1 Serving: Calories 290 (Calories from Fat 55); Fat 6g (Saturated 2g); Cholesterol 35mg; Sodium 285mg; Carbohydrate 42g (Dietary Fiber 2g); Protein 19g
% Daily Value: Vitamin A 6%; Vitamin C 10%; Calcium 4%; Iron 14%
Diet Exchanges: 3 starch, $1^1/2$ lean meat

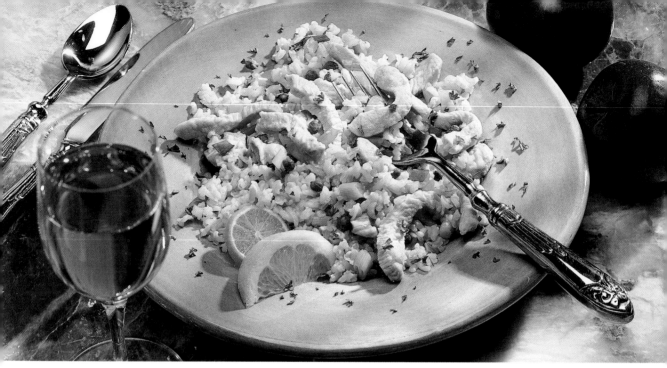

Lemon Rice with Turkey

Lemon Rice with Turkey

LO CAL / LO FAT

PREP: 20 MIN; COOK: 10 MIN

6 SERVINGS

Brown rice is unpolished, meaning the outer hull has been removed but the germ and bran layers have not been "polished" off. This gives a subtle nutty flavor and chewier texture than white rice. It is also a source of fiber and thiamin.

16	medium green onions, chopped (1 cup)
1	cup chicken broth
2	cloves garlic, finely chopped
1½	pounds uncooked turkey breast slices, cut into 3 × ¼ × ¼-inch strips
3	cups cooked brown or white rice
2	teaspoons grated lemon peel
⅓	cup lemon juice
1	tablespoon capers, rinsed and drained
¼	teaspoon pepper
3	tablespoons chopped fresh parsley

Cook onions, broth and garlic in 12-inch nonstick skillet over medium heat 3 minutes, stirring occasionally, until onions are tender. Stir in turkey. Cook 3 minutes.

Stir in remaining ingredients except parsley. Cook about 3 minutes or until rice is hot and turkey is no longer pink in center; remove from heat. Stir in parsley.

1 Serving: Calories 230 (Calories from Fat 20); Fat 2g (Saturated 1g); Cholesterol 75mg; Sodium 270mg; Carbohydrate 25g (Dietary Fiber 2g); Protein 30g
% Daily Value: Vitamin A 2%; Vitamin C 8%; Calcium 4%; Iron 12%
Diet Exchanges: 1 starch, 3 very lean meat, 2 vegetable

Fruity Turkey-Rice Pilaf

LO CAL / LO FAT / LO SODIUM / HI FIB

PREP: 10 MIN; COOK: 18 MIN

4 SERVINGS

By taking advantage of a fast-cooking long grain and wild rice mix, you can have this family-pleasing saucepan supper on the table in next to no time.

- ½   pound ground turkey breast
- 4   medium green onions, sliced (¼ cup)
- 2   cups water
- 1   package (6¾ ounces) quick-cooking long grain and wild rice mix seasoned with herbs
- ½   cups dried cherries or cranberries
- ½   cup chopped dried peaches or apricots
- ¼   teaspoon ground nutmeg or cinnamon

Spray 3-quart saucepan with cooking spray; heat over medium heat. Cook turkey and onions in saucepan about 8 minutes, stirring occasionally, until turkey is no longer pink. Stir in water and seasoning packet from rice mix. Heat to boiling, stirring occasionally; reduce heat to low.

Stir in rice, cherries, peaches and nutmeg. Cover and simmer about 5 minutes or until rice is tender and fruits are heated through.

1 Serving: Calories 230 (Calories from Fat 35); Fat 4g (Saturated 1g); Cholesterol 40mg; Sodium 40mg; Carbohydrate 42g (Dietary Fiber 8g); Protein 15g
% Daily Value: Vitamin A 6%; Vitamin C 16%; Calcium 4%; Iron 12%
Diet Exchanges: 2 starch, 1 very lean meat, 1 fruit

Risotto with Shrimp

LO CAL / LO FAT

PREP: 15 MIN; COOK: 40 MIN

6 SERVINGS

Shrimp is unique in that it is the only seafood that contains cholesterol; 1½ pounds has about 160 milligrams of cholesterol.

-   1 tablespoon margarine
-   1 medium onion, thinly sliced
-   1 pound uncooked medium shrimp, peeled and deveined
-   ½ cup dry white wine or vegetable broth
-   1½ cups uncooked Arborio rice or regular medium-grain white rice
-   1 can (14½ ounces) ready-to-serve vegetable or chicken broth
-   1 cup water
-   ¼ cup freshly grated Parmesan cheese
    Freshly ground pepper

Melt margarine in 12-inch nonstick skillet or Dutch oven over medium-high heat. Cook onion in margarine 8 to 10 minutes, stirring frequently, until tender; reduce heat to medium.

Stir in shrimp. Cook uncovered about 5 minutes, stirring frequently, until shrimp are pink and firm. Remove mixture from skillet; keep warm.

Add wine to skillet; cook until liquid has evaporated. Stir in rice. Cook uncovered over medium heat, stirring frequently, until rice begins to brown. Mix broth and water; pour ½ cup broth mixture over rice. Cook 15 to 20 minutes, adding broth ½ cup at a time and stirring occasionally, until rice is tender and creamy. Stir in shrimp mixture. Sprinkle with cheese and pepper.

1 Serving: Calories 255 (Calories from Fat 35); Fat 4g (Saturated 2g); Cholesterol 75mg; Sodium 460mg; Carbohydrate 43g (Dietary Fiber 1g); Protein 13g
% Daily Value: Vitamin A 10%; Vitamin C 2%; Calcium 8%; Iron 16%
Diet Exchanges: 2 starch, 1 lean meat, 2 vegetable

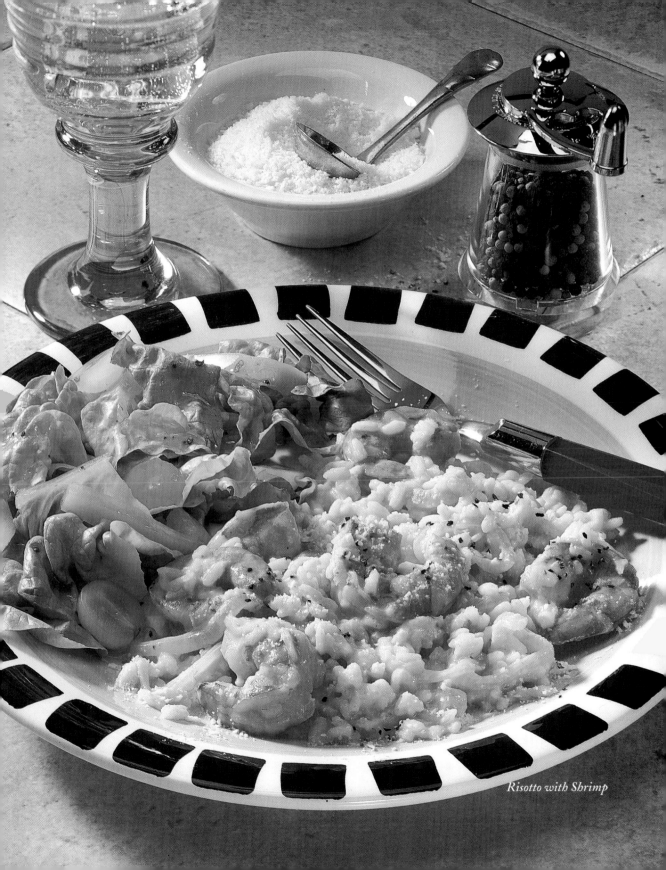

Risotto with Shrimp

Polenta Squares with Spaghetti Sauce

LO CAL / LO FAT / LO CHOL / HI FIB

PREP: 25 MIN; CHILL: 1 HR; BROIL: 6 MIN

4 SERVINGS

Polenta is a thick, creamy Italian dish that is also called cornmeal mush. Serve with a salad of mixed greens splashed with a low-fat Italian dressing and a twist of freshly ground pepper.

1 cup cornmeal

1 cup chicken broth, vegetable broth or water

3 cups boiling water

1/2 teaspoon salt

2 tablespoons grated Parmesan cheese
Cooking spray

1 cup fat-free spaghetti sauce

2 tablespoons chopped fresh or 1 teaspoon dried basil leaves

1/2 cup shredded reduced-fat mozzarella cheese (2 ounces)

Mix cornmeal and broth in 2-quart saucepan. Stir in boiling water and salt. Cook over medium-high heat, stirring constantly, until mixture thickens and boils; reduce heat. Cover and simmer 10 minutes, stirring frequently; remove from heat. Stir in Parmesan cheese.

Spread polenta in ungreased nonstick square pan, 8 × 8 × 2 inches. Cover and refrigerate about 1 hour or until firm.

Set oven control to broil. Line broiler pan with aluminum foil. Cut polenta into 4 squares. Spray both sides of polenta squares with cooking spray; place in broiler pan. Broil with tops about 4 inches from heat about 2 minutes on each side or until light brown.

Spoon spaghetti sauce over polenta squares in pan. Sprinkle with basil and mozzarella cheese. Broil about 2 minutes or until cheese is melted.

1 Serving: Calories 190 (Calories from Fat 35); Fat 4g (Saturated 2g); Cholesterol 10mg; Sodium 870mg; Carbohydrate 33g (Dietary Fiber 3g); Protein 9g
% Daily Value: Vitamin A 6%; Vitamin C 2%; Calcium 14%; Iron 10%
Diet Exchanges: 2 starch, 1 vegetable

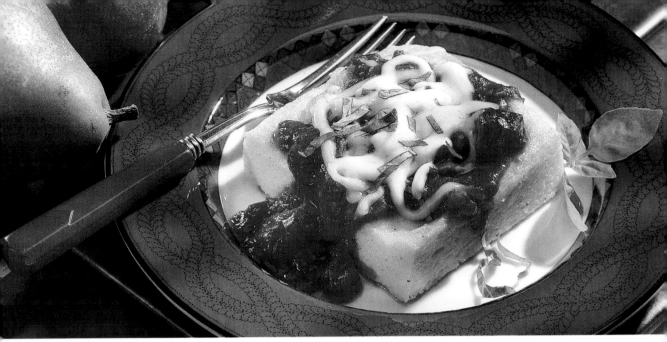

Polenta Squares with Spaghetti Sauce

Polenta Sauté

LO CAL / LO FAT / LO CHOL / HI FIB

PREP: 35 MIN; CHILL: 1 HR; COOK: 20 MIN

4 SERVINGS

Either yellow or white cornmeal can be used in this polenta. Serve polenta with salsa, reduced-fat sour cream and some sliced ripe olives.

1	cup whole kernel corn
4	cups water
1	teaspoon margarine
½	teaspoon salt
¼	teaspoon pepper
1	cup cornmeal

Spray rectangular baking dish, 11 × 7 × 1½ inches, with cooking spray. Heat all ingredients except cornmeal to boiling in 2-quart saucepan. Gradually add cornmeal, stirring constantly; reduce heat to medium-low. Cook 8 to 12 minutes, stirring occasionally, until mixture pulls away from side of saucepan. Pour into baking dish. Cool 15 minutes. Cover and refrigerate about 1 hour or until firm.

Heat oven to 250°. Cut polenta into 8 pieces. Spray 10-inch nonstick skillet with cooking spray; heat over medium heat. Cook 4 pieces polenta at a time in skillet about 5 minutes on each side or until light brown. Place on ungreased cookie sheet; keep warm in oven while cooking remaining pieces.

1 Serving: Calories 160 (Calories from Fat 20); Fat 2g (Saturated 0g); Cholesterol 0mg; Sodium 390mg; Carbohydrate 35g (Dietary Fiber 3g); Protein 4g
% Daily Value: Vitamin A 2%; Vitamin C 2%; Calcium 0%; Iron 10%
Diet Exchanges: 2 starch, 1 vegetable

Cheese Grits

LO CAL / LO FAT

PREP: 20 MIN; BAKE: 40 MIN; STAND: 10 MIN

8 SERVINGS

Hominy grits are the ground kernels of dried white or yellow corn from which the hull and germ have been removed (grits are not the same thing as cornmeal). Grits are usually available in fine, medium and coarse grinds; use the one you like best.

2	cups skim milk
2	cups water
1/2	teaspoon salt
1/4	teaspoon pepper
1	cup uncooked white hominy quick grits
1 1/2	cups shredded reduced-fat Cheddar cheese (6 ounces)
4	medium green onions, sliced (1/4 cup)
1	egg plus 2 egg whites, slightly beaten
1	tablespoon margarine
1/4	teaspoon paprika

Heat oven to 350°. Grease 1 1/2-quart casserole. Heat milk, water, salt and pepper to boiling in 2-quart saucepan. Gradually add grits, stirring constantly; reduce heat. Simmer uncovered about 5 minutes, stirring frequently, until thick. Stir in cheese and onions.

Stir 1 cup of the hot mixture into eggs; stir back into remaining hot mixture in saucepan. Pour into casserole. Dot with margarine. Sprinkle with paprika. Bake uncovered 35 to 40 minutes or until set. Let stand 10 minutes before serving.

1 Serving: Calories 160 (Calories from Fat 35); Fat 4g (Saturated 2g); Cholesterol 30mg; Sodium 350mg; Carbohydrate 20g (Dietary Fiber 0g); Protein 11g
% Daily Value: Vitamin A 8%; Vitamin C 0%; Calcium 16%; Iron 6%
Diet Exchanges: 1 starch, 1/2 skim milk, 1 fat

Toasted Barley with Mixed Vegetables

LO CAL / LO FAT / LO CHOL / HI FIB

PREP: 10 MIN; COOK: 1 HR

4 SERVINGS

Barley was one of the first grains ever cultivated, and with good reason. One cup of cooked barley provides the same amount of protein as a glass of milk. It also contains niacin, thiamin and potassium.

- 1/2 cup uncooked quick-cooking barley
- 1 can (14 1/2 ounces) ready-to-serve chicken broth
- 1 large onion, chopped (1 cup)
- 1 package (8 ounces) sliced mushrooms (3 cups)
- 2 medium carrots, thinly sliced (1 cup)
- 1 small green bell pepper, coarsely chopped (1/2 cup)
- 1 tablespoon chopped fresh or 2 teaspoons dried dill weed
- 1/4 teaspoon pepper
- 4 medium green onions, chopped (1/4 cup)

Heat oven to 350°. Spray 10-inch nonstick skillet with cooking spray. Cook barley in skillet over medium heat 3 to 7 minutes, stirring frequently until barley begins to brown, then stirring constantly until golden brown. Stir in remaining ingredients except green onions; heat to boiling. Transfer mixture to ungreased 2-quart casserole.

Cover and bake 30 minutes. Uncover and bake about 20 minutes longer or until carrots and barley are tender and most of the liquid is absorbed. Sprinkle with green onions.

1 Serving: Calories 135 (Calories from Fat 10); Fat 1g (Saturated 0g); Cholesterol 0mg; Sodium 600mg; Carbohydrate 31g (Dietary Fiber 7g); Protein 7g
% Daily Value: Vitamin A 48%; Vitamin C 20%; Calcium 4%; Iron 10%
Diet Exchanges: 2 starch, 1 vegetable

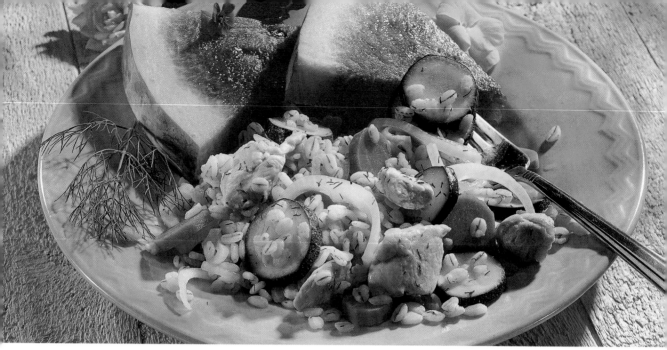

Barley-Chicken Medley

Barley-Chicken Medley

LO CAL / HI FIB

PREP: 10 MIN; COOK: 15 MIN

4 SERVINGS

Make this satisfying chicken stir-fry more colorful by using a mixture of zucchini and carrot.

$\frac{1}{2}$	pound skinless, boneless chicken breast halves
2	cups chicken broth
1	cup uncooked quick-cooking barley
$\frac{1}{2}$	teaspoon dried dill weed
$\frac{1}{2}$	teaspoon garlic salt
2	teaspoons vegetable oil
$2\frac{1}{2}$	cups thinly sliced zucchini or carrot
1	medium onion, cut lengthwise in half, then cut crosswise into thin slices

Remove fat from chicken. Cut chicken into $\frac{3}{4}$-inch pieces. Heat broth to boiling in $1\frac{1}{2}$-quart saucepan. Stir in barley, dill weed and garlic salt; reduce heat to low. Cover and simmer about 10 minutes or until barley is tender; remove from heat. Let stand covered 5 minutes.

While barley is cooking, spray 10-inch nonstick skillet with cooking spray; heat over medium-high heat. Add chicken; stir-fry about 4 minutes or until no longer pink in center. Remove chicken from skillet; keep warm.

Add oil to skillet; rotate skillet to coat with oil. Add zucchini and onion; stir-fry about 4 minutes or until vegetables are crisp-tender. Stir in chicken. Toss with cooked barley.

1 Serving: Calories 320 (Calories from Fat 65); Fat 7g (Saturated 2g); Cholesterol 55mg; Sodium 700mg; Carbohydrate 44g (Dietary Fiber 9g); Protein 29g
% Daily Value: Vitamin A 2%; Vitamin C 6%; Calcium 4%; Iron 14%
Diet Exchanges: 2 starch, 2 lean meat, 2 vegetable

Bulgur and Orange Salad

LO CAL / LO FAT / LO CHOL / HI FIB

PREP: 20 MIN; CHILL: 2 HR

4 SERVINGS

Bulgur, also spelled bulgar, *is whole wheat that has been cooked, dried and then broken into coarse fragments. It's different from cracked wheat in that it is pre-cooked. Bulgur supplies phosphorus and potassium and also contains some iron, thiamin and riboflavin.*

$1/3$ cup uncooked bulgur

1 large orange, peeled and chopped ($3/4$ cup)

1 medium onion, chopped ($1/2$ cup)

1 small tomato, chopped ($1/2$ cup)

$3/4$ cup chopped fresh parsley

2 tablespoons lemon juice

2 teaspoons grated orange peel

2 teaspoons olive or vegetable oil

$1/2$ teaspoon salt

$1/4$ teaspoon pepper

$1/8$ teaspoon crushed red pepper

Cook bulgur as directed on package—except omit salt. Toss bulgur and remaining ingredients in glass or plastic bowl. Cover and refrigerate about 2 hours or until chilled.

1 Serving: Calories 100 (Calories from Fat 25); Fat 3g (Saturated 1g); Cholesterol 0mg; Sodium 310mg; Carbohydrate 19g (Dietary Fiber 4g); Protein 3g
% Daily Value: Vitamin A 8%; Vitamin C 80%; Calcium 4%; Iron 6%
Diet Exchanges: 1 starch, 1 vegetable

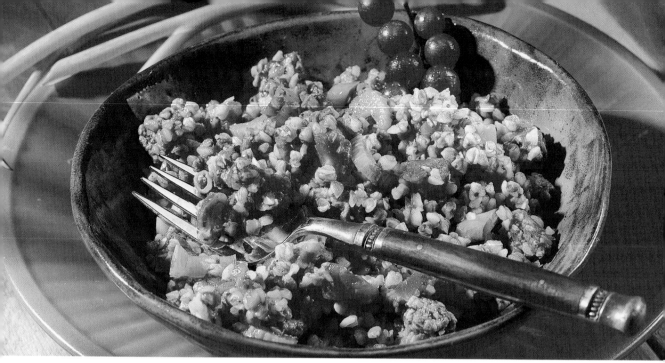

Kasha and Beef Supper

Kasha and Beef Supper

LO CAL / HI FIB

PREP: 10 MIN; COOK: 15 MIN

4 SERVINGS

Look for kasha, which may be labeled "roasted buckwheat groats," in the rice and grain section of your supermarket. These roasted kernels have a distinctive nutty flavor that blends deliciously with the ground beef and tomatoes in this skillet meal.

2	cups beef broth
1	cup uncooked kasha (roasted buckwheat groats)
1/2	pound diet-lean or extra-lean ground beef
4	medium green onions, sliced (1/4 cup)
1	medium stalk celery, sliced (1/2 cup)

1 can (14 1/2 ounces) diced tomatoes with crushed red pepper and basil, undrained

1/4 teaspoon pepper

Heat broth to boiling in 2-quart saucepan. Stir in kasha. Cover and cook over medium heat about 7 minutes or until tender; drain if needed.

While kasha is cooking, cook beef, onions and celery in 10-inch nonstick skillet over medium heat about 6 minutes, stirring occasionally, until beef is brown; drain.

Stir tomatoes and pepper into beef mixture. Heat to boiling; reduce heat. Cover and simmer 5 minutes. Stir in kasha; heat through.

1 Serving: Calories 230 (Calories from Fat 70); Fat 8g (Saturated 3g); Cholesterol 35mg; Sodium 710mg; Carbohydrate 26g (Dietary Fiber 4g); Protein 17g
% Daily Value: Vitamin A 6%; Vitamin C 14%; Calcium 6%; Iron 16%
Diet Exchanges: 1 1/2 starch, 1 1/2 lean meat, 1 vegetable

Golden Millet with Ham

LO CAL / LO FAT / LO CHOL / HI FIB

PREP: 10 MIN; COOK: 25 MIN

4 SERVINGS

Resembling mustard seed, when cooked, whole millet has a chewy texture and mild flavor similar to brown rice.

- 2   cups chicken broth
- 1   cup uncooked millet
- 1   medium yellow bell pepper, chopped (1 cup)
- 4   medium green onions, sliced ($^1/_4$ cup)
- 1   cup cubed fully cooked fat-free ham
- $^1/_2$ cup golden raisins
- $^1/_2$ cup chopped dried apricots
- $^1/_4$ teaspoon ground cinnamon

Heat broth to boiling in $1^1/_2$-quart saucepan. Stir in millet. Cover and cook over medium heat 15 minutes.

Stir in remaining ingredients. Heat to boiling; reduce heat to low. Cover and simmer about 5 minutes or until millet is tender and broth is absorbed.

1 Serving: Calories 350 (Calories from Fat 45); Fat 5g (Saturated 1g); Cholesterol 15mg; Sodium 930mg; Carbohydrate 66g (Dietary Fiber 7g); Protein 17g
% Daily Value: Vitamin A 12%; Vitamin C 48%; Calcium 4%; Iron 20%
Diet Exchanges: $3^1/_2$ starch, 1 very lean meat, 1 fruit

Oriental Stir-Fry with Millet

LO CAL / LO FAT / HI FIB

PREP: 10 MIN; COOK: 25 MIN

6 SERVINGS

2¼ cups chicken broth

1 cup uncooked millet

2 bags (16 ounces each) frozen broccoli, red peppers, onions and mushrooms, thawed

1⅓ cups apple juice

¼ cup reduced-sodium soy sauce

2 tablespoons cornstarch

½ teaspoon ground ginger

2 cups cut-up cooked chicken or turkey

Heat broth to boiling in 1½-quart saucepan; reduce heat. Stir in millet. Cover and simmer 20 minutes.

While millet is cooking, spray 12-inch nonstick skillet with cooking spray; heat over medium-high heat. Add vegetables; stir-fry 2 minutes. Stir in ⅓ cup of the apple juice. Cover and cook over medium heat about 3 minutes or until vegetables are crisp-tender.

While vegetables are cooking, mix remaining 1 cup apple juice, the soy sauce, cornstarch and ginger in small bowl. Gradually stir into vegetable mixture. Heat to boiling, stirring constantly. Boil and stir 1 minute. Stir in chicken; heat through. Toss with cooked millet.

1 Serving: Calories 290 (Calories from Fat 55); Fat 6g (Saturated 1g); Cholesterol 40mg; Sodium 800mg; Carbohydrate 43g (Dietary Fiber 6g); Protein 22g
% Daily Value: Vitamin A 34%; Vitamin C 84%; Calcium 6%; Iron 16%
Diet Exchanges: 2½ starch, 2 lean meat, 1 vegetable

Mediterranean Couscous

LO CAL / LO FAT / LO CHOL / HI FIB

PREP: 15 MIN; COOK: 5 MIN; STAND: 5 MIN

4 SERVINGS

2 teaspoons margarine

5 medium green onions, chopped (⅓ cup)

1 clove garlic, finely chopped

1½ cups water

½ teaspoon reduced-sodium chicken bouillon granules

1 cup uncooked couscous

¼ cup chopped fresh parsley

1 tablespoon chopped fresh or ½ teaspoon dried basil leaves

¼ teaspoon pepper

1 medium yellow summer squash, chopped (1½ cups)

1 medium tomato, chopped (¾ cup)

Melt margarine in 2-quart nonstick saucepan over medium-high heat. Cook onions and garlic in margarine, stirring frequently, until onions are tender. Stir in water and bouillon granules. Heat to boiling; remove from heat.

Stir in remaining ingredients. Cover and let stand about 5 minutes or until liquid is absorbed. Fluff lightly with fork.

1 Serving: Calories 205 (Calories from Fat 25); Fat 3g (Saturated 1g); Cholesterol 0mg; Sodium 35mg; Carbohydrate 40g (Dietary Fiber 3g); Protein 7g
% Daily Value: Vitamin A 8%; Vitamin C 14%; Calcium 4%; Iron 6%
Diet Exchanges: 2 starch, 2 vegetable

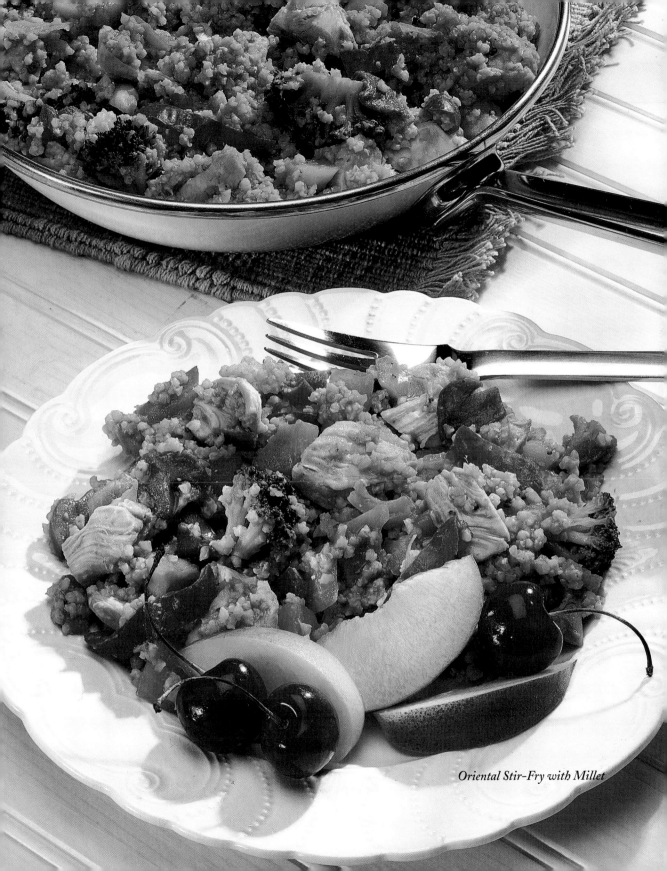

Oriental Stir-Fry with Millet

Creamy Quinoa Primavera

LO CAL / LO CHOL / HI FIB

PREP: 10 MIN; COOK: 15 MIN

6 SERVINGS

Quinoa ("keen-wa") was once a staple food of the Inca Indians in Peru. It is a small grain with a soft crunch and can be used in any recipe calling for rice. Be sure to rinse it well before using to remove the bitter-tasting, naturally occurring saponin (nature's insect repellent) that forms on the outside of the kernel. This grain provides B vitamins, calcium, iron, phosphorus and magnesium.

1½ cups uncooked quinoa

3 cups chicken broth

2 ounces reduced-fat cream cheese (Neufchâtel)

1 tablespoon chopped fresh or 1 teaspoon dried basil leaves

2 teaspoons margarine

2 cloves garlic, finely chopped

5 cups thinly sliced or bite-size pieces assorted vegetables (asparagus, broccoli, carrots, zucchini)

2 tablespoons grated Romano cheese

Rinse quinoa thoroughly; drain. Heat quinoa and broth to boiling in 2-quart saucepan; reduce heat. Cover and simmer 10 to 15 minutes or until all broth is absorbed. Stir in cream cheese and basil.

Melt margarine in 10-inch nonstick skillet over medium-high heat. Cook garlic in margarine about 30 seconds, stirring frequently, until golden. Stir in vegetables. Cook about 2 minutes, stirring frequently, until vegetables are crisp-tender. Toss vegetables and quinoa mixture. Sprinkle with Romano cheese.

1 Serving: Calories 240 (Calories from Fat 65); Fat 7g (Saturated 2g); Cholesterol 5mg; Sodium 630mg; Carbohydrate 36g (Dietary Fiber 4g); Protein 11g
% Daily Value: Vitamin A 42%; Vitamin C 26%; Calcium 8%; Iron 26%
Diet Exchanges: 2 starch, 1 vegetable, 1 fat

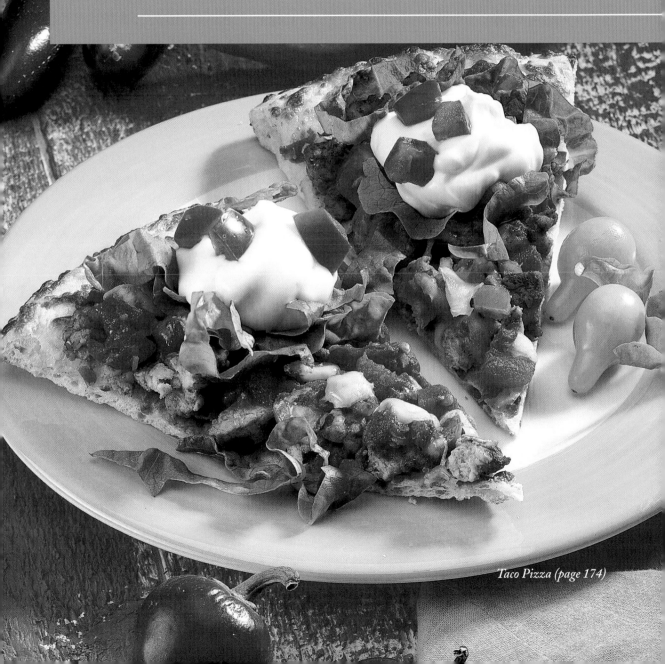

Taco Pizza (page 174)

Easy Macaroni and Cheese

LO CAL / LO CHOL

PREP: 5 MIN; COOK: 20 MIN

4 SERVINGS

Traditional macaroni and cheese tips the scales at 450 calories and 25 grams of fat. A serving of our version trims the calories to 330 and cuts the fat to 9 grams.

- 1 package (7 ounces) pasta shells
- 2 tablespoons all-purpose flour
- 1 tablespoon margarine, melted
- 1/4 teaspoon salt
- 1/4 teaspoon ground mustard (dry)
- 1/8 teaspoon pepper
- 1 cup skim milk
- 1 cup shredded reduced-fat Cheddar cheese (4 ounces)
- 2 medium green onions, sliced (2 tablespoons)
- 2 tablespoons chopped red bell pepper

Cook and drain pasta as directed on package—except omit salt. Combine flour, margarine, salt, mustard and pepper in 3-quart nonstick saucepan. Cook over low heat, stirring constantly, until margarine is absorbed; remove from heat. Gradually stir in milk. Heat to boiling, stirring constantly. Boil and stir 1 minute. Stir in cheese until melted.

Stir pasta, onions and bell pepper into sauce. Cook, stirring constantly, until hot.

1 Serving: Calories 330 (Calories from Fat 80); Fat 9g (Saturated 4g); Cholesterol 15mg; Sodium 350mg; Carbohydrate 46g (Dietary Fiber 1g); Protein 17g
% Daily Value: Vitamin A 12%; Vitamin C 6%; Calcium 30%; Iron 12%
Diet Exchanges: 2 starch, 1 vegetable, 1 skim milk, 1 fat

Wild Rice and White Bean Medley

LO CAL / LO FAT / LO CHOL / HI FIB

PREP: 5 MIN; COOK: 10 MIN

4 SERVINGS

By using the long grain and wild rice mix and cannellini beans, this creative recipe gives conventional beans and rice a whole new look and taste.

- 1 can (14 1/2 ounces) ready-to-serve chicken broth
- 1 package (6 3/4 ounces) quick-cooking long grain and wild rice mix seasoned with herbs
- 1 can (15 to 16 ounces) cannellini or great northern beans, rinsed and drained
- 1 can (8 ounces) sliced water chestnuts, drained
- 6 medium green onions, sliced (6 tablespoons)

Heat broth and rice seasoning packet to boiling in 3-quart saucepan, stirring occasionally; reduce heat.

Stir in rice and remaining ingredients. Cover and simmer about 5 minutes or until rice is tender and beans are heated through.

1 Serving: Calories 220 (Calories from Fat 10); Fat 1g (Saturated 0g); Cholesterol 0mg; Sodium 620mg; Carbohydrate 47g (Dietary Fiber 9g); Protein 15g
% Daily Value: Vitamin A 0%; Vitamin C 6%; Calcium 12%; Iron 28%
Diet Exchanges: 2 starch, 1 very lean meat, 3 vegetable

Home-Style Scrambled Eggs

LO CAL / LO FAT / LO CHOL

PREP: 10 MIN; COOK: 10 MIN

4 SERVINGS

Do your scrambled eggs end up looking more like rice or peas than the eggs from a restaurant? The trick is to avoid stirring them as much as possible while they cook.

1¹⁄₂ cups fat-free cholesterol-free egg product

³⁄₄ teaspoon salt

3 tablespoons water

1 tablespoon margarine

1 cup refrigerated diced potatoes with onions or frozen hash brown potatoes

1 small zucchini, chopped (1 cup)

1 medium tomato, seeded and chopped (³⁄₄ cup)

Mix egg product, salt and water.

Spray 10-inch nonstick skillet with cooking spray, and add margarine. Melt margarine over medium heat. Cook potatoes, zucchini and tomato in margarine, stirring occasionally, until hot.

Pour egg product mixture over vegetable mixture. As mixture begins to set at bottom and side, gently lift cooked portions with spatula so that thin, uncooked portion can flow to bottom. Avoid constant stirring. Cook 3 to 4 minutes or until eggs are thickened throughout but still moist.

1 Serving: Calories 100 (Calories from Fat 25); Fat 3g (Saturated 1g); Cholesterol 0mg; Sodium 600mg; Carbohydrate 11g (Dietary Fiber 2g); Protein 9g
% Daily Value: Vitamin A 10%; Vitamin C 8%; Calcium 4%; Iron 10%
Diet Exchanges: 1 lean meat, 2 vegetable

Roasted Pepper and Chèvre Focaccia Pizza

LO CHOL / HI FIB

PREP: 5 MIN; BAKE: 12 MIN

5 SERVINGS

Chèvre, a white goat's-milk cheese, comes in a range of textures, from creamy to dry and slightly firm. The creamy type laced with garlic and herbs is what makes this pizza a culinary masterpiece.

1 round thin Italian bread shell (12 inches in diameter)

¹⁄₂ package (4 ounces) fresh chèvre (goat) cheese with garlic and herbs, softened

3 ounces reduced-fat cream cheese (Neufchâtel), softened

1 jar (7¹⁄₄ ounces) roasted red bell peppers, drained and coarsely chopped

1 cup shredded reduced-fat mozzarella cheese (4 ounces)

Heat oven to 425°. Place bread on 12-inch pizza pan or cookie sheet.

Mix chèvre and cream cheese until well blended; spread over bread. Top with bell peppers. Sprinkle with mozzarella cheese. Bake about 12 minutes or until cheese is melted and bell peppers are heated through.

1 Serving: Calories 420 (Calories from Fat 145); Fat 16g (Saturated 5g); Cholesterol 15mg; Sodium 1150mg; Carbohydrate 56g (Dietary Fiber 3g); Protein 16g
% Daily Value: Vitamin A 24%; Vitamin C 46%; Calcium 20%; Iron 20%
Diet Exchanges: 3¹⁄₂ starch, 1 high-fat meat, 1 fat

Peanut Butter and Fruit Wraps

LO CAL / LO CHOL / HI FIB

PREP: 10 MIN

4 SERVINGS

Make lunchtime more fun by letting the youngsters spread, top and roll up their own wraps.

- 4 fat-free flour tortillas (6 to 8 inches in diameter)
- 1/2 cup reduced-fat peanut butter spread
- 1/4 cup strawberry or pineapple spreadable fruit
- 2 medium bananas, thinly sliced (2 cups)
- 1/4 cup reduced-fat granola

Spread tortillas with peanut butter, then with spreadable fruit. Top with bananas. Sprinkle with granola. Roll up tortillas.

1 Serving: Calories 325 (Calories from Fat 65); Fat 7g (Saturated 1g); Cholesterol 0mg; Sodium 85mg; Carbohydrate 61g (Dietary Fiber 4g); Protein 9g
% Daily Value: Vitamin A 4%; Vitamin C 12%; Calcium 2%; Iron 6%
Diet Exchanges: 3 starch, 1 fruit, 1 fat

Easy Dilled Tomato Bisque

LO CAL / LO FAT / LO CHOL

PREP: 5 MIN; COOK: 5 MIN

4 SERVINGS

Serve with crusty rolls and a crisp tossed-lettuce salad.

- 3 cans (11 ounces each) condensed tomato bisque or 3 cans (10 3/4 ounces each) condensed tomato soup
- 1 tablespoon chopped fresh or 1 teaspoon dried dill weed
- 8 slices lemon

Prepare soup as directed on can. Stir in dill weed. Garnish with lemon slices.

1 Serving: Calories 115 (Calories from Fat 30); Fat 3g (Saturated 1g); Cholesterol 5mg; Sodium 840mg; Carbohydrate 22g (Dietary Fiber 1g); Protein 2g
% Daily Value: Vitamin A 4%; Vitamin C 0%; Calcium 4%; Iron 4%
Diet Exchanges: 1 1/2 starch

Chicken Picante

LO CAL / LO FAT / HI FIB

PREP: 10 MIN; COOK: 15 MIN

4 SERVINGS

Serve this zesty chicken mixture over split corn muffins or hot cooked couscous. Fresh fruit or cut-up raw vegetables as a side dish would add a refreshing crunch.

- 1 pound skinless, boneless chicken breast halves
- 1 medium zucchini, sliced (2 cups)
- 1 cup sliced mushrooms (3 ounces)
- 2 1/2 cups picante sauce or salsa
- 2 teaspoons sugar

Remove fat from chicken. Cut chicken into 1-inch pieces. Spray 10-inch nonstick skillet with cooking spray; heat over medium heat. Cook chicken in skillet 3 to 4 minutes, stirring frequently, until no longer pink in center.

Stir in zucchini and mushrooms. Cook, stirring occasionally, until vegetables are crisp-tender. Stir in picante sauce and sugar. Cook about 5 minutes, stirring occasionally, until hot.

1 Serving: Calories 185 (Calories from Fat 35); Fat 4g (Saturated 1g); Cholesterol 70mg; Sodium 520mg; Carbohydrate 13g (Dietary Fiber 4g); Protein 28g
% Daily Value: Vitamin A 14%; Vitamin C 34%; Calcium 10%; Iron 14%
Diet Exchanges: 3 very lean meat, 3 vegetable

Fiesta Chicken and Rice

LO CAL / LO FAT

PREP: 5 MIN; COOK: 15 MIN

4 SERVINGS

The next time you roast or grill chicken, cook a few extra pieces so you'll have leftovers for this saucy chicken-and-rice skillet meal.

- 1 1/4 cups water
- 1 can (5 1/2 ounces) spicy eight-vegetable juice
- 1 package (4.9 ounces) rice and vermicelli mix with chicken broth and broccoli
- 1 1/2 cups cubed cooked chicken or turkey
- 1 cup frozen chopped bell peppers (from 10-ounce bag), thawed

Heat water, vegetable juice and rice-vermicelli mix and seasoning packet to boiling in 3-quart saucepan, stirring occasionally; reduce heat.

Simmer covered 15 to 20 minutes, stirring occasionally. Stir in chicken and bell peppers; heat through.

1 Serving: Calories 145 (Calories from Fat 35); Fat 4g (Saturated 1g); Cholesterol 45mg; Sodium 280mg; Carbohydrate 12g (Dietary Fiber 1g); Protein 16g
% Daily Value: Vitamin A 8%; Vitamin C 36%; Calcium 2%; Iron 6%
Diet Exchanges: 1 starch, 2 very lean meat

Spicy Mexican Skillet Chicken

LO CAL / HI FIB

PREP: 5 MIN; COOK: 15 MIN

4 SERVINGS

Black beans can be hard to find; sometimes they're shelved with other canned beans and other times with the Mexican ingredients. If you can't find them in either location, you can use kidney or pinto beans instead.

4	skinless, boneless chicken breast halves (about 1 pound)
1 to 2	teaspoons chili powder
1/4	teaspoon salt
1/4	teaspoon pepper
1	tablespoon vegetable oil
1	can (15 ounces) black beans, rinsed and drained
1	cup frozen whole kernel corn
1/3	cup thick-and-chunky salsa
	Chopped fresh cilantro, if desired
	Red chile slices, if desired

Remove fat from chicken. Mix chili powder, salt and pepper. Sprinkle evenly over both sides of chicken breast halves. Heat oil in 10-inch nonstick skillet over medium heat. Cook chicken in oil 8 to 10 minutes, turning once, until juice is no longer pink when centers of thickest pieces are cut.

Stir in beans, corn and salsa. Heat to boiling; reduce heat. Cover and simmer 3 to 5 minutes or until vegetables are hot. Sprinkle with cilantro and chile slices.

1 Serving: Calories 290 (Calories from Fat 70); Fat 8g (Saturated 2g); Cholesterol 70mg; Sodium 550mg; Carbohydrate 28g (Dietary Fiber 6g); Protein 32g
% Daily Value: Vitamin A 4%; Vitamin C 4%; Calcium 8%; Iron 16%
Diet Exchanges: 2 starch, 4 very lean meat

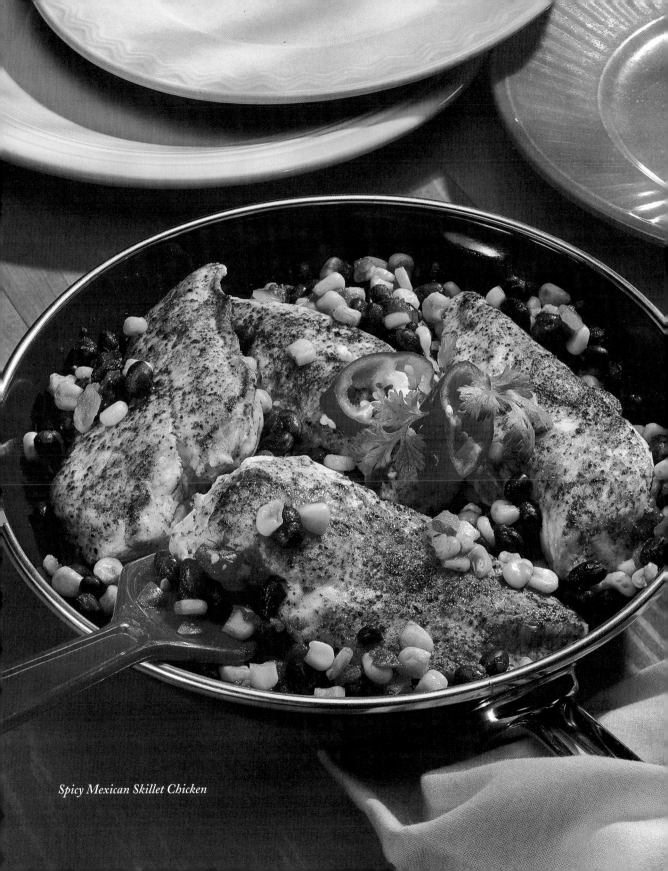

Spicy Mexican Skillet Chicken

Slim and Trim Jambalaya

LO CAL / LO FAT / HI FIB

PREP: 5 MIN; COOK: 10 MIN

4 SERVINGS

Improvise a completely new dish by replacing the chicken or turkey with ham and using chunky Italian-style or salsa tomato sauce in place of the chili-style sauce.

- 1 bag (16 ounces) frozen small whole onions, thawed
- 1 can (14½ ounces) ready-to-serve chicken broth
- 1 can (14½ ounces) chunky chili tomato sauce or regular tomato sauce
- 1½ cups cubed cooked chicken or turkey
- 1½ cups uncooked instant rice

Heat onions, broth and tomato sauce to boiling in 3-quart saucepan, stirring occasionally; reduce heat.

Stir in chicken and rice; reduce heat to low. Cover and cook about 5 minutes, stirring occasionally, until rice is tender and chicken is heated through.

1 Serving: Calories 340 (Calories from Fat 45); Fat 5g (Saturated 1g); Cholesterol 45mg; Sodium 940mg; Carbohydrate 55g (Dietary Fiber 4g); Protein 23g
% Daily Value: Vitamin A 6%; Vitamin C 20%; Calcium 8%; Iron 18%
Diet Exchanges: 3 starch, 2 very lean meat, 2 vegetable

Teriyaki Chicken Stir-Fry

LO CAL / LO FAT / HI FIB

PREP: 5 MIN; COOK: 10 MIN

4 SERVINGS

Teriyaki baste and glaze is a thick and brown-colored sauce; do not confuse it with teriyaki sauce or marinade, which has a watery consistency. You can find teriyaki baste and glaze in the Asian foods section of your supermarket.

- 1 pound cut-cup chicken breast for stir-fry
- ½ cup teriyaki baste and glaze
- 3 tablespoons lemon juice
- 1 bag (16 ounces) frozen broccoli, carrots, water chestnuts and red peppers

  Hot cooked couscous, rice or noodles, if desired

Spray 12-inch nonstick skillet with cooking spray; heat over medium-high heat. Add chicken; stir-fry 3 to 4 minutes until no longer pink in center.

Stir in remaining ingredients except couscous. Heat to boiling, stirring constantly; reduce heat. Cover and simmer about 6 minutes or until vegetables are crisp-tender. Serve with couscous.

1 Serving: Calories 205 (Calories from Fat 35); Fat 4g (Saturated 1g); Cholesterol 70mg; Sodium 1470mg; Carbohydrate 16g (Dietary Fiber 3g); Protein 29g
% Daily Value: Vitamin A 62%; Vitamin C 72%; Calcium 6%; Iron 12%
Diet Exchanges: 1 starch, 4 very lean meat

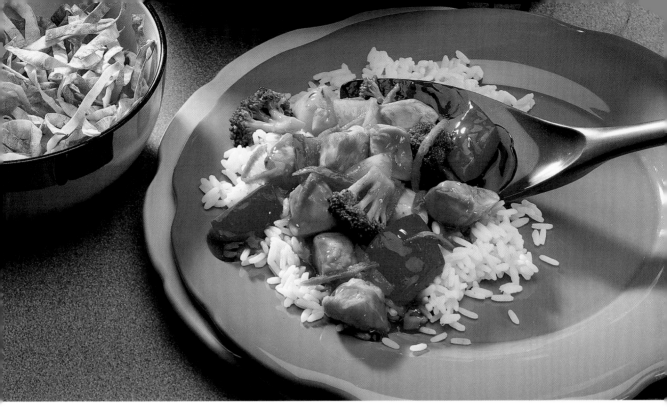

Vegetable-Chicken Stir-Fry

LO CAL / LO FAT / HI FIB

PREP: 10 MIN; COOK: 10 MIN

4 SERVINGS

Add toasty crunch with toasted wonton skins! Cut wonton skins into thin strips, and bake on an ungreased cookie sheet at 350° for 5 to 7 minutes or until light golden brown. Top each serving of this stir-fry with whole or broken toasted wonton strips.

1   pound skinless, boneless chicken breast halves or thighs

4   cups cut-up assorted vegetables (bell peppers, broccoli flowerets, shredded carrots)

1   clove garlic, finely chopped

½   cup stir-fry sauce

Remove fat from chicken. Cut chicken into 1-inch pieces. Spray 12-inch nonstick skillet with cooking spray; heat over medium-high heat. Add chicken; stir-fry about 3 minutes until no longer pink in center. Remove chicken from skillet.

Spray skillet with cooking spray. Add vegetables and garlic; stir-fry about 2 minutes or until vegetables are crisp-tender. Add chicken and stir-fry sauce. Cook and stir about 2 minutes or until hot.

1 Serving: Calories 190 (Calories from Fat 36); Fat 4g (Saturated 1g); Cholesterol 70mg; Sodium 1460mg; Carbohydrate 13g (Dietary Fiber 2g); Protein 28g
% Daily Value: Vitamin A 64%; Vitamin C 70%; Calcium 4%; Iron 10%
Diet Exchanges: 2 starch, 3 very lean meat, 1 fat

Easy Curried Chicken and Couscous

LO CAL / HI FIB

PREP: 10 MIN; COOK: 5 MIN

4 SERVINGS

Round this meal out with an easy, low-fat dessert. Slice a purchased angel food cake loaf into slices. Top with berries or sliced fruit such as peaches or nectarines.

1¾	cups water
1	cup uncooked couscous
1	can (10¾ ounces) condensed reduced-fat cream of chicken soup
½	cup water
1½	teaspoons curry powder
1½	cups cut-up cooked chicken
2	cups frozen mixed vegetables, thawed

Heat 1¾ cups water to boiling in 10-inch nonstick skillet. Stir in couscous; remove from heat. Cover and let stand about 5 minutes or until water is absorbed. Remove couscous to large serving platter; keep warm.

Heat soup, ½ cup water, the curry powder, chicken and vegetables to boiling in same skillet; reduce heat. Cover and simmer 3 to 5 minutes or until vegetables are tender. Pour chicken mixture over couscous.

1 Serving: Calories 345 (Calories from Fat 65); Fat 7g (Saturated 2g); Cholesterol 50mg; Sodium 670mg; Carbohydrate 51g (Dietary Fiber 6g); Protein 25g
% Daily Value: Vitamin A 42%; Vitamin C 2%; Calcium 4%; Iron 12%
Diet Exchanges: 3 starch, 1½ lean meat, 1 vegetable

Sweet-and-Sour Chicken

LO CAL / LO FAT / HI FIB

PREP: 10 MIN; COOK: 7 MIN

4 SERVINGS

Chow mein noodles are deep-fat fried, making them very crisp but adding extra fat. We've listed them in the recipe as an optional ingredient, so if you can't do without them, just use less than you normally would.

1	pound skinless, boneless chicken breast halves
4	cups cut-up assorted vegetables (bell peppers, carrots, tomatoes)
1	can (8 ounces) pineapple chunks in juice, drained
½	cup sweet-and-sour sauce
	Chow mein noodles, if desired

Remove fat from chicken. Cut chicken into 1-inch pieces. Spray 12-inch nonstick skillet with cooking spray; heat over medium-high heat. Add chicken; stir-fry 3 to 4 minutes until no longer pink in center.

Add vegetables; stir-fry about 2 minutes or until crisp-tender. Stir in pineapple and sweet-and-sour sauce; cook and stir 1 minute. Serve over noodles.

1 Serving: Calories 230 (Calories from Fat 45); Fat 5g (Saturated 1g); Cholesterol 70mg; Sodium 190mg; Carbohydrate 23g (Dietary Fiber 3g); Protein 26g
% Daily Value: Vitamin A 66%; Vitamin C 66%; Calcium 4%; Iron 10%
Diet Exchanges: 2½ lean meat, 1 vegetable, 1 fruit

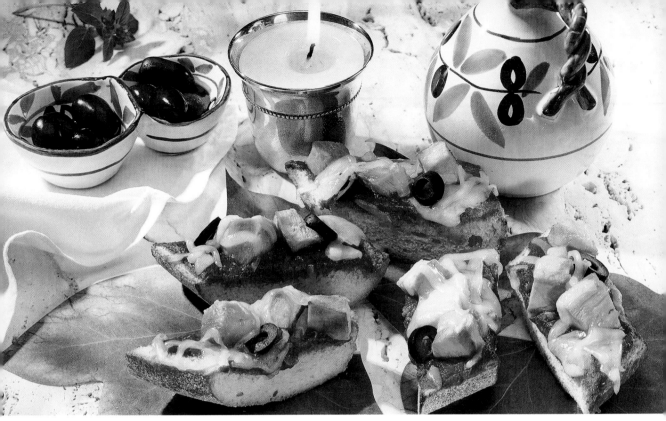

Chicken French-Bread Pizza

Chicken French-Bread Pizza

LO CAL / HI FIB

PREP: 5 MIN; BAKE: 12 MIN

6 SERVINGS

At your next party, cut thin slices of this chicken- and olive-laden pizza to serve as appetizers.

1 loaf (1 pound) unsliced French bread

1 can (8 ounces) pizza sauce

2 cups cubed cooked chicken or turkey

1 can (2¼ ounces) sliced ripe olives, drained

1 cup shredded reduced-fat mozzarella cheese (4 ounces)

Heat oven to 425°. Split bread horizontally in half. Place bread, cut sides up, on cookie sheet.

Spread pizza sauce over bread. Top with chicken and olives. Sprinkle with cheese. Bake about 12 minutes or until cheese is melted and chicken is heated through.

1 Serving: Calories 305 (Calories from Fat 110); Fat 12g (Saturated 5g); Cholesterol 60mg; Sodium 660mg; Carbohydrate 29g (Dietary Fiber 2g); Protein 22g
% Daily Value: Vitamin A 10%; Vitamin C 8%; Calcium 20%; Iron 14%
Diet Exchanges: 2 starch, 2 lean meat, 1 fat

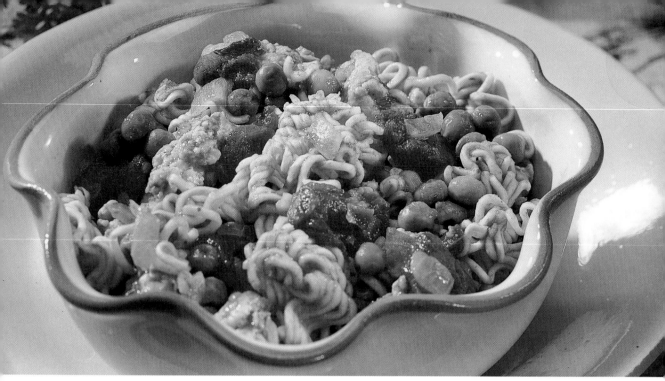

Take-It-Easy Noodle Dinner

Take-It-Easy Noodle Dinner

LO CAL / LO FAT / HI FIB

PREP: 5 MIN; COOK: 15 MIN

4 SERVINGS

Does your taste run more to beef? Then simmer this quick skillet dish with extra-lean ground beef and beef-flavor ramen noodle soup mix.

1   **pound ground turkey breast**

1   **medium onion, coarsely chopped ($^1/_2$ cup)**

1   **can (14$^1/_2$ ounces) stewed tomatoes, undrained**

1   **package (10 ounces) frozen green peas, thawed**

1   **package (3 ounces) chicken-flavor reduced-fat baked ramen noodle soup mix**

Cook turkey and onion in 12-inch nonstick skillet over medium heat about 8 minutes, stirring occasionally, until turkey is no longer pink.

Stir in tomatoes, peas and seasoning packet from soup mix. Break up noodles; stir into turkey mixture. Heat to boiling, stirring occasionally; reduce heat. Cover and simmer about 6 minutes, stirring occasionally to separate noodles, until noodles are tender.

1 Serving: Calories 190 (Calories from Fat 10); Fat 1g (Saturated 0g); Cholesterol 75mg; Sodium 340mg; Carbohydrate 19g (Dietary Fiber 5g); Protein 31g
% Daily Value: Vitamin A 10%; Vitamin C 18%; Calcium 6%; Iron 16%
Diet Exchanges: 1 starch, 4 very lean meat

Mozzarella-Topped Chicken and Eggplant

LO CAL / HI FIB

PREP: 5 MIN; COOK: 13 MIN

4 SERVINGS

Mamma mia! This slimmed-down version of chicken and eggplant parmigiana truly saves calories and time. It cuts calories by starting with unbreaded chicken, omitting olive oil for sautéing and using reduced-fat mozzarella. The recipe conserves your time by simmering everything quickly in a skillet and taking advantage of Italian-style tomato sauce.

- 8 skinless, boneless chicken thighs (about 1⅓ pounds)
- 1 small eggplant, peeled and cut into 1-inch cubes (4 cups)
- 1 can (15 ounces) Italian-style tomato sauce
- ½ teaspoon cracked black pepper
- ½ cup shredded reduced-fat mozzarella cheese (2 ounces)

Remove fat from chicken. Spray 12-inch nonstick skillet with cooking spray. Cook eggplant and chicken in skillet over medium heat about 10 minutes, stirring frequently, until juice of chicken is no longer pink when centers of thickest pieces are cut.

Stir in tomato sauce and pepper; heat through. Remove from heat. Sprinkle with cheese.

1 Serving: Calories 310 (Calories from Fat 125); Fat 14g (Saturated 5g); Cholesterol 90mg; Sodium 800mg; Carbohydrate 15g (Dietary Fiber 4g); Protein 35g
% Daily Value: Vitamin A 12%; Vitamin C 12%; Calcium 16%; Iron 20%
Diet Exchanges: ½ starch, 4 lean meat, 2 vegetable

Turkey and Tomato-Rice Stew

LO CAL / LO FAT / HI FIB

PREP: 5 MIN; COOK: 15 MIN

6 SERVINGS

To keep the fat to a minimum, be sure to buy ground turkey breast. Because it's all white meat and includes no turkey skin, it's lower in fat than regular ground turkey. If ground turkey breast isn't available, use extra-lean ground beef.

- 1 pound ground turkey breast
- 1 bag (16 ounces) frozen broccoli, red peppers, onions and mushrooms, thawed
- 1 can (14½ ounces) Mexican-style diced tomatoes with chili spices or Mexican-style stewed tomatoes, undrained
- 1 can (14½ ounces) ready-to-serve chicken broth
- 1 can (11 ounces) condensed old-fashioned tomato rice soup

Spray 3-quart saucepan with cooking spray. Cook turkey in saucepan over medium heat about 8 minutes, stirring occasionally, until no longer pink.

Stir in remaining ingredients. Heat to boiling; reduce heat. Simmer uncovered 5 minutes, stirring occasionally.

1 Serving: Calories 160 (Calories from Fat 20); Fat 2g (Saturated 1g); Cholesterol 50mg; Sodium 870mg; Carbohydrate 19g (Dietary Fiber 3g); Protein 22g
% Daily Value: Vitamin A 22%; Vitamin C 50%; Calcium 6%; Iron 12%
Diet Exchanges: 1 starch, 2 very lean meat, 1 vegetable

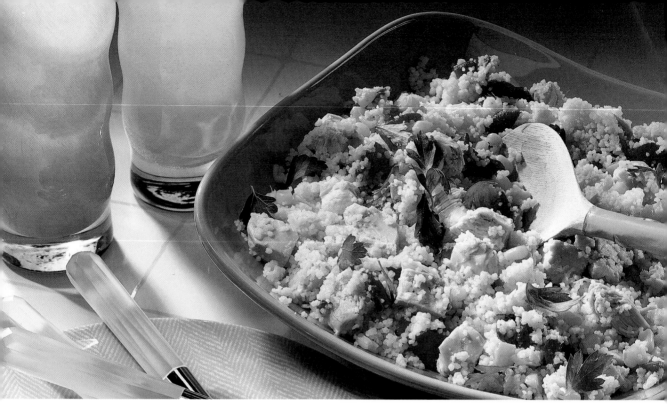

Turkey with Roasted Peppers and Couscous

Turkey with Roasted Peppers and Couscous

LO FAT / HI FIB

PREP: 5 MIN; COOK: 8 MIN

4 SERVINGS

When you have only minutes to rustle up dinner, this quick-cooking turkey-and-couscous medley can be a life-saver.

1   can (14¹/₂ ounces) ready-to-serve chicken broth

1   package (10 ounces) frozen whole kernel corn, thawed

1¹/₂   cups cubed cooked turkey or chicken

1¹/₄   cups uncooked couscous

1   jar (7 to 7¹/₄ ounces) roasted red bell peppers, drained and coarsely chopped

Heat broth and corn to boiling in 3-quart saucepan; reduce heat to low. Stir in remaining ingredients.

Cover and simmer about 3 minutes, stirring occasionally, until couscous is tender and turkey is heated through.

1 Serving: Calories 360 (Calories from Fat 45); Fat 5g (Saturated 1g); Cholesterol 45mg; Sodium 520mg; Carbohydrate 58g (Dietary Fiber 5g); Protein 26g
% Daily Value: Vitamin A 16%; Vitamin C 58%; Calcium 2%; Iron 10%
Diet Exchanges: 4 starch, 2 very lean meat

Turkey and Fruit Tossed Salad

LO CAL / LO FAT / HI FIB

PREP: 10 MIN

6 SERVINGS

Although any assortment of greens will taste great in this salad, the slightly bitter tang of an Italian-style mix with romaine and radicchio is especially nice with the chicken, dried fruit and subtly sweet French dressing.

1   bag (10 ounces) salad mix

2½ cups cubed cooked turkey or chicken

1   package (6 ounces) diced dried fruits and raisins (about 1¼ cups)

1   medium stalk celery, sliced (½ cup)

½   cup fat-free sweet-spicy French dressing

Place salad mix, chicken, dried fruits and celery in large bowl. Pour dressing over mixture; toss lightly to coat.

1 Serving: Calories 200 (Calories from Fat 35); Fat 4g (Saturated 1g); Cholesterol 50mg; Sodium 270mg; Carbohydrate 26g (Dietary Fiber 3g); Protein 18g
% Daily Value: Vitamin A 8%; Vitamin C 2%; Calcium 4%; Iron 10%
Diet Exchanges: 1 starch, 2 very lean meat, 1 vegetable, ½ fruit

Italian Turkey-Couscous Salad

LO CAL / LO FAT / HI FIB

PREP: 15 MIN

6 SERVINGS

This salad is as simple as heating chicken broth. All you have to do is heat the broth to boiling, then stir in the couscous, and toss it with the other ingredients.

2   cups chicken broth

1   package (10 ounces) couscous (1⅓ cups)

1   bag (16 ounces) frozen broccoli, carrots, onions, red peppers, celery, water chestnuts and mushrooms, thawed

3   cups cubed cooked turkey or chicken

1   bottle (8 ounces) fat-free creamy Italian dressing (¾ cup)

Lettuce leaves, if desired

Heat broth to boiling in 1½-quart saucepan; reduce heat. Stir in couscous; remove from heat. Cover and let stand 5 minutes.

Mix couscous, vegetables and chicken in large bowl. Pour dressing over mixture; toss lightly to coat. Line 6 salad plates with lettuce. Spoon salad onto lettuce.

1 Serving: Calories 300 (Calories from Fat 55); Fat 6g (Saturated 2g); Cholesterol 60mg; Sodium 620mg; Carbohydrate 38g (Dietary Fiber 4g); Protein 27g
% Daily Value: Vitamin A 10%; Vitamin C 20%; Calcium 4%; Iron 12%
Diet Exchanges: 2 starch, 3 very lean meat, 1½ vegetable

Chili Dogs

LO CAL / LO FAT / LO CHOL / HI FIB

PREP: 5 MIN; COOK: 10 MIN

6 SERVINGS

If you like, top this dinner favorite with some shredded reduced-fat or fat-free Cheddar cheese.

- 6   cooked fat-free turkey franks
- 1   can (15 ounces) chunky tomato sauce with onions, celery and green bell peppers
- 1   can (8 ounces) kidney beans, rinsed and drained
- 1   teaspoon chili powder
- 6   hot dog buns, split
    Chopped red onion, if desired

Heat franks, tomato sauce, beans and chili powder to boiling in 10-inch nonstick skillet; reduce heat. Simmer uncovered 5 minutes, stirring occasionally.

Place franks in buns. Top with bean mixture. Serve with onion.

1 Serving: Calories 260 (Calories from Fat 45); Fat 5g (Saturated 1g); Cholesterol 15mg; Sodium 1130mg; Carbohydrate 46g (Dietary Fiber 5g); Protein 13g
% Daily Value: Vitamin A 6%; Vitamin C 8%; Calcium 8%; Iron 18%
Diet Exchanges: 3 starch, 1 very lean meat

Speedy Cassoulet

LO CAL / HI FIB

PREP: 5 MIN; COOK: 10 MIN

4 SERVINGS

Traditional French cassoulet is a slow-cooking white bean stew made with a variety of meats, such as sausage, pork, duck or goose. This version is adapted to fit today's busy schedules and health concerns. It shaves time, fat and calories off this classic recipe.

- 1   can (15 to 16 ounces) cannellini or great northern beans, rinsed and drained
- 1   can (14½ ounces) diced tomatoes with roasted garlic, undrained
- 1   can (14½ ounces) ready-to-serve chicken broth
- ½   pound fully cooked turkey kielbasa (Polish sausage), cut into ½-inch slices (1½ cups)
- 1½ cups frozen chopped bell peppers (from 10-ounce bag), thawed
    Seasoned bread crumbs, if desired

Heat beans, tomatoes, broth and turkey kielbasa to boiling in 3-quart saucepan, stirring occasionally; reduce heat.

Stir in bell peppers. Simmer uncovered 5 minutes, stirring occasionally. Sprinkle with bread crumbs.

1 Serving: Calories 345 (Calories from Fat 155); Fat 17g (Saturated 6g); Cholesterol 35mg; Sodium 1200mg; Carbohydrate 36g (Dietary Fiber 9g); Protein 21g
% Daily Value: Vitamin A 10%; Vitamin C 52%; Calcium 14%; Iron 30%
Diet Exchanges: 2 starch, 2½ medium-fat meat, 1 vegetable

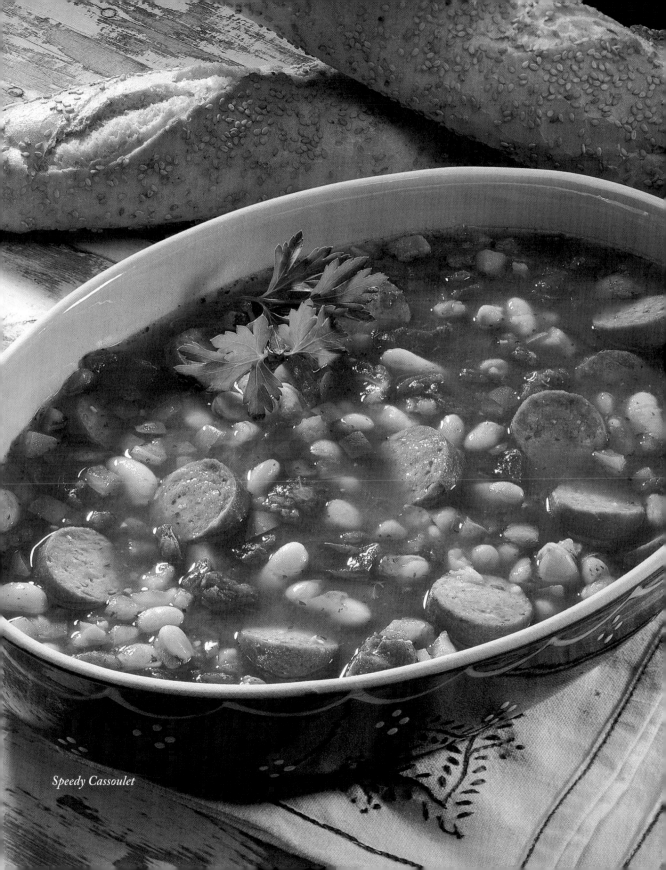

Speedy Cassoulet

Turkey Pastrami Reubens

LO CAL / HI FIB

PREP: 5 MIN; COOK: 8 MIN

4 SERVINGS

This newfangled version of the classic sandwich skimps on the fat and calories but not on the flavor. It has only 350 calories and 12 grams of fat versus 595 calories and 45 grams of fat in the traditional sandwich. For a change of pace, use smoked turkey in place of the turkey pastrami.

- 8 slices dark rye or pumpernickel bread
- 1/3 cup fat-free Thousand Island dressing
- 4 slices (1 1/2 ounces each) reduced-fat natural Swiss cheese
- 6 ounces cooked fat-free turkey pastrami, thinly sliced
- 1 cup sauerkraut, rinsed and well drained

Spread one side of each bread slice with dressing. Top 4 of the bread slices with cheese, turkey pastrami and sauerkraut. Top with remaining bread slices.

Spray 12-inch nonstick skillet with cooking spray. Heat sandwiches in skillet over medium heat 4 minutes; turn. Heat about 4 minutes longer or until bread is toasted and cheese is melted.

1 Serving: Calories 350 (Calories from Fat 110); Fat 12g (Saturated 6g); Cholesterol 45mg; Sodium 1500mg; Carbohydrate 37g (Dietary Fiber 4g); Protein 28g
% Daily Value: Vitamin A 10%; Vitamin C 6%; Calcium 60%; Iron 18%
Diet Exchanges: 2 1/2 starch, 3 lean meat

Sausage with Fettuccine

LO CAL / LO FAT / HI FIB

PREP: 5 MIN; COOK: 8 MIN

4 SERVINGS

For an eye-catching main dish, ladle this ruby red sauce over spinach fettuccine.

- 1 package (9 ounces) refrigerated fettuccine
- 2 cans (15 ounces each) chunky garlic-and-herb tomato sauce
- 1 bag (16 ounces) frozen stir-fry bell peppers and onions, thawed
- 1 ring (1 pound) fully cooked fat-free Polish or kielbasa sausage, cut into 1/2-inch pieces
  Finely shredded Parmesan cheese, if desired

Cook and drain fettuccine as directed on package; keep warm.

Heat tomato sauce, pepper mixture and sausage to boiling in same saucepan. Stir in fettuccine; heat through. Serve with cheese.

1 Serving: Calories 340 (Calories from Fat 35); Fat 4g (Saturated 1g); Cholesterol 85mg; Sodium 950mg; Carbohydrate 61g (Dietary Fiber 6g); Protein 21g
% Daily Value: Vitamin A 16%; Vitamin C 70%; Calcium 10%; Iron 26%
Diet Exchanges: 3 starch, 1 lean meat, 3 vegetable

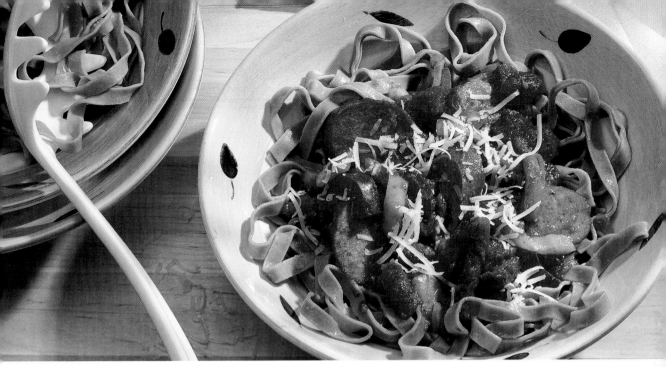

Sausage with Fettuccine

Fix-It-Fast Vegetable and Tuna Chowder

LO CAL / LO FAT / LO CHOL / HI FIB

PREP: 5 MIN; COOK: 10 MIN

6 SERVINGS

When your family's busy schedule starts to get the best of you, whip together this tasty tuna chowder. All you need do is measure the half-and-half, mix the ingredients, heat and serve. It's ready in just 15 minutes!

1 bag (16 ounces) frozen petite peas, baby whole carrots, snow peas and baby cob corn, thawed

1 can (14¾ ounces) cream-style corn

1 can (14½ ounces) ready-to-serve chicken broth

2 cans (6 ounces each) tuna in water, drained

1½ cups fat-free half-and-half or refrigerated fat-free nondairy creamer

Heat all ingredients to boiling in 3-quart saucepan, stirring occasionally; reduce heat. Simmer uncovered 5 minutes, stirring occasionally.

1 Serving: Calories 225 (Calories from Fat 25); Fat 3g (Saturated 1g); Cholesterol 15mg; Sodium 690mg; Carbohydrate 31g (Dietary Fiber 4g); Protein 20g
% Daily Value: Vitamin A 48%; Vitamin C 14%; Calcium 2%; Iron 12%
Diet Exchanges: 2 starch, 1 very lean meat, 1 vegetable

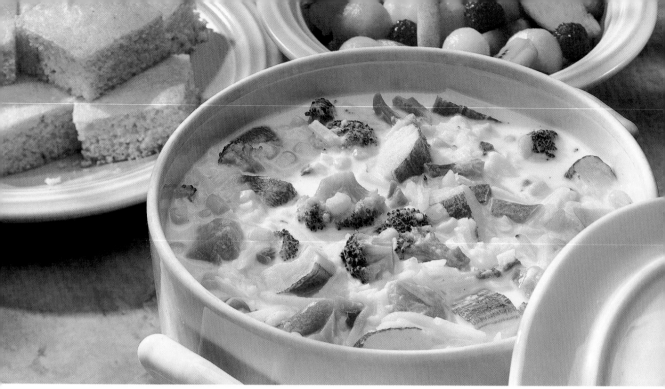

Hearty Potato Chowder with Crab

Hearty Potato Chowder with Crab

LO CAL / LO FAT / LO CHOL / HI FIB

PREP: 5 MIN; COOK: 13 MIN

6 SERVINGS

Serve bowls of this steaming hearty crab chowder with squares of freshly baked corn bread and a mixed-fruit salad.

1 bag (24 ounces) frozen country-style hash brown or O'Brien potatoes, thawed

1 bag (16 ounces) frozen broccoli, corn and red peppers, thawed

1 can (14½ ounces) ready-to-serve chicken broth

2 cups fat-free half-and-half or refrigerated fat-free nondairy creamer

1 package (16 ounces) refrigerated imitation crabmeat chunks

¼ teaspoon pepper, if desired

Heat potatoes, vegetables and broth to boiling in Dutch oven, stirring occasionally; reduce heat. Cover and simmer 5 minutes. Stir in remaining ingredients; heat through.

1 Serving: Calories 280 (Calories from Fat 20); Fat 2g (Saturated 0g); Cholesterol 25mg; Sodium 1440mg; Carbohydrate 52g (Dietary Fiber 5g); Protein 18g
% Daily Value: Vitamin A 26%; Vitamin C 30%; Calcium 4%; Iron 6%
Diet Exchanges: 3 starch, 1½ very lean meat, 1 vegetable

Broiled Lemon Pepper-Salmon Patties

LOW CALORIE

PREP: 5 MIN; FREEZE: 8 MIN; BROIL: 8 MIN

4 SERVINGS

If you love salmon but still want to watch the fat in your diet, pink or chum salmon are good choices.

- 1 cup soft bread crumbs (about $1^1/_2$ slices bread)
- $^1/_4$ cup reduced-fat mayonnaise or salad dressing
- 1 egg white, slightly beaten
- $^1/_2$ teaspoon lemon pepper
- 1 can ($7^1/_2$ ounces) skinless boneless pink salmon, drained and flaked
  Tartar sauce, if desired

Mix bread crumbs, mayonnaise, egg white and lemon pepper in medium bowl. Mix in salmon. Spoon salmon mixture into 4 mounds onto cookie sheet lined with waxed paper. Freeze about 8 minutes or until firm enough to shape into patties.

Set oven control to broil. Spray broiler pan rack with cooking spray. Pat salmon mixture into 3-inch round patties. Place on rack in broiler pan.

Broil patties with tops 4 to 5 inches from heat 6 minutes. Carefully turn patties, using a wide spatula. Broil about 2 minutes longer or until golden brown. Serve with tartar sauce.

1 Serving: Calories 150 (Calories from Fat 80); Fat 8g (Saturated 1g); Cholesterol 30mg; Sodium 550mg; Carbohydrate 6g (Dietary Fiber 0g); Protein 11g
% Daily Value: Vitamin A 0%; Vitamin C 0%; Calcium 10%; Iron 4%
Diet Exchanges: $^1/_2$ starch, $1^1/_2$ medium-fat meat

Caesar Salad with Lobster

LO CAL / LO FAT

PREP: 10 MIN

4 SERVINGS

Cooked chicken or imitation crabmeat chunks are equally delicious in place of the lobster chunks in this fruit-accented tossed salad.

- 1 bag (10 ounces) salad mix
- 1 can (11 ounces) mandarin orange segments, chilled and drained
- 1 package (8 ounces) refrigerated imitation lobster chunks
- 1 small unpeeled cucumber, cut into $^1/_4$-inch slices
- $^1/_3$ cup fat-free Caesar or ranch dressing
  Sliced almonds, if desired

Place all ingredients except almonds in large bowl; toss lightly to coat. Sprinkle with almonds.

1 Serving: Calories 120 (Calories from Fat 10); Fat 1g (Saturated 0g); Cholesterol 40mg; Sodium 480mg; Carbohydrate 17g (Dietary Fiber 2g); Protein 13g
% Daily Value: Vitamin A 4%; Vitamin C 18%; Calcium 6%; Iron 6%
Diet Exchanges: $1^1/_2$ very lean meat, $^1/_2$ vegetable, 1 fruit

Shrimp Carbonara with White Cheddar Sauce

HIGH FIBER

PREP: 5 MIN; COOK: 20 MIN

4 SERVINGS

The vegetable broth gives this special-occasion pasta a full-bodied vegetable flavor, but if you don't have any on hand, substitute chicken broth.

1   can (14½ ounces) ready-to-serve vegetable broth

1   package (6.2 ounces) shell-shaped pasta and white Cheddar sauce mix

1   cup skim milk

1   bag (16 ounces) frozen shoepeg corn, broccoli flowerets, baby corn cob and carrots, thawed

1   package (12 ounces) frozen uncooked peeled deveined medium shrimp, thawed

Freshly ground pepper, if desired

Heat broth to boiling in 3-quart saucepan. Stir in pasta; reduce heat. Simmer uncovered about 12 minutes, stirring frequently, until most of the broth is absorbed. Stir in skim milk and pasta seasoning packet. Heat to boiling; reduce heat.

Stir in vegetables and shrimp. Simmer uncovered about 3 minutes, stirring occasionally, until shrimp are pink and firm and vegetables are heated through; remove from heat. Let stand about 3 minutes or until sauce is thickened. Serve with pepper.

1 Serving: Calories 410 (Calories from Fat 65); Fat 7g (Saturated 3g); Cholesterol 125mg; Sodium 1530mg; Carbohydrate 65g (Dietary Fiber 5g); Protein 27g
% Daily Value: Vitamin A 22%; Vitamin C 16%; Calcium 12%; Iron 14%
Diet Exchanges: 4 starch, 2 very lean meat, 1 vegetable

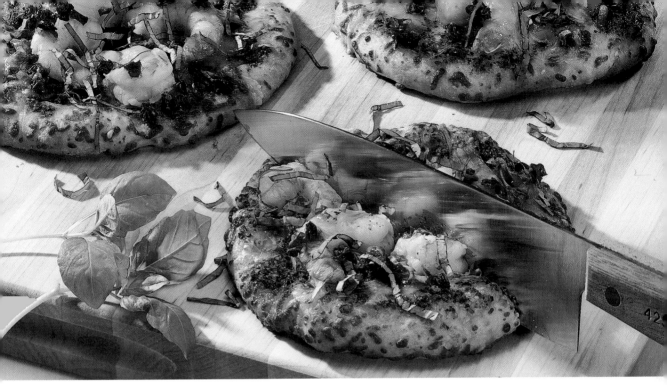

Shrimp-Pesto Pizzas

Shrimp-Pesto Pizzas

LOW CALORIE

PREP: 10 MIN; BAKE: 12 MIN

4 SERVINGS

Shrimp, pesto and sun-dried tomatoes top this pizza; serve it with a tossed spinach salad.

- ¼ cup finely chopped sun-dried tomatoes (not oil-packed)
- 4 rounds focaccia bread or Italian bread shells (6 inches in diameter)
- ¼ cup basil pesto
- ¾ pound cooked peeled deveined medium shrimp, thawed if frozen
- ½ cup shredded reduced-fat mozzarella cheese (2 ounces)

  Chopped fresh basil, if desired

Heat oven to 425°. Pour boiling water over sun-dried tomatoes. Let stand 3 minutes; drain.

Place breads on cookie sheet. Spread pesto over breads. Top with shrimp and tomatoes. Sprinkle with cheese. Bake about 12 minutes or until cheese is melted and shrimp are heated through. Sprinkle with basil.

1 Serving: Calories 285 (Calories from Fat 125); Fat 14g (Saturated 4g); Cholesterol 130mg; Sodium 700mg; Carbohydrate 20g (Dietary Fiber 1g); Protein 21g
% Daily Value: Vitamin A 6%; Vitamin C 2%; Calcium 18%; Iron 20%
Diet Exchanges: 1½ starch, 2½ medium-fat meat

Mediterranean Shrimp with Tomato and Feta

LO CAL / LO FAT / HI FIB

PREP: 5 MIN; COOK: 8 MIN

6 SERVINGS

Go on a culinary journey to Greece with this beguiling, yet simply prepared, shrimp main dish. The feta accent adds Mediterranean flair. If you like, substitute 1½ cups of cooked chicken for the shrimp.

- 2 cans (15 ounces each) chunky garlic-and-herb tomato sauce
- 1 bag (16 ounces) frozen small whole onions, thawed
- ½ cup dry white wine or vegetable broth
- ¾ pound cooked peeled deveined medium shrimp, thawed if frozen
- 1 package (4 ounces) feta cheese, crumbled (⅔ cup)

  Hot cooked couscous or linguine, if desired

Heat tomato sauce, onions and wine to boiling in 3-quart saucepan, stirring occasionally; reduce heat.

Stir in shrimp; heat through. Remove from heat. Stir in cheese. Serve over couscous.

1 Serving: Calories 160 (Calories from Fat 45); Fat 5g (Saturated 3g); Cholesterol 100mg; Sodium 1170mg; Carbohydrate 18g (Dietary Fiber 3g); Protein 14g
% Daily Value: Vitamin A 18%; Vitamin C 20%; Calcium 14%; Iron 14%
Diet Exchanges: 1 starch, 2 very lean meat, 1 vegetable

Spicy Pepper Steak

LOW CALORIE

PREP: 10 MIN; COOK: 5 MIN

4 SERVINGS

Chili oil may also be called hot chili oil, hot oil or hot stir-fry oil. This is a fiery-hot vegetable or sesame oil infused with the flavors of hot chili peppers. You can find it in the Asian foods section of the supermarket.

- 1 tablespoon chili oil or vegetable oil
- 1 pound cut-up beef for stir-fry
- 1 large bell pepper, cut into ¾-inch squares
- 1 medium onion, sliced
- ¼ cup hoisin sauce

  Hot cooked noodles or rice, if desired

Heat oil in 12-inch nonstick skillet over medium-high heat. Add beef; cook about 2 minutes or until brown.

Add bell pepper and onion; stir-fry about 1 minute or until vegetables are crisp-tender. Stir in hoisin sauce; cook and stir about 30 seconds or until hot. Serve with noodles.

1 Serving: Calories 185 (Calories from Fat 65); Fat 7g (Saturated 2g); Cholesterol 55mg; Sodium 300mg; Carbohydrate 11g (Dietary Fiber 1g); Protein 21g
% Daily Value: Vitamin A 4%; Vitamin C 24%; Calcium 2%; Iron 12%
Diet Exchanges: 2½ lean meat, 2 vegetable

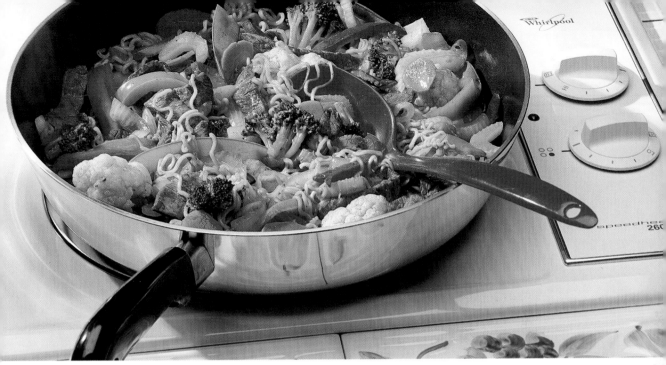

Ramen Stir-Fry

Ramen Stir-Fry

LO CAL / HI FIB

PREP: 5 MIN; COOK: 20 MIN

4 SERVINGS

You will find the beef easier to cut in this recipe if it's partially frozen, about 1½ hours.

1   **pound beef boneless sirloin**

2   **cups water**

1   **package (3 ounces) Oriental-flavor ramen soup mix**

1   **bag (16 ounces) fresh (refrigerated) stir-fry vegetables**

¼   **cup stir-fry sauce**

Remove fat from beef. Cut beef into thin strips. Spray 12-inch nonstick skillet with cooking spray; heat over medium-high heat. Cook beef in skillet 3 to 5 minutes, stirring occasionally, until brown. Remove beef from skillet.

Heat water to boiling in skillet. Break up noodles from soup mix into water; stir until slightly softened. Stir in vegetables.

Heat to boiling. Boil 5 to 7 minutes, stirring occasionally, until vegetables are crisp-tender. Stir in contents of seasoning packet from soup mix, stir-fry sauce and beef. Cook 3 to 5 minutes, stirring frequently, until hot.

1 Serving: Calories 260 (Calories from Fat 80); Fat 9g (Saturated 2g); Cholesterol 55mg; Sodium 1490mg; Carbohydrate 23g (Dietary Fiber 4g); Protein 26g
% Daily Value: Vitamin A 14%; Vitamin C 30%; Calcium 4%; Iron 20%
Diet Exchanges: 1 starch, 2½ lean meat, 2 vegetable

Quick Beef Tips and Vegetables

LO CAL / LO FAT

PREP: 5 MIN; COOK: 10 MIN

4 SERVINGS

When using frozen stir-fry vegetables, look for snap pea pods instead of snow (Chinese) pea pods. Snap pea pods retain their crispness through freezing and stir-frying.

1/2 **pound beef boneless sirloin tip steak**

1 **bag (16 ounces) frozen mixed vegetables with snap pea pods**

1 **tablespoon water**

1/4 **cup stir-fry sauce with garlic and ginger**

2 **cups hot cooked rice**

Remove fat from beef. Cut beef into 1/2-inch cubes.

Spray 12-inch nonstick skillet with cooking spray; heat over medium-high heat. Add beef; stir-fry about 2 minutes or until brown. Add vegetables and water; stir-fry 1 minute.

Stir in stir-fry sauce until well mixed; reduce heat to medium. Cover and cook 5 to 7 minutes, stirring frequently, until vegetables are crisp-tender. Serve over rice.

1 Serving: Calories 215 (Calories from Fat 45); Fat 5g (Saturated 2g); Cholesterol 40mg; Sodium 190mg; Carbohydrate 27g (Dietary Fiber 1g); Protein 16g
% Daily Value: Vitamin A 2%; Vitamin C 22%; Calcium 2%; Iron 12%
Diet Exchanges: 2 lean meat, 2 vegetable, 1 fruit

Quick Beef and Noodle Dinner

LOW CALORIE

PREP: 5 MIN; COOK: 12 MIN

4 SERVINGS

For a chill-chasing, stick-to-the-ribs meal, try these beef cubed steaks nestled in a bed of noodles with rich mushroom gravy. Cut down on dishwashing time by bringing the steaks to the table right in the skillet.

1/2 **pound beef, boneless sirloin steak**

1 **can (14 1/2 ounces) ready-to-serve beef broth**

1 **jar (12 ounces) mushroom gravy**

1 **jar (4 1/2 ounces) sliced mushrooms, drained**

2 **cups uncooked extra-wide egg noodles (4 ounces)**

Remove fat from beef. Cut beef into 1/2-inch cubes.

Spray 12-inch nonstick skillet with cooking spray; heat over medium-high heat. Add beef; cook about 2 minutes or until brown.

Mix broth, gravy and mushrooms in same skillet. Heat to boiling. Stir in noodles. Top with beef; reduce heat. Cover and simmer 8 to 10 minutes, stirring occasionally, until noodles are tender.

1 Serving: Calories 285 (Calories from Fat 180); Fat 15g (Saturated 5g); Cholesterol 60mg; Sodium 1210mg; Carbohydrate 21g (Dietary Fiber 2g); Protein 18g
% Daily Value: Vitamin A 0%; Vitamin C 0%; Calcium 6%; Iron 16%
Diet Exchanges: 1 starch, 2 meat, 2 fat

Veal with Asparagus

LO CAL / LO FAT

PREP: 10 MIN; COOK: 20 MIN

4 SERVINGS

Veal, like other meats, is a source of the mineral iron. Iron is important for oxygen transfer to our cells, and it helps prevent anemia.

1 teaspoon vegetable oil

1 tablespoon finely chopped shallot or onion

1 clove garlic, finely chopped

$3/4$ pound thin slices lean veal round steak or veal for scaloppine

$3/4$ pound asparagus spears, cut into 1-inch pieces*

1 package (8 ounces) sliced mushrooms (3 cups)

$1/3$ cup dry white wine or chicken broth

2 teaspoons chopped fresh or $1/2$ teaspoon dried thyme leaves

Heat oil in 10-inch nonstick skillet over medium-high heat. Cook shallot and garlic in oil, stirring frequently, until garlic is golden; reduce heat to medium. Add veal. Cook about 3 minutes, turning once, until light brown.

Stir in remaining ingredients. Heat to boiling; reduce heat. Cover and simmer about 12 minutes, stirring occasionally, until asparagus is crisp-tender.

*1 package (10 ounces) frozen asparagus cuts, thawed, can be substituted for the fresh asparagus.

1 Serving: Calories 125 (Calories from Fat 45); Fat 5g (Saturated 2g); Cholesterol 55mg; Sodium 50mg; Carbohydrate 5g (Dietary Fiber 1g); Protein 16g
% Daily Value: Vitamin A 4%; Vitamin C 10%; Calcium 2%; Iron 10%
Diet Exchanges: 2 lean meat, 1 vegetable

Old-Time Beef and Vegetable Stew

LO CAL / LO FAT / HI FIB

PREP: 5 MIN; COOK: 10 MIN

6 SERVINGS

Frozen stew vegetables and spicy eight-vegetable juice let you cook up this old-fashioned family pleaser in a flash.

1 pound lean beef boneless sirloin

1 bag (16 ounces) frozen stew vegetables, thawed

1 can (15 ounces) chunky garlic-and-herb tomato sauce

1 can ($14^{1}/_2$ ounces) ready-to-serve beef broth

2 cans ($5^{1}/_2$ ounces each) spicy eight-vegetable juice

Corn bread, if desired

Remove fat from beef. Cut beef into $1/2$-inch cubes. Spray 10-inch nonstick skillet with cooking spray; heat over medium-high heat. Cook beef in skillet, stirring occasionally, until brown.

Stir in remaining ingredients except corn bread. Heat to boiling; reduce heat. Simmer uncovered 5 minutes, stirring occasionally. Serve with corn bread.

1 Serving: Calories 250 (Calories from Fat 55); Fat 6g (Saturated 2g); Cholesterol 65mg; Sodium 860mg; Carbohydrate 25g (Dietary Fiber 3g); Protein 27g
% Daily Value: Vitamin A 14%; Vitamin C 24%; Calcium 4%; Iron 18%
Diet Exchanges: 1 starch, 3 lean meat, 2 vegetable, $1/2$ fat

Taco Pizza

HIGH FIBER

PREP: 15 MIN; BAKE: 12 MIN

4 SERVINGS

Italian bread shells have many names, including "Italian flatbread" and "ready-to-serve pizza crust" (photo, page 147).

- 1 round focaccia bread or Italian bread shell (12 inches in diameter)
- $3/4$ pound diet-lean or extra-lean ground beef
- $1/2$ envelope (1$1/4$-ounce size) taco seasoning mix (about 2 tablespoons)
- 1 can (10 ounces) diced tomatoes and green chilies, drained
- $1/2$ cup shredded reduced-fat Cheddar cheese (2 ounces)

    Shredded lettuce, if desired

    Reduced-fat sour cream, if desired

    Chopped tomatoes, if desired

Heat oven to 425°. Place bread on 12-inch pizza pan or cookie sheet.

Cook beef in 10-inch nonstick skillet over medium heat about 6 minutes, stirring occasionally, until brown; drain. Stir in taco seasoning mix; stir in half the amount of water as directed on package. Simmer uncovered 5 minutes.

Spoon beef mixture over bread. Top with tomatoes. Sprinkle with cheese. Bake about 12 minutes or until cheese is melted and tomatoes are heated through. Serve topped with lettuce, sour cream and tomatoes.

1 Serving: Calories 585 (Calories from Fat 180); Fat 20g (Saturated 5g); Cholesterol 50mg; Sodium 1600mg; Carbohydrate 73g (Dietary Fiber 4g); Protein 32g
% Daily Value: Vitamin A 8%; Vitamin C 8%; Calcium 10%; Iron 36%
Diet Exchanges: 5 starch, 2 lean meat, 2 fat

Philadelphia Cheese Steak Sandwiches

LOW CALORIE

PREP: 5 MIN; COOK: 7 MIN; BROIL: 3 MIN

4 SERVINGS

Ask Philadelphians what their favorite food from back home is, and the cheese steak sandwich is sure to be mentioned. Some like it with sliced beef; others with shaved beef. But no matter how you cut it, the sandwich has to have cheese—and lots of it.

- 2 medium onions, cut lengthwise in half, then cut crosswise into thin slices
- $3/4$ pound thinly sliced cooked lean roast beef
- 4 French-style rolls or hoagie buns (about 6 inches long), split
- $1/4$ cup fat-free Italian dressing
- 4 slices ($3/4$ ounce each) reduced-fat process American-flavored cheese product

Spray 10-inch nonstick skillet with cooking spray; heat over medium heat. Cook onions in skillet about 5 minutes, stirring frequently, until tender. Stir in beef; heat through.

Set oven control to broil. Place rolls cut side up on cookie sheet; brush with dressing. Broil with tops 4 to 5 inches from heat 2 minutes.

Divide beef mixture among rolls. Top with cheese. Broil about 1 minute or until cheese is melted. Serve immediately.

1 Serving: Calories 340 (Calories from Fat 115); Fat 13g (Saturated 5g); Cholesterol 60mg; Sodium 770mg; Carbohydrate 32g (Dietary Fiber 2g); Protein 26g
% Daily Value: Vitamin A 6%; Vitamin C 2%; Calcium 14%; Iron 18%
Diet Exchanges: 2 starch, 3 lean meat

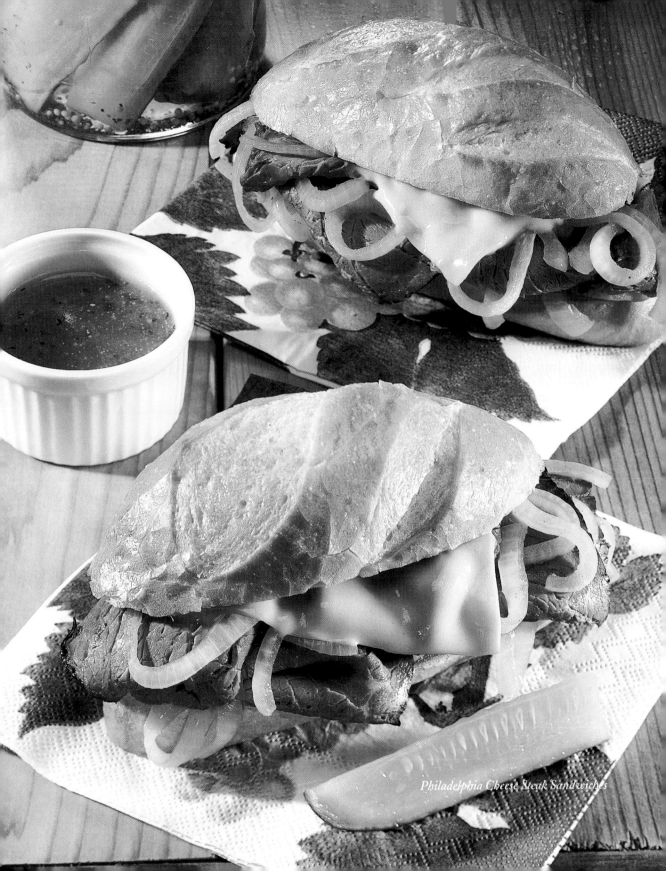

Philadelphia Cheese Steak Sandwiches

Stir-Fried Beef and Vegetable Soup

LO CAL / LO FAT / LO CHOL

PREP: 10 MIN; COOK: 10 MIN

4 SERVINGS

Use wonton skins to make fun, crisp crackers to go with this soup! Cut wonton skins diagonally in half, and arrange in a single layer on ungreased cookie sheet. Spray with cooking spray. Bake in 350° oven 5 to 8 minutes or until crisp and golden brown.

1/2   pound beef boneless sirloin steak

1   bag (16 ounces) fresh (refrigerated) stir-fry vegetables

1   bag (about 7 ounces) fresh (refrigerated) stir-fry noodles with soy sauce-flavored sauce

1   can (14 1/2 ounces) ready-to-serve beef or Oriental broth

3   cups water

Remove fat from beef. Cut beef into 1/4-inch slices. (Beef is easier to cut if partially frozen, about 1 1/2 hours.)

Spray 12-inch nonstick skillet with cooking spray; heat over medium-high heat. Add beef; stir-fry about 2 minutes or until brown. Stir in remaining ingredients; heat to boiling. Boil about 5 minutes, stirring occasionally, until vegetables are crisp-tender.

1 Serving: Calories 145 (Calories from Fat 35); Fat 4g (Saturated 2g); Cholesterol 20mg; Sodium 230mg; Carbohydrate 18g (Dietary Fiber 2g); Protein 11g
% Daily Value: Vitamin A 24%; Vitamin C 20%; Calcium 4%; Iron 8%
Diet Exchanges: 1 starch, 1 lean meat

Deli Beef and Bean Tossed Salad

LO CAL / LO FAT / LO CHOL / HI FIB

PREP: 10 MIN

6 SERVINGS

Toss and tumble your way to a top-notch meal with this five-ingredient salad that goes together in only 10 minutes. For a colorful presentation, select a salad mix that contains lettuce, shredded carrot and shredded red cabbage.

1   bag (10 ounces) salad mix

1   pint (2 cups) deli three-bean salad or 1 can (15 to 17 ounces) three-bean salad, chilled

1/4   pound deli cooked lean beef, turkey or ham, cut into julienne strips (3/4 cup)

1   cup shredded reduced-fat Cheddar or Swiss cheese (4 ounces)

12   cherry tomatoes, cut in half

Place all ingredients in large bowl; toss lightly to mix.

1 Serving: Calories 100 (Calories from Fat 20); Fat 2g (Saturated 1g); Cholesterol 15mg; Sodium 590mg; Carbohydrate 13g (Dietary Fiber 3g); Protein 10g
% Daily Value: Vitamin A 6%; Vitamin C 12%; Calcium 10%; Iron 8%
Diet Exchanges: 1/2 starch, 1 very lean meat, 1 vegetable

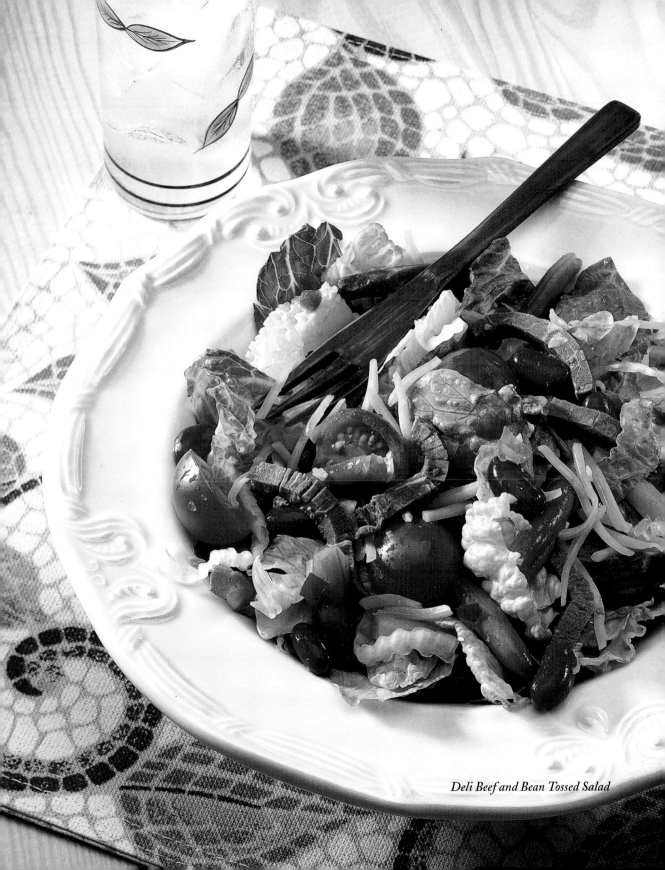

Deli Beef and Bean Tossed Salad

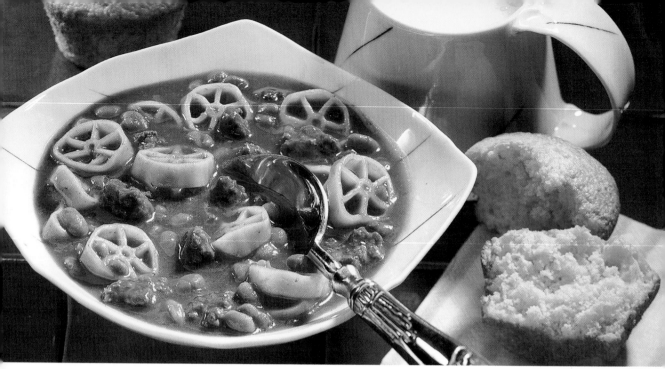

Chuck Wagon Chili

Chuck Wagon Chili

HIGH FIBER

PREP: 5 MIN; COOK: 20 MIN

4 SERVINGS

Bring this pasta and chili combo to the table, and all the cowpokes at your house will beg for seconds. Bow-tie pasta or medium shells also are attractive alternatives to the wagon-wheel pasta or elbow macaroni.

$^{1}/_{2}$ **pound diet-lean or extra-lean ground beef**

1   **can (16 ounces) vegetarian beans in tomato sauce**

1   **can (14$^{1}/_{2}$ ounces) ready-to-serve beef broth**

1   **can (10$^{3}/_{4}$ ounces) condensed tomato soup**

1   **cup uncooked wagon wheel pasta or elbow macaroni**

Cook beef in 3-quart saucepan over medium heat about 6 minutes, stirring occasionally, until brown; drain. Stir in beans, broth and soup. Heat to boiling, stirring occasionally; reduce heat.

Stir in pasta. Cover and simmer about 10 minutes, stirring frequently, until pasta is tender.

1 Serving: Calories 380 (Calories from Fat 80); Fat 9g (Saturated 3g); Cholesterol 34mg; Sodium 1520mg; Carbohydrate 57g (Dietary Fiber 7g); Protein 25g
% Daily Value: Vitamin A 2%; Vitamin C 10%; Calcium 8%; Iron 28%
Diet Exchanges: 3$^{1}/_{2}$ starch, 2 lean meat

Pork Chop Dinner with Rice and Vegetables

HIGH FIBER

PREP: 5 MIN; COOK: 20 MIN

6 SERVINGS

You'll find a pork chop-and-rice bake or skillet dinner in many a community cookbook, but this wholesome version skips some of the customary high-fat, high-calorie ingredients and retains all of the traditional flavor.

- 3 pork boneless butterfly loin chops, 1/2 inch thick (about 1/2 pound), halved
- 2 cans (10 3/4 ounces each) reduced-fat condensed cream of mushroom soup
- 1 bag (16 ounces) frozen broccoli, red peppers, onions and mushrooms, thawed
- 1 can (14 1/2 ounces) ready-to-serve chicken broth
- 2 cups uncooked instant brown rice

Remove fat from pork. Spray 12-inch nonstick skillet with cooking spray. Cook pork in skillet over medium heat about 5 minutes, turning once, until brown. Remove pork from skillet.

Heat soup, vegetables and broth to boiling in same skillet, stirring occasionally. Stir in rice; reduce heat. Cover and simmer 5 minutes. Top with pork. Cover and simmer about 5 minutes longer or until pork is slightly pink in center and rice is tender.

1 Serving: Calories 375 (Calories from Fat 80); Fat 9g (Saturated 3g); Cholesterol 40mg; Sodium 780mg; Carbohydrate 57g (Dietary Fiber 5g); Protein 22g
% Daily Value: Vitamin A 16%; Vitamin C 40%; Calcium 6%; Iron 10%
Diet Exchanges: 3 starch, 1 1/2 lean meat, 2 vegetable

Tortellini Primavera with Ham

LO CAL / HI FIB

PREP: 5 MIN; COOK: 12 MIN

6 SERVINGS

In Italian, primavera means "spring style" and usually refers to foods cooked with fresh or cooked vegetables. This colorful ham- and vegetable-studded dish is a superb example.

- 2 packages (9 ounces each) refrigerated cheese-filled tortellini
- 1 jar (24 to 28 ounces) fat-free spaghetti sauce
- 1 bag (16 ounces) frozen broccoli, cauliflower and carrots, thawed
- 1 1/2 cups cubed fully cooked fat-free ham
- 1/3 cup finely shredded Parmesan cheese

Cook and drain tortellini as directed on package; keep warm.

Heat spaghetti sauce, vegetables and ham to boiling in same saucepan, stirring occasionally. Stir in tortellini and cheese; heat through.

1 Serving: Calories 240 (Calories from Fat 70); Fat 8g (Saturated 4g); Cholesterol 95mg; Sodium 920mg; Carbohydrate 28g (Dietary Fiber 3g); Protein 17g
% Daily Value: Vitamin A 34%; Vitamin C 24%; Calcium 18%; Iron 12%
Diet Exchanges: 1 1/2 starch, 2 lean meat, 1 vegetable

Skillet Ham and Vegetables au Gratin

LO CAL / LO FAT / HI FIB

PREP: 10 MIN; COOK: 30 MIN

6 SERVINGS

For a change of pace, stir in a 4-ounce can of diced green chilies or a 2-ounce jar of diced pimientos (drained) with the potatoes.

1½ cups cut-up fully cooked ham

1 large onion, chopped (1 cup)

1 package (5.25 ounces) au gratin potato mix

2½ cups hot water

¼ teaspoon pepper

1 bag (16 ounces) frozen broccoli, cauliflower and carrots, thawed

1 cup shredded reduced-fat Cheddar cheese (4 ounces)

Spray 10-inch nonstick skillet with cooking spray; heat over medium-high heat. Cook ham and onion in skillet about 5 minutes, stirring frequently, until onion is tender.

Stir in potatoes and sauce mix from potato mix, the hot water and pepper. Heat to boiling; reduce heat. Cover and simmer 10 minutes, stirring occasionally. Stir in vegetables. Cover and simmer about 10 minutes or until potatoes are tender. Sprinkle with cheese.

1 Serving: Calories 255 (Calories from Fat 45); Fat 5g (Saturated 2g); Cholesterol 25mg; Sodium 1090mg; Carbohydrate 39g (Dietary Fiber 3g); Protein 16g
% Daily Value: Vitamin A 24%; Vitamin C 22%; Calcium 12%; Iron 6%
Diet Exchanges: 2 starch, 1 lean meat, 2 vegetable

Deli Ham Pita Sandwiches

LO CAL / LO FAT / LO CHOL / HI FIB

PREP: 10 MIN

4 SERVINGS

Create a deli full of new sandwiches by mixing and matching the meats and cheeses in this recipe. Next time, try cold sliced roast beef, smoked turkey or turkey pastrami with reduced-fat Cheddar or Swiss cheese.

4 fat-free whole wheat pita breads (6 inches in diameter), cut in half to form pockets

8 small lettuce leaves

¼ pound thinly sliced fully cooked fat-free ham

½ cup shredded reduced-fat mozzarella cheese

½ pint (1 cup) deli marinated mixed-vegetable salad, drained

Line pita breads with lettuce leaves. Place ham and cheese in pita breads. Spoon in vegetable salad.

1 Serving: Calories 230 (Calories from Fat 55); Fat 6g (Saturated 2g); Cholesterol 17mg; Sodium 840mg; Carbohydrate 36g (Dietary Fiber 5g); Protein 13g
% Daily Value: Vitamin A 4%; Vitamin C 10%; Calcium 12%; Iron 12%
Diet Exchanges: 2 starch, 1 medium-fat meat, 1 vegetable

Lickety-Split Ham and Corn Chowder

LO CAL / LO FAT / HI FIB

PREP: 5 MIN; COOK: 10 MIN

4 SERVINGS

If you don't have cream of potato soup on hand, substitute cream of mushroom or cream of celery soup.

1½   cups cubed fully cooked fat-free ham

1½   cups fat-free half-and-half or refrigerated fat-free nondairy creamer

1   can (10¾ ounces) condensed cream of potato soup

1   package (10 ounces) frozen whole kernel corn

1   jar (2 ounces) diced pimientos, drained

     Shredded reduced-fat Swiss cheese, if desired

Heat all ingredients except cheese to boiling in 2½-quart saucepan, stirring occasionally; reduce heat. Simmer uncovered 5 minutes, stirring occasionally. Sprinkle with cheese.

1 Serving: Calories 250 (Calories from Fat 55); Fat 6g (Saturated 2g); Cholesterol 30mg; Sodium 1170mg; Carbohydrate 37g (Dietary Fiber 3g); Protein 15g
% Daily Value: Vitamin A 6%; Vitamin C 14%; Calcium 4%; Iron 8%
Diet Exchanges: 2½ starch, 1½ very lean meat

Ham and Slaw Salad

LO CAL / HI FIB

PREP: 12 MIN

4 SERVINGS

When the weather's so hot you don't want to heat up the kitchen, stay cool with this refreshing slaw. Cut slices of crusty French bread, and pour tall glasses of lemonade or iced tea to go with it.

1   pint (2 cups) deli coleslaw (creamy style)

2   cans (8 ounces each) tropical fruit salad, chilled and drained

½   cup golden raisins

     Lettuce leaves, if desired

1½   cups cubed fully cooked fat-free ham

If coleslaw is very wet, drain off excess liquid. Mix coleslaw, fruit salad and raisins in large bowl.

Line 4 salad plates with lettuce. Spoon coleslaw mixture into center of each plate. Make indentation in center of each mound of coleslaw mixture; fill with ham.

1 Serving: Calories 275 (Calories from Fat 115); Fat 13g (Saturated 2g); Cholesterol 25mg; Sodium 750mg; Carbohydrate 34g (Dietary Fiber 3g); Protein 8g
% Daily Value: Vitamin A 18%; Vitamin C 12%; Calcium 4%; Iron 8%
Diet Exchanges: 1 starch, 1 very lean meat, 1 fruit, 2 fat

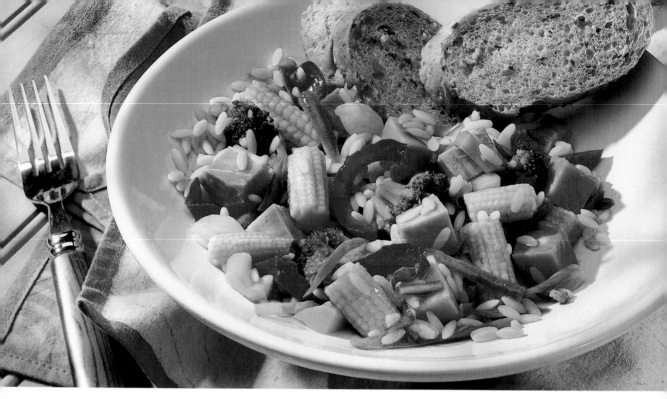

Sweet-and-Sour Pasta Salad

Sweet-and-Sour Pasta Salad

LO CAL / LO FAT / LO CHOL / HI FIB

PREP: 20 MIN

6 SERVINGS

Here's a refreshing salad for summer entertaining. Serve it with a crispy baguette and iced tea.

1   cup uncooked rosamarina (orzo) pasta (6 ounces)

1   bag (16 ounces) frozen stir-fry vegetables

1   can (14 ounces) baby corn nuggets, drained

1¹⁄₂   cups cubed fully cooked ham

³⁄₄   cup sweet-and-sour sauce

Cook pasta as directed on package—except omit salt and do not drain. Place frozen vegetables in colander. To drain pasta, pour hot water over frozen vegetables in colander. Let stand until vegetables are thawed.

Place vegetables and pasta in large bowl. Add corn, ham and sweet-and-sour sauce; toss.

1 Serving: Calories 250 (Calories from Fat 45); Fat 5g (Saturated 2g); Cholesterol 20mg; Sodium 730mg; Carbohydrate 41g (Dietary Fiber 3g); Protein 13g
% Daily Value: Vitamin A 2%; Vitamin C 28%; Calcium 2%; Iron 14%
Diet Exchanges: 1 starch, 1 lean meat, 2 vegetable, 1 fruit

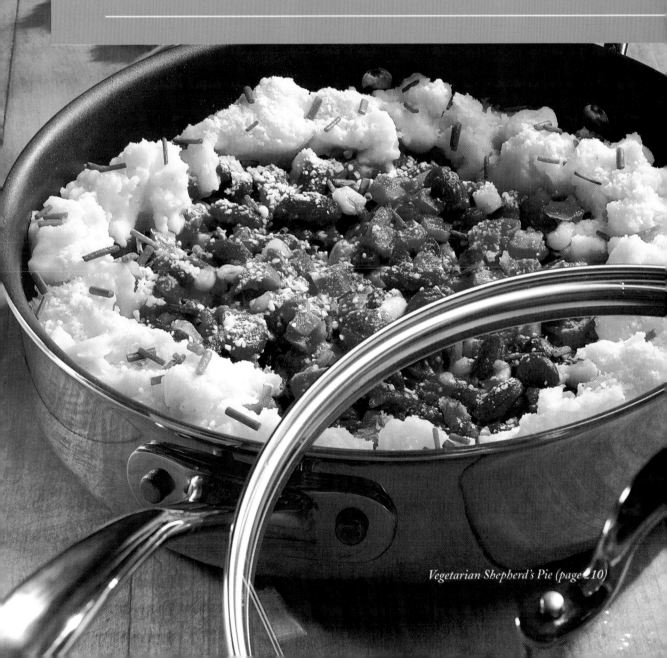

MEATLESS
MAIN DISHES

Vegetarian Shepherd's Pie (page 210)

Vegetarian Stir-Fry

LO CAL / LO CHOL / HI FIB

PREP: 20 MIN; COOK: 7 MIN

4 SERVINGS

Apple juice, soy sauce and garlic give this intriguing stir-fry wonderful gusto. Add extra color and flavor by using a combination of vegetables.

¾ cup apple juice

2 tablespoons cornstarch

3 tablespoons reduced-sodium soy sauce

2 tablespoons vegetable oil

6 cups cut-up vegetables (such as 1-inch pieces asparagus, sliced zucchini, cauliflowerets or broccoli flowerets)

1 medium onion, cut lengthwise in half, then cut crosswise into thin slices

1 clove garlic, finely chopped

3 tablespoons apple juice

1 can (15 to 16 ounces) garbanzo beans, rinsed and drained

Mix ¾ cup apple juice, the cornstarch and soy sauce; set aside.

Heat wok or 12-inch nonstick skillet over medium-high heat. Add oil; rotate wok to coat side. Add vegetables, onion and garlic; stir-fry 1 minute. Add 3 tablespoons apple juice. Cover and cook about 3 minutes or until vegetables are tender.

Stir in beans and soy sauce mixture; reduce heat to medium. Cook about 3 minutes, stirring frequently, until sauce is thickened.

1 Serving: Calories 300 (Calories from Fat 90); Fat 10g (Saturated 1g); Cholesterol 0mg; Sodium 570mg; Carbohydrate 50g (Dietary Fiber 12g); Protein 14g
% Daily Value: Vitamin A 10%; Vitamin C 56%; Calcium 10%; Iron 24%
Diet Exchanges: 2 starch, 4 vegetable, 2 fat

Vegetable Kung Pao

LO CAL / LO FAT / LO CHOL / HI FIB

PREP: 5 MIN; COOK: 10 MIN

4 SERVINGS

Peanuts are bursting with folic acid, which is particularly important for pregnant women because it helps to prevent birth defects of the brain and spinal cord. Other sources of folic acid are dark green and orange vegetables and fortified cereals.

½	cup dry-roasted peanuts
	Cooking spray
1	tablespoon cornstarch
1	teaspoon sugar
1	tablespoon cold water
½	cup chicken broth
1	teaspoon chili puree with garlic
1	bag (16 ounces) frozen whole carrots, green beans and yellow (wax) beans
	Hot cooked rice, if desired

Spray nonstick wok or 12-inch nonstick skillet with cooking spray; heat over medium-high heat. Spread peanuts in single layer on paper towel; lightly spray with cooking spray, about 2 seconds. Add peanuts to wok; stir-fry about 1 minute or until toasted. Immediately remove from wok; cool.

Mix cornstarch, sugar and cold water; set aside. Mix broth and chili puree in wok; heat to boiling. Stir in vegetables. Heat to boiling; reduce heat to medium-low. Cover and cook 5 minutes, stirring occasionally.

Move vegetables to side of wok. Stir cornstarch mixture into liquid in wok. Cook and stir vegetables and sauce over high heat about 1 minute or until sauce is thickened. Stir in peanuts. Serve with rice.

1 Serving: Calories 95 (Calories from Fat 35); Fat 4g (Saturated 2g); Cholesterol 0mg; Sodium 190mg; Carbohydrate 11g (Dietary Fiber 3g); Protein 7g
% Daily Value: Vitamin A 36%; Vitamin C 30%; Calcium 4%; Iron 4%
Diet Exchanges: 1 lean meat, 2 vegetable

Moroccan Spiced Vegetables and Couscous

LO FAT / LO CHOL / HI FIB

PREP: 15 MIN; COOK: 5 MIN; STAND: 5 MIN

4 SERVINGS

Sweet potatoes are heads and shoulders above ordinary potatoes. They offer loads of beta-carotene, a form of vitamin A that works as an antioxidant and protects our cells from damage.

1 tablespoon olive or vegetable oil

1 large onion, chopped (1 cup)

2 cloves garlic, finely chopped

1 can (14¹/₂ ounces) ready-to-serve chicken broth

1 can (23 ounces) sweet potatoes, cut into pieces

2 cups frozen cut leaf spinach (from 16-ounce bag), thawed and squeezed to drain

¹/₂ cup raisins

1 teaspoon ground cumin

¹/₂ teaspoon ground cinnamon

¹/₂ teaspoon salt

1 cup uncooked couscous

Heat oil in Dutch oven over medium-high heat. Cook onion and garlic in oil 2 to 3 minutes, stirring frequently, until onion is tender.

Stir in remaining ingredients except couscous; heat to boiling. Stir in couscous; reduce heat to low. Cover and simmer about 5 minutes or until all liquid is absorbed. Fluff with fork.

1 Serving: Calories 425 (Calories from Fat 45); Fat 5g (Saturated 1g); Cholesterol 0mg; Sodium 840mg; Carbohydrate 92g (Dietary Fiber 9g); Protein 12g
% Daily Value: Vitamin A 100%; Vitamin C 20%; Calcium 14%; Iron 20%
Diet Exchanges: 4¹/₂ starch, 1 fruit

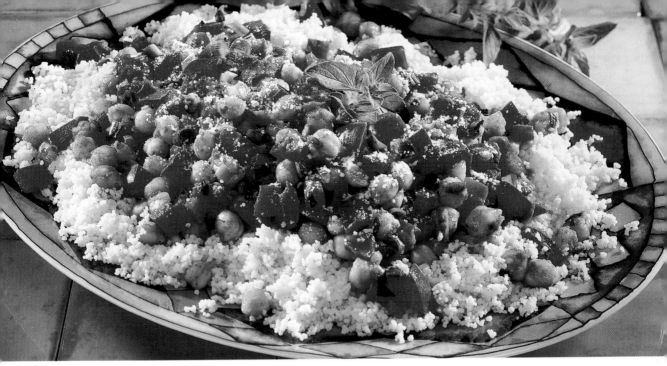

Vegetable Couscous

LO CAL / LO FAT / LO CHOL / HI FIB

PREP: 15 MIN; COOK: 5 MIN

6 SERVINGS

Although many kinds of flavored couscous are available, the plain variety will highlight the fresh flavors in this dish.

1 can (15 to 16 ounces) garbanzo beans, rinsed and drained

2 large tomatoes, chopped (2 cups)

1 small red bell pepper, chopped (¹/₂ cup)

4 medium green onions, chopped (¹/₄ cup)

1 clove garlic, finely chopped

1 tablespoon chopped fresh or 1 teaspoon dried oregano leaves

1 teaspoon paprika

1 teaspoon olive or vegetable oil

5 cups hot cooked couscous

¹/₄ cup grated Parmesan cheese

Heat all ingredients except couscous and cheese to boiling in 2-quart saucepan. Serve over couscous. Sprinkle with cheese.

1 Serving: Calories 280 (Calories from Fat 35); Fat 4g (Saturated 1g); Cholesterol 5mg; Sodium 500mg; Carbohydrate 56g (Dietary Fiber 8g); Protein 13g
% Daily Value: Vitamin A 14%; Vitamin C 30%; Calcium 10%; Iron 16%
Diet Exchanges: 3 starch, 2 vegetable

Polenta with Italian Vegetables

LO CAL / LO FAT / LO CHOL / HI FIB

PREP: 15 MIN; COOK: 15 MIN

6 SERVINGS

Whisking the cornmeal into the cold water first will help keep your polenta free of lumps.

1	cup yellow cornmeal
3/4	cup cold water
2 1/2	cups boiling water
1/2	teaspoon salt
2/3	cup shredded Swiss cheese
2	teaspoons olive or vegetable oil
2	medium zucchini or yellow summer squash sliced, (4 cups)
1	medium red bell pepper, chopped (1 cup)
1	small onion, chopped (1/4 cup)
1	clove garlic, finely chopped
1/4	cup chopped fresh or 1 tablespoon dried basil leaves
1	can (14 ounces) artichoke heart quarters, drained

Beat cornmeal and cold water in 2-quart saucepan with wire whisk. Stir in boiling water and salt. Cook over medium-high heat, stirring constantly, until mixture thickens and boils; reduce heat to low. Cover and simmer 10 minutes, stirring occasionally. Stir in cheese until smooth; keep polenta warm.

Heat oil in 10-inch nonstick skillet over medium-high heat. Cook zucchini, bell pepper, onion and garlic in oil about 5 minutes, stirring occasionally, until vegetables are crisp-tender. Stir in basil and artichoke hearts. Serve vegetable mixture over polenta.

1 Serving: Calories 170 (Calories from Fat 45); Fat 5g (Saturated 2g); Cholesterol 10mg; Sodium 370mg; Carbohydrate 28g (Dietary Fiber 5g); Protein 8g
% Daily Value: Vitamin A 18%; Vitamin C 40%; Calcium 16%; Iron 10%
Diet Exchanges: 1 starch, 1 lean meat, 2 vegetable

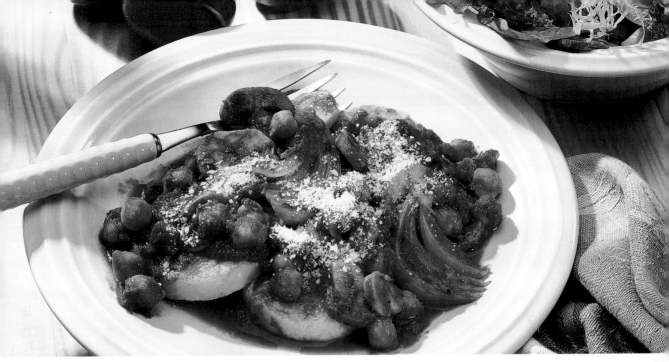

Garbanzo and Vegetable Sauce with Polenta

Garbanzo and Vegetable Sauce with Polenta

LO CAL / LO FAT / LO CHOL / HI FIB

PREP: 10 MIN; COOK: 15 MIN

4 SERVINGS

Tubes of refrigerated polenta can be found in the produce section of the supermarket, or make a batch of Polenta Sauté (page 137).

1   tube (16 to 24 ounces) refrigerated polenta

1   jar (26 to 28 ounces) fat-free chunky spaghetti sauce

1   can (15 to 16 ounces) garbanzo beans, rinsed and drained

1   medium yellow summer squash, thinly sliced (2 cups)

1   medium onion, cut into 8 wedges

1½   cups sliced mushrooms (4 ounces)

½   cup dry red wine or grape juice

2   tablespoons grated Parmesan cheese

Prepare polenta as directed on tube. Heat remaining ingredients except cheese to boiling in Dutch oven over medium heat, stirring occasionally; reduce heat to low. Cover and simmer 10 minutes.

Serve vegetable mixture over polenta slices. Sprinkle with cheese.

1 Serving: Calories 285 (Calories from Fat 25); Fat 3g (Saturated 1g); Cholesterol 2mg; Sodium 1180mg; Carbohydrate 63g (Dietary Fiber 11g); Protein 13g
% Daily Value: Vitamin A 12%; Vitamin C 14%; Calcium 10%; Iron 28%
Diet Exchanges: 4 starch

Hoppin' John with Corn Muffins

LO CAL / LO FAT / LO CHOL / HI FIB

PREP: 15 MIN; COOK: 15 MIN; STAND: 5 MIN

6 SERVINGS

The hint of sweetness from the corn muffins brings out the best in this tomato and black-eyed pea combo. If you prefer, buy corn muffins at your local bakery instead of making them from the mix.

1   pouch (6.5 ounces) golden corn bread and muffin mix

1/3   cup milk

2   tablespoons margarine, melted

1   egg

1   medium green bell pepper, coarsely chopped (1 cup)

1   medium onion, coarsely chopped (1/2 cup)

2   cloves garlic, finely chopped

1/2   cup uncooked instant rice

1   teaspoon red pepper sauce

2   medium tomatoes, chopped (1 1/2 cups)

1   can (15 to 16 ounces) black-eyed peas, undrained

Prepare and bake corn muffins as directed on package, using milk, margarine and egg; keep warm.

While muffins are baking, spray 2-quart saucepan with cooking spray; heat over medium heat. Cook bell pepper, onion and garlic in saucepan about 5 minutes, stirring frequently, until onion is tender.

Stir in remaining ingredients. Heat to boiling; reduce heat to medium. Cover and cook 5 minutes; remove from heat. Let stand covered 5 minutes.

Split each muffin in half, and place on dinner plate. Spoon black-eyed pea mixture over muffins.

1 Serving: Calories 215 (Calories from Fat 35); Fat 4g (Saturated 2g); Cholesterol 15mg; Sodium 420mg; Carbohydrate 43g (Dietary Fiber 7g); Protein 9g
% Daily Value: Vitamin A 4%; Vitamin C 22%; Calcium 8%; Iron 16%
Diet Exchanges: 2 starch, 3 vegetable

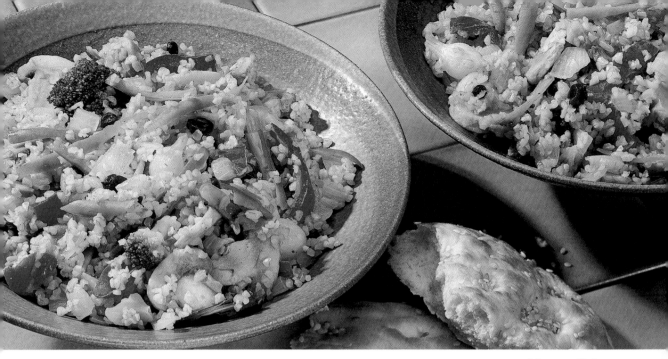

Moroccan Bulgur

Moroccan Bulgur

LO CAL / LO FAT / LO CHOL / HI FIB

PREP: 10 MIN; COOK: 15 MIN; STAND 20 MIN

4 SERVINGS

Bulgur is whole wheat that has been cooked, dried and broken into coarse fragments. It is a good source of potassium, a nutrient needed for water balance and proper nerve and muscle function.

3	cups sliced mushrooms (8 ounces)
2	large onions, chopped (2 cups)
2	cloves garlic, finely chopped
1	package (16 ounces) frozen broccoli, green beans, pearl onions and red bell peppers
1 1/2	cups uncooked bulgur
1/4	cup currants or raisins
2	teaspoons curry powder
1/2	teaspoon salt
2	cups water

Spray 10-inch nonstick skillet with cooking spray; heat over medium-high heat. Cook mushrooms, onions and garlic in skillet about 8 minutes, stirring occasionally, until onions are tender.

Stir in remaining ingredients except water. Cook 2 minutes, stirring occasionally. Stir in water. Heat to boiling; remove from heat. Cover and let stand 15 to 20 minutes or until water is absorbed.

1 Serving: Calories 240 (Calories from Fat 10); Fat 1g (Saturated 0g); Cholesterol 0mg; Sodium 330mg; Carbohydrate 61g (Dietary Fiber 14g); Protein 11g
% Daily Value: Vitamin A 24%; Vitamin C 26%; Calcium 8%; Iron 16%
Diet Exchanges: 2 starch, 3 vegetable, 1 fruit

Indian Lentils and Rice

LO CAL / LO FAT / LO CHOL / HI FIB

PREP: 15 MIN; COOK: 40 MIN

6 SERVINGS

Yogurt is a terrific addition to Indian foods, plus many brands of yogurt contain live and active cultures that can help keep your digestive system healthy. Check the container label for the "live and active cultures" seal.

4	medium green onions, chopped (¹/₄ cup)
1	tablespoon finely chopped gingerroot
¹/₈	teaspoon crushed red pepper
2	cloves garlic, finely chopped
1	can (49¹/₂ ounces) or 3 cans (14¹/₂ ounces each) ready-to-serve vegetable broth
1¹/₂	cups dried lentils (12 ounces), sorted and rinsed
1	teaspoon ground turmeric
¹/₂	teaspoon salt
1	large tomato, chopped (1 cup)
¹/₄	cup shredded coconut
2	tablespoons chopped fresh or 2 teaspoons dried mint leaves
3	cups hot cooked rice
1¹/₂	cups plain fat-free yogurt

Spray 3-quart saucepan with cooking spray. Cook onions, gingerroot, red pepper and garlic in saucepan over medium heat 3 to 5 minutes, stirring occasionally, until onions are tender.

Stir in 5 cups of the broth, the lentils, turmeric and salt. Heat to boiling; reduce heat. Cover and simmer 25 to 30 minutes, adding remaining broth if needed, until lentils are tender. Stir in tomato, coconut and mint. Serve over rice with yogurt.

1 Serving: Calories 290 (Calories from Fat 20); Fat 2g (Saturated 1g); Cholesterol 0mg; Sodium 1120mg; Carbohydrate 61g (Dietary Fiber 11g); Protein 18g
% Daily Value: Vitamin A 16%; Vitamin C 10%; Calcium 16%; Iron 32%
Diet Exchanges: 3¹/₂ starch

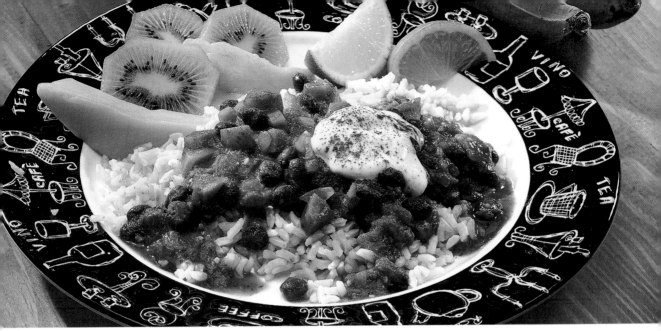

Cuban Black Beans and Rice

Cuban Black Beans and Rice

LO CAL / LO FAT / LO CHOL / HI FIB

PREP: 15 MIN; COOK: 55 MIN

6 SERVINGS

1   large onion, chopped (1 cup)

1   medium green bell pepper, chopped (1 cup)

2   medium carrots, chopped (³/₄ cup)

1   cup orange juice

2   teaspoons paprika

1   teaspoon ground coriander

¹/₈   teaspoon crushed red pepper

1   can (14¹/₂ ounces) whole tomatoes, undrained

2   cloves garlic, finely chopped

1   can (15 ounces) black beans, rinsed and drained

4   cups hot cooked brown rice

1   cup plain fat-free yogurt

Paprika, if desired

1   lime, cut into wedges

Heat onion, bell pepper, carrots, orange juice, paprika, coriander, red pepper, tomatoes and garlic to boiling in 2-quart saucepan; reduce heat. Cover and simmer about 45 minutes, stirring occasionally, until thickened; remove from heat. Stir in beans.

Place 1 cup of the bean mixture in blender or food processor. Cover and blend on medium speed about 30 seconds or until smooth. Stir blended mixture into bean mixture in saucepan. Cook over medium heat about 3 minutes or until hot. Serve over rice with yogurt. Sprinkle with paprika. Serve with lime wedges.

1 Serving: Calories 280 (Calories from Fat 20); Fat 2g (Saturated 1g); Cholesterol 0mg; Sodium 150mg; Carbohydrate 61g (Dietary Fiber 8g); Protein 12g
% Daily Value: Vitamin A 34%; Vitamin C 38%; Calcium 16%; Iron 16%
Diet Exchanges: 3¹/₂ starch

Herbed Red Beans and Rice Skillet Dinner

LO CHOL / HI FIB

PREP: 10 MIN; COOK: 15 MIN

4 SERVINGS

There's no need to take the time to chop vegetables for this great-tasting one-dish meal. The frozen vegetables are ready to cook, and the fresh mushrooms are sautéed whole.

1	teaspoon margarine
1	package (8 ounces) whole mushrooms
1	cup chicken broth
2	teaspoons dried basil leaves
1	jar (23 ounces) ready-to-heat cream of mushroom soup
1	bag (16 ounces) frozen corn, broccoli and red peppers, thawed
1	can (15 to 16 ounces) red beans or red kidney beans, rinsed and drained
1 1/2	cups uncooked instant brown rice

Melt margarine in 12-inch nonstick skillet over medium heat. Cook mushrooms in margarine 3 minutes, stirring occasionally.

Stir in remaining ingredients except rice. Heat to boiling, stirring occasionally. Stir in rice; reduce heat to low. Cover about 10 minutes or until rice is tender.

1 Serving: Calories 390 (Calories from Fat 80); Fat 9g (Saturated 2g); Cholesterol 5mg; Sodium 870mg; Carbohydrate 73g (Dietary Fiber 8g); Protein 12g
% Daily Value: Vitamin A 30%; Vitamin C 72%; Calcium 10%; Iron 16%
Diet Exchanges: 4 starch, 2 1/2 vegetable, 1/2 fat

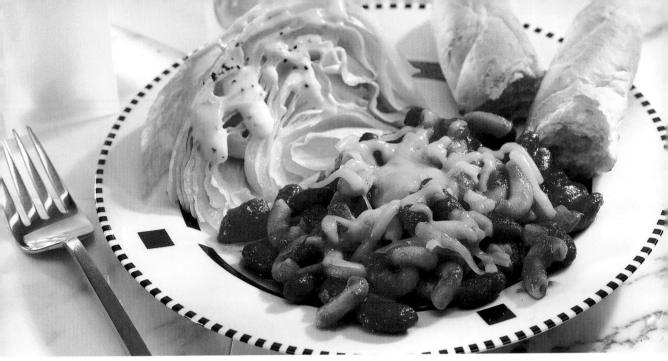

Macaroni-Bean Skillet

Macaroni-Bean Skillet

LO CAL / LO FAT / LO CHOL / HI FIB

PREP: 10 MIN; COOK: 18 MIN

4 SERVINGS

Round out this hearty kidney bean and macaroni medley with crusty breadsticks and lettuce wedges drizzled with your favorite fat-free dressing.

- 1   cup salsa
- $^2/_3$ cup uncooked elbow macaroni (2 ounces)
- $^3/_4$ cup water
- 2   teaspoons chili powder
- 1   can (15 or 16 ounces) kidney beans, rinsed and drained
- 1   can (8 ounces) reduced-sodium tomato sauce
- $^1/_2$ cup shredded reduced-fat Cheddar cheese (2 ounces)

Heat all ingredients except cheese to boiling in 10-inch nonstick skillet; reduce heat to low. Cover and simmer about 15 minutes, stirring frequently, until macaroni is just tender. Sprinkle with cheese.

1 Serving: Calories 270 (Calories from Fat 20); Fat 2g (Saturated 1g); Cholesterol 3mg; Sodium 540mg; Carbohydrate 49g (Dietary Fiber 10g); Protein 17g
% Daily Value: Vitamin A 14%; Vitamin C 18%; Calcium 14%; Iron 12%
Diet Exchanges: 3 starch, 1 very lean meat

Crunchy Bean Skillet

LO CHOL / HI FIB

PREP: 15 MIN; COOK: 10 MIN

6 SERVINGS

Toasting the walnuts before sprinkling them on top will heighten their flavor and give this dish added crunch. See directions for toasting on page 242.

- 3 cans (15 to 16 ounces each) cannellini beans, rinsed and drained
- 1 jar (14 ounces) spaghetti sauce
- 2 medium stalks celery, sliced (1 cup)
- 4 medium green onions, sliced ($^1/_4$ cup)
- 1 teaspoon parsley flakes
- 1 teaspoon dried basil leaves
- $^1/_2$ teaspoon dried oregano leaves
- 1 cup shredded reduced-fat mozzarella cheese (4 ounces)
- $^1/_2$ cup coarsely chopped walnuts

Mix all ingredients except cheese and walnuts in 10-inch nonstick skillet. Heat to boiling; reduce heat. Sprinkle with cheese. Cover and simmer 3 to 5 minutes or just until cheese is melted. Sprinkle with walnuts.

1 Serving: Calories 395 (Calories from Fat 145); Fat 16g (Saturated 4g); Cholesterol 10mg; Sodium 650mg; Carbohydrate 56g (Dietary Fiber 13g); Protein 20g
% Daily Value: Vitamin A 8%; Vitamin C 12%; Calcium 24%; Iron 28%
Diet Exchanges: 3 starch, 1 lean meat, 2 vegetable, 1 fat

Hearty Bean and Macaroni Stew

LO CAL / LO FAT / LO CHOL / HI FIB

PREP: 10 MIN; COOK: 20 MIN

4 SERVINGS

Even if you're tempted, don't let this stew simmer all day. Pasta can turn mushy if left in liquid for too long.

- 1 cup uncooked medium macaroni shells ($3^1/_2$ ounces)
- $^1/_4$ cup chopped green bell pepper
- 1 tablespoon chopped fresh or 1 teaspoon dried basil leaves
- 1 teaspoon Worcestershire sauce
- 1 clove garlic, finely chopped
- 1 large tomato, coarsely chopped (1 cup)
- 1 small onion, chopped ($^1/_4$ cup)
- 1 can (15 to 16 ounces) kidney beans, drained
- $^1/_2$ can (15- to 16-ounce size) garbanzo beans, drained
- 1 can ($14^1/_2$ ounces) ready-to-serve vegetable broth

Mix all ingredients in 2-quart saucepan. Heat to boiling, stirring occasionally; reduce heat. Cover and simmer about 15 minutes, stirring occasionally, until macaroni is tender.

1 Serving: Calories 265 (Calories from Fat 20); Fat 2g (Saturated 0g); Cholesterol 0mg; Sodium 730mg; Carbohydrate 57g (Dietary Fiber 11g); Protein 16g
% Daily Value: Vitamin A 10%; Vitamin C 16%; Calcium 6%; Iron 28%
Diet Exchanges: 3 starch, 1 vegetable

Three-Squash Stew

LO CAL / LO FAT / LO CHOL / HI FIB

PREP: 20 MIN; COOK: 17 MIN

6 SERVINGS

Pattypan squash are small and slightly rounded, with a scalloped edge. If you can't find them in your supermarket, just increase the amount of sliced zucchini and yellow squash.

1   tablespoon olive or vegetable oil

1   large onion, sliced (1 cup)

1   clove garlic, crushed

1   jalapeño chili, finely chopped

2   medium yellow summer squash, sliced (4 cups)

2   medium zucchini, sliced (4 cups)

4   cups 1-inch pieces pattypan squash

3   cups 1-inch pieces green beans

1   cup fresh or frozen whole kernel corn

1   tablespoon chopped fresh or 1 teaspoon dried thyme leaves

2   cans (15 to 16 ounces each) kidney beans, undrained

Heat oil in Dutch oven over medium-high heat. Cook onion, garlic and chili in oil about 2 minutes, stirring occasionally until tender.

Stir in remaining ingredients. Cook over low heat 10 to 15 minutes, stirring frequently, until squash is tender.

1 Serving: Calories 250 (Calories from Fat 35); Fat 4g (Saturated 1g); Cholesterol 0mg; Sodium 360mg; Carbohydrate 51g (Dietary Fiber 15g); Protein 17g
% Daily Value: Vitamin A 18%; Vitamin C 34%; Calcium 10%; Iron 32%
Diet Exchanges: 3 starch, 1 vegetable

Bean-Pasta Stew

LO CAL / LO FAT / LO CHOL / HI FIB

PREP: 10 MIN; COOK: 25 MIN

4 SERVINGS

Anything goes when it comes to choosing the beans in this stew. You can use the pinto or navy beans suggested, or try lima, cannellini, garbanzo, butter or kidney beans. If you like, use a can each of two different kinds.

2   cans (15 to 16 ounces each) pinto or navy beans, rinsed and drained

1   can (14$\frac{1}{2}$ ounces) Italian-style stewed tomatoes, undrained

1   can (14$\frac{1}{2}$ ounces) ready-to-serve chicken broth

1   package (10 ounces) frozen cut green beans, thawed

2   medium stalks celery, sliced (1 cup)

1$\frac{1}{2}$ teaspoons Italian seasoning

$\frac{1}{2}$ cup uncooked small pasta shells or elbow macaroni (2 ounces)

Grated Parmesan cheese, if desired

Heat all ingredients except pasta and cheese to boiling in 3-quart saucepan; reduce heat to low. Stir in pasta. Cover and simmer about 15 minutes, stirring occasionally, until pasta is tender. Serve with cheese.

1 Serving: Calories 350 (Calories from Fat 20); Fat 2g (Saturated 1g); Cholesterol 0mg; Sodium 1130mg; Carbohydrate 81g (Dietary Fiber 22g); Protein 24g
% Daily Value: Vitamin A 6%; Vitamin C 18%; Calcium 18%; Iron 42%
Diet Exchanges: 4 starch, 4 vegetable

African Vegetable Stew

LO CAL / LO FAT / LO CHOL / HI FIB

PREP: 15 MIN; COOK: 1 HR

6 SERVINGS

This is a great do-ahead dish. Make the stew the day before, and refrigerate overnight. Not only does this save time later, it will also give the flavors in the stew a chance to blend and intensify.

2	tablespoons margarine
1	large onion, chopped (1 cup)
1/2	cup chopped fresh parsley
2	cloves garlic, finely chopped
1	teaspoon ground cinnamon
1/2	teaspoon ground turmeric
1/2	teaspoon pepper
1/4	teaspoon ground ginger
5	cups water
2	medium carrots, sliced (1 cup)
1/2	cup dried lentils (4 ounces), sorted and rinsed
1	cup uncooked regular long grain rice
1	can (15 ounces) whole tomatoes, undrained
3/4	teaspoon salt
1	package (10 ounces) frozen green peas
1	package (9 ounces) frozen sliced green beans
3	sprigs mint, chopped
3/4	cup plain fat-free yogurt

Melt margarine in Dutch oven over medium heat. Cook onion, parsley, garlic, cinnamon, turmeric, pepper and ginger in margarine, stirring occasionally, until onion is tender. Stir in water, carrots and lentils. Heat to boiling; reduce heat. Cover and simmer 25 minutes.

Stir in rice, tomatoes and salt, breaking up tomatoes. Heat to boiling; reduce heat. Cover and simmer 20 minutes.

Stir in peas, green beans and mint. Heat to boiling; reduce heat. Cover and simmer about 5 minutes or until peas and beans are tender. Serve with yogurt.

1 Serving: Calories 275 (Calories from Fat 45); Fat 5g (Saturated 1g); Cholesterol 0mg; Sodium 540mg; Carbohydrate 56g (Dietary Fiber 10g); Protein 12g
% Daily Value: Vitamin A 70%; Vitamin C 20%; Calcium 16%; Iron 28%
Diet Exchanges: 3 starch, 1 vegetable, 1 fat

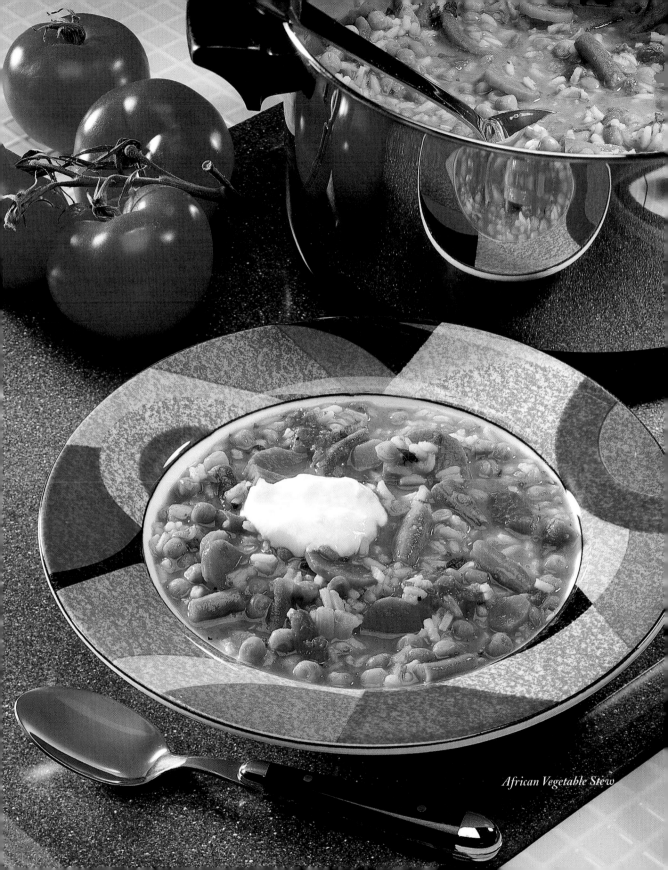

African Vegetable Stew

Mixed-Bean Stew with Cottage Dumplings

LO CAL / LO FAT / LO CHOL / HI FIB

PREP: 15 MIN; COOK: 25 MIN

6 SERVINGS

If you're watching your salt intake, look for low-sodium tomato sauce on your supermarket shelves.

Cottage Dumplings (right)

1   can (15 to 16 ounces) great northern, cannellini or navy beans, rinsed and drained

1   can (15 ounces) black beans, rinsed and drained

1   can (15 ounces) tomato sauce

1   medium red bell pepper, chopped (1 cup)

2   cloves garlic, finely chopped

2   tablespoons chopped fresh or 2 teaspoons dried basil leaves

2   teaspoons olive or vegetable oil

1/4   teaspoon pepper

Prepare Cottage Dumplings. Heat remaining ingredients to boiling in 3-quart saucepan; reduce heat. Shape dumpling mixture into 12 balls, using about 2 tablespoons each. Carefully slide balls onto beans in simmering stew (do not drop directly into liquid). Cook uncovered 10 minutes. Cover and cook about 10 minutes longer or until dumplings are firm.

Cottage Dumplings

1   cup shredded reduced-fat Monterey Jack cheese (4 ounces)

2/3   cup frozen (thawed) or canned (drained) whole kernel corn

1/2   cup fat-free small-curd cottage cheese

1/3   cup soft whole-grain or white bread crumbs

1/3   cup yellow cornmeal

1/4   cup fat-free cholesterol-free egg product or 2 egg whites

Mix all ingredients.

1 Serving: Calories 350 (Calories from Fat 55); Fat 6g (Saturated 3g); Cholesterol 10mg; Sodium 720mg; Carbohydrate 60g (Dietary Fiber 10g); Protein 24g
% Daily Value: Vitamin A 24%; Vitamin C 40%; Calcium 30%; Iron 30%
Diet Exchanges: 4 starch, 1 very lean meat

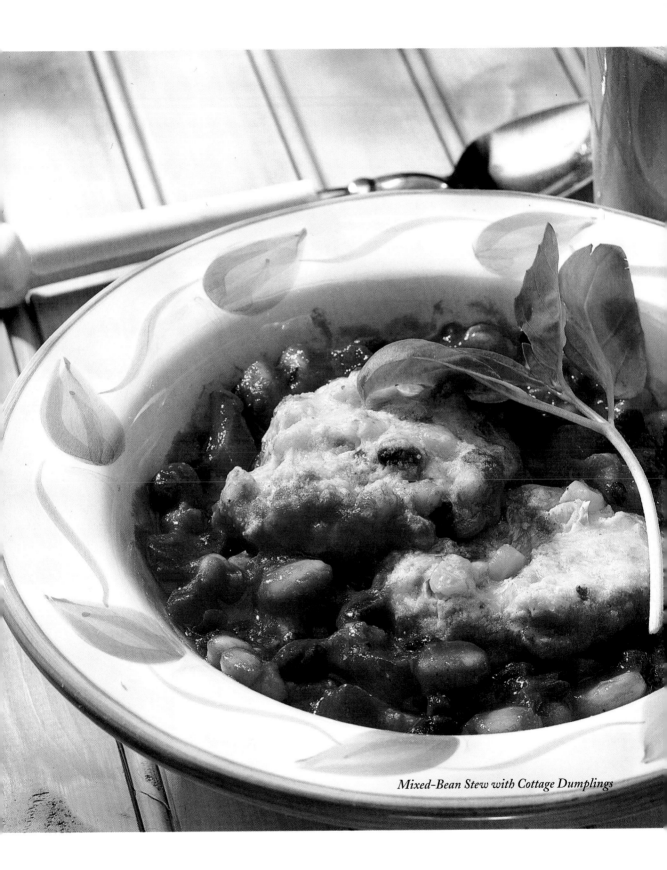

Mixed-Bean Stew with Cottage Dumplings

Hearty Vegetable Stew

LO CAL / LO FAT / LO CHOL / HI FIB

PREP: 10 MIN; COOK: 13 MIN

6 SERVINGS

Crisp, tart citrus flavors complement this one-dish meal. Add a squirt of lemon or lime juice to the stew just before serving, or pass around a bowl of fresh lemon wedges and let your guests help themselves.

1   medium onion, cut lengthwise in half, then cut crosswise into thin slices

1   bag (16 ounces) coleslaw mix or broccoli slaw (6 cups)

2   cans (15 to 16 ounces each) cannellini, navy or great northern beans, rinsed and drained

2   cans (14½ ounces each) Italian-style stewed tomatoes, undrained

1   medium zucchini or yellow summer squash, thinly sliced (2 cups)

2   teaspoons Italian seasoning

¾   teaspoon garlic salt

Spray Dutch oven with cooking spray; heat over medium heat. Cook onion in Dutch oven about 5 minutes, stirring occasionally, until tender.

Stir in remaining ingredients. Heat to boiling; reduce heat to low. Cover and simmer about 5 minutes, stirring occasionally, until vegetables are tender.

1 Serving: Calories 240 (Calories from Fat 10); Fat 1g (Saturated 0g); Cholesterol 0mg; Sodium 540mg; Carbohydrate 53g (Dietary Fiber 13g); Protein 17g
% Daily Value: Vitamin A 8%; Vitamin C 40%; Calcium 22%; Iron 38%
Diet Exchanges: 2 starch, 4 vegetable

Lentil Stew

LO CAL / LO FAT / LO CHOL / HI FIB

PREP: 15 MIN; COOK: 50 MIN

6 SERVINGS

Lentils are a super source of soluble fiber, a type of fiber that when included as part of a low-fat diet may help to lower blood cholesterol.

    2   teaspoons vegetable oil
    1   large onion, chopped (1 cup)
    1   clove garlic, finely chopped
    1   cup dried lentils (8 ounces), sorted and rinsed
  1/4   cup chopped fresh parsley
    3   cups water
  1/2   teaspoon ground cumin
  1/2   teaspoon salt
  1/4   teaspoon pepper
  1/4   teaspoon ground mace
    2   medium baking potatoes, coarsely chopped
    1   package (8 ounces) small white mushrooms, cut in half
    1   can (28 ounces) whole tomatoes, undrained

Heat oil in Dutch oven over medium-high heat. Cook onion and garlic in oil, stirring frequently, until onion is tender.

Stir in remaining ingredients, breaking up tomatoes. Heat to boiling; reduce heat. Cover and simmer about 40 minutes, stirring occasionally, until potatoes are tender.

1 Serving: Calories 160 (Calories from Fat 20); Fat 2g (Saturated 0g); Cholesterol 0mg; Sodium 400mg; Carbohydrate 35g (Dietary Fiber 10g); Protein 11g
% Daily Value: Vitamin A 8%; Vitamin C 24%; Calcium 6%; Iron 24%
Diet Exchanges: 2 starch

Savory Black-Eyed Peas

LO CAL / LO FAT / LO CHOL / HI FIB

PREP: 15 MIN; COOK: 15 MIN

4 SERVINGS

The mild, peppery flavor of fresh savory is a cross between mint and thyme.

    1   cup chicken broth
    3   medium carrots, thinly sliced (1 1/2 cups)
    2   medium stalks celery, sliced (1 cup)
    1   large onion, chopped (1 cup)
1 1/2   tablespoons chopped fresh or
        1 1/2 teaspoons dried savory or basil leaves
    1   clove garlic, finely chopped
    1   can (15 to 16 ounces) black-eyed peas, rinsed and drained
  1/2   cup shredded reduced-fat Monterey Jack cheese (2 ounces)

Heat broth, carrots, celery, onion, savory and garlic to boiling in 10-inch nonstick skillet; reduce heat to medium. Cook 8 to 10 minutes, stirring occasionally, until vegetables are tender. Stir in peas. Cook, stirring occasionally, until hot. Sprinkle with cheese.

1 Serving: Calories 160 (Calories from Fat 25); Fat 3g (Saturated 2g); Cholesterol 10mg; Sodium 440mg; Carbohydrate 29g (Dietary Fiber 8g); Protein 12g
% Daily Value: Vitamin A 86%; Vitamin C 8%; Calcium 16%; Iron 16%
Diet Exchanges: 2 starch

Vegetable Tortillas

LO CAL / LO FAT / LO CHOL

PREP: 10 MIN; COOK: 20 MIN

6 SERVINGS

Chayote, a fruit that resembles a large pear in size and shape, is an interesting change of pace from the usual zucchini and yellow squash. Chayote are most widely available during the winter months, but you may be able to find them in some supermarkets all year long.

- 1 small red bell pepper, chopped ($^1/_2$ cup)
- 1 small yellow bell pepper, chopped ($^1/_2$ cup)
- $^1/_2$ cup chopped chayote or zucchini
- 6 fat-free flour tortillas (6 to 8 inches in diameter)
- $1^1/_2$ cups shredded reduced-fat Monterey Jack cheese (6 ounces)

  Cooking spray

Mix bell peppers and chayote. Spoon $^1/_4$ cup of the vegetable mixture onto center of each tortilla. Top each with $^1/_4$ cup of the cheese. Roll tortilla tightly around vegetable mixture.

Spray 10-inch nonstick skillet with cooking spray; heat over medium heat. Cook 2 filled tortillas, seam sides down, in skillet about 3 minutes or until bottoms are light brown. Spray tops of tortillas lightly with cooking spray; turn tortillas. Cook about 3 minutes longer or until bottoms are light brown. Repeat with remaining tortillas.

1 Serving: Calories 190 (Calories from Fat 45); Fat 5g (Saturated 3g); Cholesterol 15mg; Sodium 490mg; Carbohydrate 26g (Dietary Fiber 1g); Protein 11g
% Daily Value: Vitamin A 8%; Vitamin C 26%; Calcium 20%; Iron 0%
Diet Exchanges: 1 starch, 1 vegetable, $^1/_2$ skim milk, 1 fat

Portabella Mushroom Fajitas

LO CAL / LO FAT / LO CHOL

PREP: 15 MIN; COOK: 10 MIN

6 SERVINGS

Portabella mushrooms, with their hearty texture and flavor, replace the meat in this signature Mexican dish.

- 1 tablespoon vegetable oil
- 1 clove garlic, finely chopped
- 1 teaspoon ground cumin
- $^1/_2$ teaspoon salt
- $^3/_4$ pound fresh portabella mushrooms, thinly sliced (6 cups)
- 2 cups frozen stir-fry bell peppers and onions (from 16-ounce bag)
- $^1/_4$ cup chopped fresh cilantro
- 2 tablespoons lime juice
- 6 fat-free flour tortillas (6 to 8 inches in diameter)

  Reduced-fat sour cream, if desired

  Salsa, if desired

Heat oil, garlic, cumin and salt in 10-inch nonstick skillet over medium-high heat. Cook mushrooms and bell pepper mixture in oil 5 to 7 minutes, stirring frequently, until vegetables are crisp-tender. Sprinkle with cilantro and lime juice.

Spoon about $^1/_2$ cup mushroom mixture onto each tortilla; roll up. Serve with sour cream and salsa.

1 Serving: Calories 160 (Calories from Fat 25); Fat 3g (Saturated 1g); Cholesterol 0mg; Sodium 540mg; Carbohydrate 30g (Dietary Fiber 2g); Protein 5g
% Daily Value: Vitamin A 2%; Vitamin C 22%; Calcium 0%; Iron 12%
Diet Exchanges: 2 starch

Bean and Cheese Burritos

LO CAL / LO FAT / LO CHOL / HI FIB

PREP: 10 MIN; COOK: 10 MIN

4 SERVINGS

Sprinkle chopped fresh cilantro or parsley over these burritos for a splash of color and a fresh taste. For a bold flavor, use sharp reduced-fat Cheddar cheese instead of mild. For a more subtle flavor, substitute reduced-fat mozzarella cheese for the Cheddar.

8	fat-free flour tortillas (6 to 8 inches in diameter)
1/3	cup finely chopped onion
1/3	cup finely chopped green bell pepper
1	can (16 ounces) fat-free refried beans
1 1/4	cups taco sauce
1	cup shredded reduced-fat Cheddar cheese (4 ounces)
	Choice of toppings, if desired (shredded lettuce, chopped tomatoes, chopped ripe olives, plain low-fat or fat-free yogurt and/or reduced-fat sour cream)

Heat tortillas as directed on package. While tortillas are heating, spray 10-inch nonstick skillet with cooking spray; heat over medium heat. Cook onion and bell pepper in skillet about 5 minutes, stirring frequently, until vegetables are tender. Stir in refried beans and 1/4 cup of the taco sauce; heat through.

Heat remaining 1 cup taco sauce in 1-quart saucepan over medium heat about 2 minutes, stirring occasionally, until heated through. Remove from heat; cover to keep warm.

Place about 1/3 cup of bean mixture on center of each tortilla. Fold one end of tortilla up about 1 inch over filling; fold right and left sides over folded end, overlapping. Fold remaining end down.

Spoon warm taco sauce over burritos. Sprinkle with cheese. Serve with choice of toppings.

1 Serving: Calories 255 (Calories from Fat 25); Fat 3g (Saturated 1g); Cholesterol 5mg; Sodium 1160mg; Carbohydrate 49g (Dietary Fiber 9g); Protein 17g
% Daily Value: Vitamin A 8%; Vitamin C 24%; Calcium 20%; Iron 14%
Diet Exchanges: 2 starch, 1/2 very lean meat, 4 vegetable

Black Bean Tacos

LO CHOL / HI FIB

PREP: 15 MIN; COOK: 15 MIN

4 SERVINGS

In a pinch, make these tacos with canned pinto or red beans instead of the black beans.

- 2 cans (15 ounces each) black beans, rinsed and drained
- 1 medium onion, chopped (1/2 cup)
- 1 small green bell pepper, chopped (1/2 cup)
- 2 cloves garlic, finely chopped
- 1 jar (8 ounces) taco sauce or salsa (1 cup)
- 8 taco shells
- 1/2 cup shredded lettuce
- 1 small tomato, chopped (1/2 cup)
- 1/2 cup reduced-fat sour cream

Mash beans from 1 can of beans; set aside.

Spray 10-inch nonstick skillet with cooking spray; heat over medium heat. Cook onion, bell pepper and garlic in skillet about 5 minutes, stirring frequently, until vegetables are tender.

Stir in mashed beans, remaining beans and the taco sauce. Heat to boiling; reduce heat. Simmer uncovered 5 minutes.

Spoon about 1/4 cup bean mixture into each taco shell. Top with lettuce, tomato and sour cream.

1 Serving: Calories 455 (Calories from Fat 90); Fat 10g (Saturated 3g); Cholesterol 10mg; Sodium 1100mg; Carbohydrate 85g (Dietary Fiber 18g); Protein 24g
% Daily Value: Vitamin A 12%; Vitamin C 30%; Calcium 26%; Iron 36%
Diet Exchanges: 4 starch, 1 lean meat, 5 vegetable

Sautéed Bean Cakes with Tomato Salsa

LO FAT / LO CHOL / HI FIB

PREP: 5 MIN; CHILL: 1 HR; COOK: 5 MIN

6 SERVINGS

Have you noticed the Diet Exchanges information included here—and in all other recipes in the book? Developed for use by people with diabetes, the Diet Exchanges also are used in a number of weight-loss plans. See page 445 for more information on how to use these exchanges.

Tomato Salsa (right)

4 cups soft whole wheat or white bread crumbs (about 6 slices bread)

1/2 cup chopped fresh parsley

1/2 cup plain fat-free yogurt

1 tablespoon Dijon mustard

1 tablespoon lemon juice

2 medium green onions, finely chopped (2 tablespoons)

1/4 cup fat-free cholesterol-free egg product or 2 egg whites

2 cans (15 to 16 ounces each) great northern beans, rinsed, drained and mashed

2 teaspoons margarine

Prepare Tomato Salsa. Mix 3 1/2 cups of the bread crumbs, the parsley, yogurt, mustard, lemon juice, onions, egg product and beans. Shape mixture into 12 patties. Coat patties with remaining 1/2 cup bread crumbs.

Melt margarine in 10-inch nonstick skillet over medium heat. Cook patties in margarine 5 to 6 minutes, turning after 3 minutes, until golden brown. Serve with salsa.

Tomato Salsa

2 large tomatoes, chopped (2 cups)

2 tablespoons chopped fresh cilantro

2 tablespoons red wine vinegar

1/4 teaspoon salt

Mix all ingredients. Cover and refrigerate 1 hour to blend flavors.

1 Serving: Calories 445 (Calories from Fat 25); Fat 5g (Saturated 1g); Cholesterol 5mg; Sodium 900mg; Carbohydrate 79g (Dietary Fiber 9g); Protein 21g
% Daily Value: Vitamin A 8%; Vitamin C 18%; Calcium 22%; Iron 40%
Diet Exchanges: 2 starch, 3 vegetable

Cajun Bean Patties

LO CAL / LO FAT / LO CHOL / HI FIB

PREP: 10 MIN; COOK: 10 MIN

4 SERVINGS

Although Cajun seasoning may vary slightly depending on the source, it is generally a blend of garlic, onion, chilies, black pepper, mustard and celery.

Tomato-Herb Sauce (right)

2   cans (15 to 16 ounces each) dark red kidney beans, drained and rinsed

¼   cup fat-free cholesterol-free egg product or 2 egg whites

¼   cup plain dry bread crumbs

2   teaspoons Cajun or Creole seasoning

1   tablespoon vegetable oil

Reduced-fat sour cream, if desired

Prepare Tomato-Herb Sauce. Mash beans, egg product, bread crumbs and Cajun seasoning in large bowl, using potato masher or fork, until most of the beans are crushed. Shape mixture into four ½-inch-thick patties, using moist hands.

Heat oil in 10-inch nonstick skillet over medium-high heat. Cook patties in oil 3 to 4 minutes on each side or until patties are heated through and slightly crusty. Top patties with sauce. Serve with a dollop of sour cream.

Tomato-Herb Sauce

1   can (14½ ounces) stewed tomatoes

1   tablespoon cornstarch

2   tablespoons cold water

½   teaspoon dried basil leaves

¼   teaspoon dried thyme leaves

Drain tomatoes, reserving liquid. Cut up tomatoes. Mix cornstarch and cold water in 1-quart saucepan. Stir in tomatoes, tomato liquid, basil and thyme. Cook over medium heat 3 to 4 minutes, stirring occasionally, until bubbly and slightly thickened.

1 Serving: Calories 205 (Calories from Fat 55); Fat 4g (Saturated 1g); Cholesterol 0mg; Sodium 670mg; Carbohydrate 38g (Dietary Fiber 7g); Protein 11g
% Daily Value: Vitamin A 6%; Vitamin C 10%; Calcium 8%; Iron 22%
Diet Exchanges: 2 starch, 1 vegetable, 1 fat

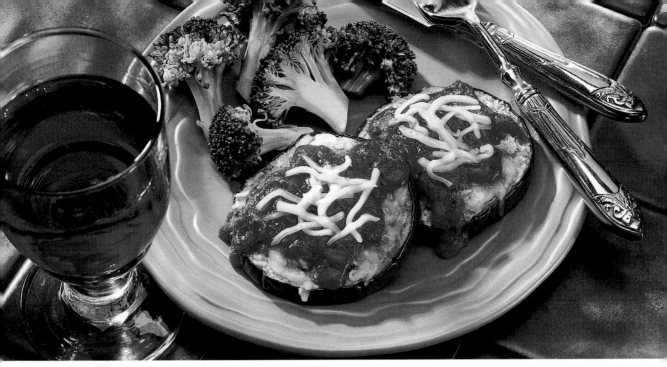

Eggplant Parmesan

Eggplant Parmesan

LO CAL / LO CHOL / HI FIB

PREP: 15 MIN; BROIL: 11 MIN

6 SERVINGS

1	medium eggplant (1½ pounds), peeled and cut into ¼-inch slices
	Cooking spray
⅓	cup finely shredded Parmesan cheese
¼	cup seasoned dry bread crumbs
2	teaspoons olive or vegetable oil
1	cup spaghetti sauce
1½	cups shredded reduced-fat mozzarella cheese (6 ounces)

Set oven control to broil. Generously spray both sides of each eggplant slice with cooking spray. Place on rack in broiler pan. Broil with tops 4 to 5 inches from heat about 10 minutes, turning once, until tender.

While eggplant is broiling, mix Parmesan cheese and bread crumbs; toss with oil.

Heat spaghetti sauce in 1-quart saucepan over medium heat about 2 minutes, stirring occasionally, until heated through. Remove from heat; cover to keep warm.

Sprinkle 1 cup of the mozzarella cheese over eggplant slices. Spoon bread crumb mixture over cheese. Broil about 1 minute or until cheese is melted and crumbs are brown. Top eggplant with spaghetti sauce and remaining ½ cup mozzarella cheese.

1 Serving: Calories 195 (Calories from Fat 90); Fat 10g (Saturated 4g); Cholesterol 20mg; Sodium 480mg; Carbohydrate 18g (Dietary Fiber 3g); Protein 11g
% Daily Value: Vitamin A 8%; Vitamin C 6%; Calcium 28%; Iron 6%
Diet Exchanges: ½ medium-fat meat, 3½ vegetable, 1½ fat

Vegetarian Shepherd's Pie

LO CAL / LO FAT / LO CHOL / HI FIB

PREP: 10 MIN; COOK: 23 MIN

6 SERVINGS

For the mashed potatoes, either use leftovers, prepare instant mashed potatoes or pick up mashed potatoes from the deli. Looking for an easy way to put the potatoes on top of this dish? A small ice-cream scoop is great for spooning on the warm mashed potatoes (photo, page 183).

2 cans (15 or 16 ounces each) kidney beans, rinsed and drained

1 jar (16 ounces) thick-and-chunky salsa (2 cups)

1 cup frozen whole kernel corn

1 medium carrot, chopped (1/2 cup)

1 1/2 cups warm mashed potatoes

2 tablespoons grated Parmesan cheese

Chopped fresh chives or parsley, if desired

Heat beans, salsa, corn and carrot to boiling in 10-inch nonstick skillet; reduce heat to low. Cover and simmer about 15 minutes or until carrot is tender.

Spoon mashed potatoes onto bean mixture around edge of skillet. Cover and simmer 5 minutes. Sprinkle with cheese and chives.

1 Serving: Calories 255 (Calories from Fat 35); Fat 4g (Saturated 1g); Cholesterol 0mg; Sodium 705mg; Carbohydrate 52g (Dietary Fiber 13g); Protein 16g
% Daily Value: Vitamin A 26%; Vitamin C 20%; Calcium 12%; Iron 28%
Diet Exchanges: 2 1/2 starch, 3 vegetable

Mushroom-Topped Baked Potatoes

LO CAL / LO FAT / LO CHOL / HI FIB

PREP: 10 MIN; COOK: 8 MIN

4 SERVINGS

When time is tight, bake the potatoes in your microwave oven—you'll have dinner on the table in less than 20 minutes. If you have more time, bake the taters in the regular oven.

4	medium unpeeled baking potatoes
1	tablespoon margarine
4	cups sliced mushrooms (10 ounces)
1	clove garlic, finely chopped
1	cup skim milk
3	tablespoons all-purpose flour
1	teaspoon freeze-dried chives
$^1\!/_2$	teaspoon chicken bouillon granules
$^1\!/_4$	teaspoon salt
$^1\!/_4$	teaspoon pepper
$^1\!/_4$	cup shredded Parmesan cheese

Pierce potatoes. Arrange potatoes about 1 inch apart in circle on microwavable paper towel in microwave oven. Microwave uncovered on High about 8 minutes or until tender.

While potatoes are cooking, melt margarine in 10-inch nonstick skillet over medium heat. Cook mushrooms and garlic in skillet about 3 minutes, stirring frequently, until mushrooms are tender.

Mix remaining ingredients except cheese; stir into mushrooms. Heat to boiling, stirring constantly. Boil and stir 1 minute; remove from heat.

Place each potato on dinner plate. Cut potatoes lengthwise in half. Spoon mushroom sauce over potatoes. Sprinkle with cheese.

1 Serving: Calories 235 (Calories from Fat 45); Fat 5g (Saturated 2g); Cholesterol 5mg; Sodium 480mg; Carbohydrate 42g (Dietary Fiber 4g); Protein 9g
% Daily Value: Vitamin A 8%; Vitamin C 16%; Calcium 16%; Iron 16%
Diet Exchanges: 2 starch, 2 vegetable, $^1\!/_2$ fat

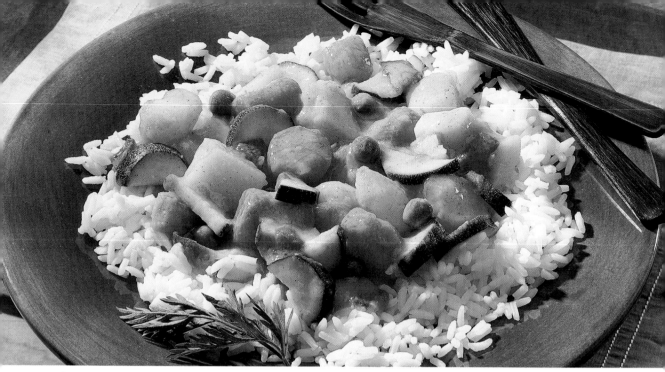

Curried Potato and Vegetable Sauce

Curried Potato and Vegetable Sauce

LO CAL / LO FAT / LO CHOL / HI FIB

PREP: 10 MIN; COOK: 15 MIN

4 SERVINGS

½ cup water

1 bag (16 ounces) frozen sweet peas, potatoes and carrots

1 medium tomato, seeded and chopped (¾ cup)

1 medium zucchini, cut lengthwise in half, then cut crosswise into slices (2 cups)

1 can (10¾ ounces) condensed cream of potato soup

¾ cup skim milk

1½ to 2 teaspoons curry powder

¼ teaspoon salt

Hot cooked rice or couscous, if desired

Heat water to boiling in 3-quart saucepan. Stir in frozen vegetables. Heat to boiling; reduce heat to low. Cover and simmer 6 to 8 minutes, stirring occasionally, until crisp-tender.

Stir in remaining ingredients except rice. Simmer uncovered 2 to 4 minutes, stirring occasionally, until zucchini is tender and mixture is hot. Serve over rice.

1 Serving: Calories 165 (Calories from Fat 20); Fat 2g (Saturated 1g); Cholesterol 5mg; Sodium 780mg; Carbohydrate 35g (Dietary Fiber 6g); Protein 8g
% Daily Value: Vitamin A 10%; Vitamin C 18%; Calcium 12%; Iron 10%
Diet Exchanges: 2 starch, 1 vegetable

Ratatouille Pizza

LO CAL / LO CHOL / HI FIB

PREP: 20 MIN; BAKE: 12 MIN

4 SERVINGS

This innovative pizza features the popular French side dish made from eggplant, zucchini, tomatoes, onion, garlic and herbs as a zesty topping for refrigerated pizza dough. For added appeal, try a combination of eggplant, zucchini and yellow summer squash.

1   can (10 ounces) refrigerated pizza crust dough*

2   cups diced peeled eggplant

2   cups diced peeled zucchini or yellow summer squash

3   medium tomatoes, chopped (2$^1/_4$ cups)

1   medium onion, cut lengthwise in half, then cut crosswise into thin slices

2   cloves garlic, finely chopped

2   tablespoons chopped fresh or 1$^1/_2$ teaspoons dried basil leaves

$^1/_4$ teaspoon ground red pepper (cayenne)

1$^1/_2$ cups shredded reduced-fat mozzarella cheese (6 ounces)

Heat oven to 425°. Grease cookie sheet or 12-inch pizza pan. Pat pizza dough into 14 × 12-inch rectangle on cookie sheet, or pat into pizza pan. Bake about 7 minutes or until light brown.

While the pizza crust is baking, heat remaining ingredients except cheese in 10-inch nonstick skillet over medium heat about 8 minutes, stirring occasionally, until vegetables are tender.

Spoon vegetable mixture onto pizza crust. Sprinkle with cheese. Bake about 5 minutes or until cheese is melted.

*If you prefer, use homemade pizza crust instead of the refrigerated product.

1 Serving: Calories 315 (Calories from Fat 70); Fat 8g (Saturated 5g); Cholesterol 20mg; Sodium 570mg; Carbohydrate 48g (Dietary Fiber 5g); Protein 18g
% Daily Value: Vitamin A 12%; Vitamin C 16%; Calcium 34%; Iron 16%
Diet Exchanges: 3 starch, 1 lean meat, 1 vegetable

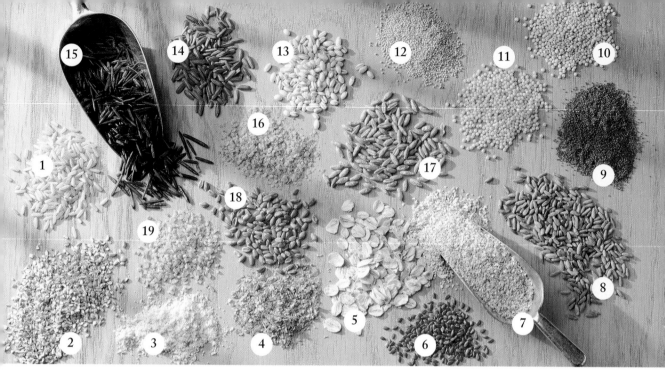

Know Your Grains: 1) brown rice; 2) kasha; 3) whole-grain cornmeal; 4) wheat bran; 5) rolled oats; 6) flaxseed; 7) oatbran; 8) rye; 9) teff; 10) quinoa; 11) millet; 12) amaranth; 13) pearled barley; 14) basmati hybrid rice; 15) wild rice; 16) toasted wheat germ; 17) triticale; 18) wheat berries; 19) bulgur

Wild Mushroom Pizza

LO CAL / LO FAT / LO CHOL / HI FIB

PREP: 15 MIN; BAKE: 10 MIN

6 SERVINGS

Clean the mushrooms just before using—simply rinse with water and blot dry. Beware—if mushrooms are soaked in water, they will lose their texture and become quite soggy.

1 tablespoon olive or vegetable oil

1 pound assorted fresh wild mushrooms (such as morel, oyster and shiitake), sliced (6 cups)

1 medium onion, chopped (½ cup)

2 cloves garlic, finely chopped

2 tablespoons chopped fresh parsley

1 package (10 ounces) thin Italian bread shell or ready-to-serve pizza crust (12 to 14 inches in diameter)

½ cup finely shredded Parmesan cheese

Heat oven to 450°. Heat oil in 12-inch nonstick skillet over high heat. Cook mushrooms, onion and garlic in oil about 5 minutes, stirring frequently, until onion is crisp-tender. Stir in parsley.

Spoon mushroom mixture over bread shell. Sprinkle with cheese. Bake 8 to 10 minutes or until cheese is melted.

1 Serving: Calories 240 (Calories from Fat 55); Fat 6g (Saturated 2g); Cholesterol 5mg; Sodium 470mg; Carbohydrate 40g (Dietary Fiber 4g); Protein 10g
% Daily Value: Vitamin A 0%; Vitamin C 4%; Calcium 10%; Iron 6%
Diet Exchanges: 2 starch, 2 vegetable, 1 fat

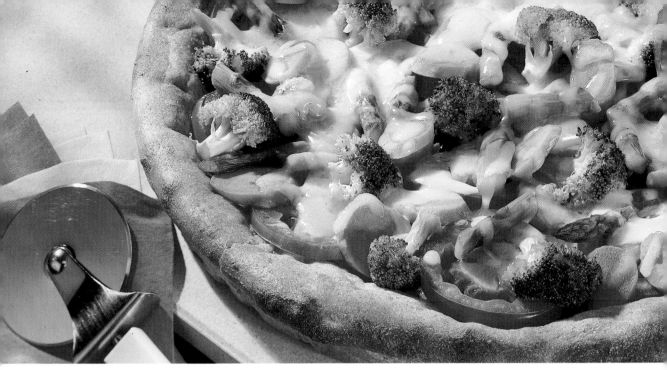

Pizza Primavera

Pizza Primavera

LO CAL / LO FAT / LO CHOL / HI FIB

PREP: 20 MIN; BAKE: 20 MIN

6 SERVINGS

Roma (plum) tomatoes are the best choice for this pizza. Why? Because they are not as juicy as regular tomatoes and they won't make the crust soggy.

1   loaf (1 pound) frozen honey-wheat or white bread dough, thawed

¹/₄   cup fat-free Italian dressing

¹/₂   pound asparagus, cut into 1-inch pieces

2   medium carrots, sliced (1 cup)

1   cup small broccoli flowerets

3   roma (plum) tomatoes, thinly sliced

1   cup shredded reduced-fat mozzarella cheese (4 ounces)

Heat oven to 450°. Spray cookie sheet with cooking spray. Pat or roll dough into 12-inch circle on cookie sheet. Prick dough thoroughly with fork. Bake 8 minutes (if dough puffs during baking, flatten with spoon).

Heat dressing to boiling in 10-inch nonstick skillet. Stir in asparagus, carrots and broccoli. Heat to boiling; reduce heat to medium. Cover and cook 3 to 4 minutes or until vegetables are crisp-tender.

Place tomato slices on partially baked crust. Spread vegetable mixture evenly over tomatoes. Sprinkle with cheese. Bake 7 to 9 minutes or until cheese is melted and crust is golden brown.

1 Serving: Calories 265 (Calories from Fat 55); Fat 6g (Saturated 2g); Cholesterol 0mg; Sodium 630mg; Carbohydrate 48g (Dietary Fiber 5g); Protein 10g
% Daily Value: Vitamin A 50%; Vitamin C 24%; Calcium 20%; Iron 16%
Diet Exchanges: 3 starch, 1 vegetable

Broccoli-Cheese Calzones

LO CAL / LO FAT / LO CHOL / HI FIB

PREP: 15 MIN; BAKE: 20 MIN

6 SERVINGS

1 container (15 ounces) fat-free ricotta cheese

1 package (10 ounces) frozen chopped broccoli, thawed

1/3 cup grated Parmesan cheese

1/4 cup fat-free cholesterol-free egg product or 2 egg whites

1 teaspoon dried basil leaves

1/4 teaspoon garlic powder

1 loaf (1 pound) frozen honey-wheat or white bread dough, thawed

1 can (8 ounces) pizza sauce

Heat oven to 375°. Grease 2 cookie sheets. Mix all ingredients except bread dough and pizza sauce.

Divide bread dough into 6 equal parts. Roll each part into 7-inch circle on lightly floured surface with floured rolling pin. Top half of each dough circle with cheese mixture to within 1 inch of edge. Carefully fold dough over filling; pinch edge or press with fork to seal securely.

Place calzones on cookie sheets. Bake about 20 minutes or until golden brown. Cool 5 minutes.

While calzones are cooling, heat pizza sauce in 1-quart saucepan over medium heat about 2 minutes, stirring occasionally, until heated through. Spoon warm sauce over calzones.

1 Serving: Calories 295 (Calories from Fat 35); Fat 4g (Saturated 2g); Cholesterol 5mg; Sodium 750mg; Carbohydrate 48g (Dietary Fiber 4g); Protein 21g
% Daily Value: Vitamin A 16%; Vitamin C 22%; Calcium 30%; Iron 18%
Diet Exchanges: 3 starch, 1 1/2 lean meat

Red Pepper-Artichoke Pizza

LO CAL / HI FIB

PREP: 10 MIN; BAKE 15 MIN

4 SERVINGS

If you have a little more time, try using your favorite homemade pizza crust instead of the refrigerated pizza dough.

1 can (10 ounces) refrigerated pizza crust dough

1 tablespoon skim milk

1/2 teaspoon garlic powder

1/2 teaspoon dried basil leaves

1 tub (8 ounces) reduced-fat cream cheese

1 jar (12 ounces) roasted red bell peppers, drained and coarsely chopped

1 jar (6 to 7 ounces) marinated artichoke hearts, drained and coarsely chopped

1 small tomato, chopped (1/2 cup)

3 medium green onions, sliced (3 tablespoons)

Heat oven to 425°. Grease cookie sheet. Pat pizza dough into 13 × 11-inch rectangle on cookie sheet. Bake about 5 minutes or until crust just starts to brown.

Mix milk, garlic powder, basil and cream cheese. Spread on partially baked crust. Top with bell peppers, artichoke hearts, tomato and onions.

Bake about 10 minutes or until vegetables are heated through and edges of crust are golden brown.

1 Serving: Calories 335 (Calories from Fat 100); Fat 11g (Saturated 6g); Cholesterol 30mg; Sodium 740mg; Carbohydrate 51g (Dietary Fiber 5g); Protein 13g
% Daily Value: Vitamin A 52%; Vitamin C 100%; Calcium 12%; Iron 20%
Diet Exchanges: 3 starch, 1 vegetable, 2 fat

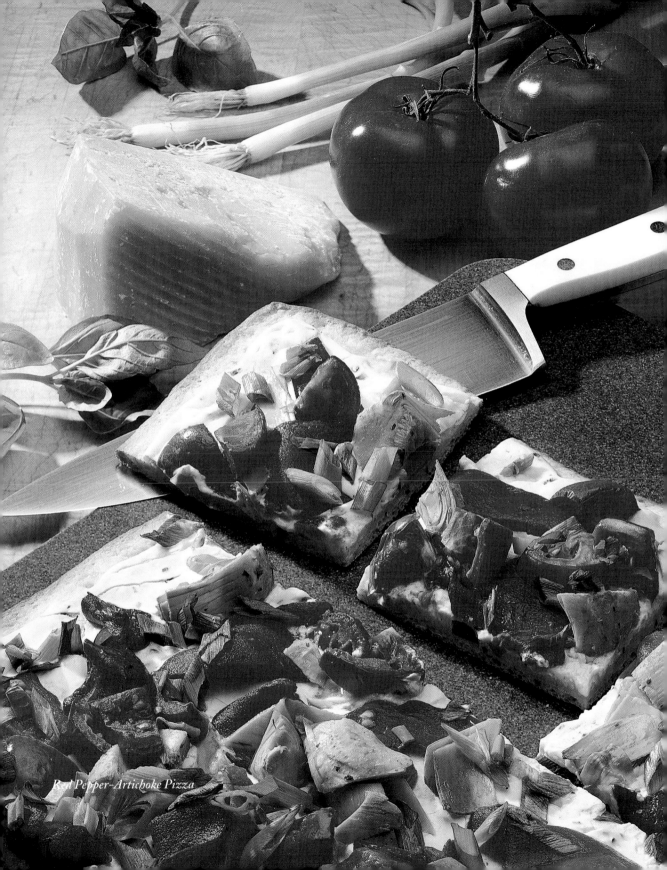

Red Pepper-Artichoke Pizza

Vegetarian Fried Rice

LO CHOL / HI FIB

PREP: 15 MIN; COOK: 10 MIN

4 SERVINGS

Brown rice contains more nutrients than white rice because it still contains some of the hull.

3	cups uncooked quick-cooking brown rice
½	cup fat-free cholesterol-free egg product
1	tablespoon vegetable oil
2	medium carrots, sliced (1 cup)
4	medium green onions, sliced (¼ cup)
1	clove garlic, finely chopped
2	cups snow (Chinese) pea pods, cut in half
1	cup bean sprouts
2	tablespoons reduced-sodium soy sauce

Cook brown rice as directed on package. While rice is cooking, spray 10-inch nonstick skillet with cooking spray; heat over medium-high heat until very hot. Pour egg product over bottom of skillet and cook until firm; remove from skillet and set aside. When eggs are cool, cut into small pieces.

Heat oil in skillet over medium-high heat. Add carrots, onions and garlic; stir-fry 1 minute. Add pea pods and bean sprouts; stir-fry 2 minutes. Stir in rice and soy sauce. Reduce heat to medium; stir-fry 2 minutes. Stir in cooked eggs; cook until heated through.

1 Serving: Calories 575 (Calories from Fat 80); Fat 9g (Saturated 2g); Cholesterol 0mg; Sodium 350mg; Carbohydrate 116g (Dietary Fiber 11g); Protein 19g
% Daily Value: Vitamin A 28%; Vitamin C 18%; Calcium 10%; Iron 22%
Diet Exchanges: 7 starch, 2 vegetable

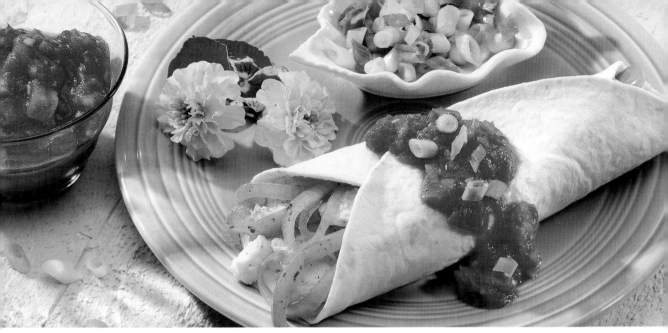

Vegetable-Egg Fajitas

Vegetable-Egg Fajitas

LO CAL / LO FAT / LO CHOL / HI FIB

PREP: 15 MIN; COOK: 10 MIN

4 SERVINGS

Finish off this spicy meal with a burst of vitamin C by serving a scoop of Pineapple Ice (page 413) for dessert.

1½   cups fat-free cholesterol-free egg product

⅓   cup skim milk

1   medium bell pepper, cut into ¼-inch strips

1   medium onion, sliced and separated into rings

1   tablespoon fajita seasoning mix (from 1.27-ounce envelope)

4   fat-free flour tortillas (6 to 8 inches in diameter)

½   cup salsa

Mix egg product and milk with fork; set aside. Spray 12-inch nonstick skillet with cooking spray; heat over medium-high heat. Mix bell pepper, onion and fajita seasoning mix in skillet. Cook, stirring occasionally, until vegetables are tender. Remove vegetables from skillet; keep warm. Wipe out skillet with paper towel.

Reduce heat; pour egg mixture into skillet. As mixture begins to set at bottom and side, gently lift cooked portions with spatula so that thin, uncooked portion can flow to bottom. Avoid constant stirring. Cook 3 to 4 minutes or until eggs are thickened throughout but still moist.

Spoon one-fourth of the egg mixture onto center of each tortilla; top with vegetables. Fold 2 sides of tortilla over filling, overlapping. Secure with toothpick. Serve each fajita topped with 2 tablespoons salsa.

1 Serving: Calories 172 (Calories from Fat 0); Fat 0g (Saturated 0g); Cholesterol 0mg; Sodium 675mg; Carbohydrate 34g (Dietary Fiber 3g); Protein 12g
% Daily Value: Vitamin A 12%; Vitamin C 30%; Calcium 8%; Iron 18%
Diet Exchanges: 2 starch, 1 very lean meat

Cheesy Scrambled Eggs

LO CAL / LO CHOL / HI FIB

PREP: 10 MIN; COOK: 8 MIN; BROIL: 2 MIN

4 SERVINGS

1½   cups fat-free cholesterol-free egg product

¼   cup skim milk

½   teaspoon salt

¼   teaspoon red pepper sauce

1   small green bell pepper, chopped (½ cup)

½   package (8-ounce size) reduced-fat cream cheese (Neufchâtel), softened

4   English muffins, split and toasted

½   cup shredded reduced-fat Cheddar cheese (2 ounces)

  Paprika, if desired

Mix egg product, milk, salt and pepper sauce; set aside.

Spray 10-inch nonstick skillet with cooking spray; heat over medium heat. Cook bell pepper in skillet about 5 minutes, stirring frequently, until tender. Pour egg mixture into skillet. As mixture begins to set on bottom and side, gently lift cooked portions with spatula so that thin, uncooked portion can flow to bottom. Avoid constant stirring. Cook about 3 minutes or until eggs are thickened throughout but still moist; remove from heat.

Spoon cream cheese over egg mixture. Gently stir cream cheese into eggs until cheese is smooth and melted. Spoon egg mixture over English muffin halves. Sprinkle with Cheddar cheese.

Set oven control to broil. Place English muffin halves on ungreased cookie sheet. Broil with tops 4 inches from heat about 2 minutes or just until cheese begins to melt. Sprinkle with paprika.

1 Serving: Calories 275 (Calories from Fat 80); Fat 9g (Saturated 5g); Cholesterol 25mg; Sodium 900mg; Carbohydrate 32g (Dietary Fiber 3g); Protein 19g
% Daily Value: Vitamin A 16%; Vitamin C 22%; Calcium 22%; Iron 18%
Diet Exchanges: 2 starch, 2 lean meat, ½ vegetable

Scrambled Eggs Rancheros

LO CAL / LO FAT / LO CHOL / HI FIB

PREP: 10 MIN; COOK: 5 MIN

4 SERVINGS

Transform this dish into a grab-and-go meal by serving the tortillas burrito style. Just fold one end of each tortilla up about 1 inch over filling; fold right and left sides over folded end, overlapping. Fold remaining end down, and you're set to go!

4	fat-free flour tortillas (6 to 8 inches in diameter)
1	cup salsa
1$\frac{1}{2}$	cups fat-free cholesterol-free egg product
$\frac{1}{4}$	cup skim milk
$\frac{1}{2}$	teaspoon onion salt
$\frac{1}{8}$	teaspoon pepper
2	teaspoons margarine
$\frac{3}{4}$	cup shredded reduced-fat Cheddar cheese (3 ounces)

Heat tortillas as directed on package. Heat salsa in 1-quart saucepan over medium heat about 2 minutes, stirring occasionally, until heated through. Remove from heat; cover to keep warm.

While salsa is heating, mix egg product, milk, onion salt and pepper. Melt margarine in 10-inch nonstick skillet over medium heat. Pour egg mixture into skillet. As mixture begins to set on bottom and side, gently lift cooked portions with spatula so that thin, uncooked portion can flow to bottom. Avoid constant stirring. Cook about 3 minutes or until eggs are thickened throughout but still moist.

Spread salsa over each tortilla. Divide scrambled eggs among tortillas. Sprinkle with cheese.

1 Serving: Calories 210 (Calories from Fat 35); Fat 4g (Saturated 1g); Cholesterol 5mg; Sodium 990mg; Carbohydrate 30g (Dietary Fiber 3g); Protein 17g
% Daily Value: Vitamin A 14%; Vitamin C 10%; Calcium 16%; Iron 12%
Diet Exchanges: 2 starch, 1$\frac{1}{2}$ very lean meat

Spinach Frittata with Creole Sauce

PREP: 20 MIN; COOK: 10 MIN

4 SERVINGS

Characterized by its heavy use of tomatoes, Creole cooking is a combination of French, Spanish and African flavors.

Creole Sauce (right)

2 teaspoons margarine

1 small onion, chopped (¹/₄ cup)

3 cups coarsely chopped spinach (4 ounces)

1¹/₂ cups fat-free cholesterol-free egg product

¹/₂ teaspoon chopped fresh or ¹/₈ teaspoon dried thyme leaves

¹/₈ teaspoon salt

¹/₈ teaspoon pepper

2 tablespoons shredded reduced-fat mozzarella cheese

Prepare Creole Sauce; keep warm. Melt margarine in 8-inch nonstick skillet over medium heat. Cook onion in margarine 3 minutes, stirring occasionally. Add spinach; toss just until spinach is wilted.

Beat egg product, thyme, salt and pepper; pour over spinach. Cover and cook over medium-low heat 5 to 7 minutes or until eggs are set and light brown on bottom. Sprinkle with cheese. Cut into wedges. Serve with sauce.

Creole Sauce

1 large tomato, coarsely chopped (1 cup)

1 small onion, chopped (¹/₄ cup)

2 tablespoons sliced celery

¹/₄ teaspoon paprika

¹/₈ teaspoon pepper

¹/₈ teaspoon red pepper sauce

Heat all ingredients to boiling in 1-quart saucepan, stirring occasionally; reduce heat. Simmer uncovered about 5 minutes, stirring occasionally, until thickened.

1 Serving: Calories 85 (Calories from Fat 25); Fat 3g (Saturated 1g); Cholesterol 2mg; Sodium 270mg; Carbohydrate 7g (Dietary Fiber 2g); Protein 10g
% Daily Value: Vitamin A 30%; Vitamin C 14%; Calcium 8%; Iron 14%
Diet Exchanges: 1 lean meat, 1 vegetable

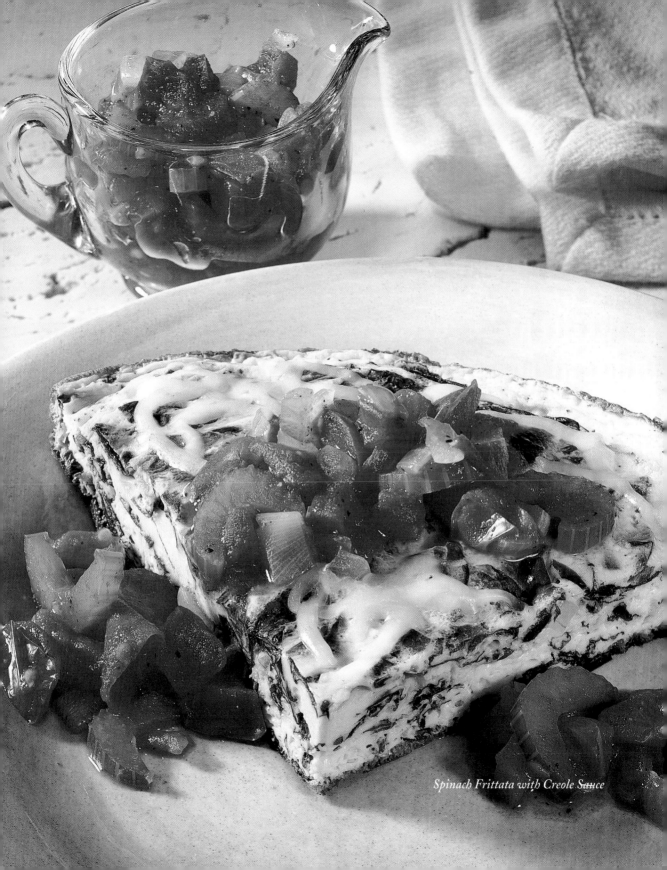

Spinach Frittata with Creole Sauce

Spaghetti Frittata

LO CAL / LO FAT / LO CHOL

PREP: 10 MIN; COOK: 10 MIN; STAND: 5 MIN

4 SERVINGS

Topped with a spoonful of tomato sauce, everyone's favorite—spaghetti—takes on a new twist.

¼	cup shredded reduced-fat mozzarella cheese (1 ounce)
¼	cup chopped fresh or 1 tablespoon dried basil leaves
1½	cups fat-free cholesterol-free egg product
½	teaspoon salt
⅛	teaspoon red pepper sauce
1	clove garlic, finely chopped
2	cups cold cooked spaghetti

Spray 10-inch nonstick skillet with cooking spray; heat until hot. Mix all ingredients except spaghetti in large bowl. Stir in spaghetti. Pour spaghetti mixture into skillet, spreading evenly. Cook uncovered over medium-low heat 5 to 6 minutes or until bottom begins to brown (shake skillet occasionally to prevent frittata from sticking).

Place large plate over skillet; invert frittata onto plate. Slide frittata, cooked side up, back into skillet. Cook about 5 minutes longer or until egg mixture is set and bottom is brown. Turn onto serving plate. Let stand 5 minutes before cutting. Cut into wedges.

1 Serving: Calories 150 (Calories from Fat 20); Fat 2g (Saturated 1g); Cholesterol 5mg; Sodium 460mg; Carbohydrate 22g (Dietary Fiber 2g); Protein 13g
% Daily Value: Vitamin A 6%; Vitamin C 0%; Calcium 8%; Iron 14%
Diet Exchanges: 1½ starch, 1 very lean meat

Hash Brown Frittata

LO CAL / LO FAT / LO CHOL / HI FIB

PREP: 10 MIN; COOK: 25 MIN

4 SERVINGS

Add some kick to this frittata by topping it off with your favorite salsa or barbecue sauce. Serve each wedge with a spoonful of sauce or 1/2 cup of salsa on the side.

2	cups refrigerated shredded hash brown potatoes (from 1-pound 4-ounce bag)
1	can (11 ounces) whole kernel corn with red and green peppers, drained
1	teaspoon onion salt
1	cup fat-free cholesterol-free egg product
1/4	cup skim milk
1/2	teaspoon dried marjoram leaves
1/2	teaspoon red pepper sauce
1/3	cup shredded reduced-fat Cheddar cheese

Mix potatoes, corn and onion salt. Spray 10-inch nonstick skillet with cooking spray; heat over medium heat. Pack potato mixture firmly into skillet, leaving 1/2-inch space around edge. Reduce heat to medium-low. Cook uncovered about 10 minutes or until bottom starts to brown.

While potato mixture is cooking, mix egg product, milk, marjoram and pepper sauce. Pour egg mixture over potato mixture. Cook uncovered over medium-low heat. As mixture begins to set on bottom and side, gently lift cooked portions with spatula so that thin, uncooked portion can flow to bottom. Avoid constant stirring. Cook about 5 minutes or until eggs are thickened throughout but still moist. Sprinkle with cheese.

Reduce heat to low. Cover and cook about 10 minutes or until center is set and cheese is bubbly. Loosen bottom of frittata with spatula. Cut frittata into 4 wedges. Serve immediately.

1 Serving: Calories 235 (Calories from Fat 20); Fat 2g (Saturated 1g); Cholesterol 2mg; Sodium 990mg; Carbohydrate 44g (Dietary Fiber 5g); Protein 12g
% Daily Value: Vitamin A 6%; Vitamin C 14%; Calcium 10%; Iron 12%
Diet Exchanges: 2 1/2 starch, 1/2 very lean meat, 1 vegetable

Savory Potato Supper Cake

LO CAL / LO FAT / LO CHOL / HI FIB

PREP: 25 MIN; BAKE: 50 MIN

6 SERVINGS

For a delicious finishing touch, top each serving with a dollop of reduced-fat sour cream and a dusting of ground nutmeg.

1	cup fat-free ricotta cheese
1/2	cup soft whole-grain or white bread crumbs
1	tablespoon chopped fresh or 1 teaspoon dried marjoram leaves
1/2	teaspoon salt
1/4	teaspoon pepper
1/3	cup fat-free cholesterol-free egg product or 3 egg whites
4	cups shredded sweet potatoes (1 pound)
4	cups shredded baking potatoes (1 pound)
3/4	cup chopped onion
	Pear Sauce (right) or 1 cup unsweetened applesauce

Heat oven to 375°. Spray rectangular pan, 13 × 9 × 2 inches, with cooking spray. Mix cheese, bread crumbs, marjoram, salt, pepper and egg whites in large bowl. Stir in potatoes and onion. Spread in pan.

Bake uncovered 45 to 50 minutes or until potatoes are tender and golden brown. While potato mixture is baking, prepare Pear Sauce. Cut potato mixture into squares. Serve with sauce.

Pear Sauce

3	medium Bosc pears, peeled and chopped (2 cups)
1/4	cup water
2	tablespoons frozen (thawed) apple juice concentrate
1	teaspoon vanilla
1/2	teaspoon ground cinnamon
1/4	teaspoon ground nutmeg

Cover and cook all ingredients in 1-quart saucepan over medium heat 10 minutes, stirring occasionally; reduce heat to medium-low. Cook about 30 minutes longer, stirring occasionally, until pears are very tender. Place mixture in blender or food processor. Cover and blend until chunky.

1 Serving: Calories 215 (Calories from Fat 10); Fat 1g (Saturated 0g); Cholesterol 0mg; Sodium 340mg; Carbohydrate 46g (Dietary Fiber 4g); Protein 10g
% Daily Value: Vitamin A 100%; Vitamin C 18%; Calcium 12%; Iron 8%
Diet Exchanges: 2 starch, 3 vegetable

Cheese and Chilies Bake

LO CAL / LO CHOL

PREP: 10 MIN; BAKE: 25 MIN

4 SERVINGS

This healthy variation of Impossible Pie has a moist texture, almost like bread pudding or spoon bread.

- ³/₄ cup shredded reduced-fat Cheddar cheese (3 ounces)
- ³/₄ cup shredded reduced-fat mozzarella cheese (3 ounces)
- 1 can (4 ounces) chopped green chilies, drained
- 1 cup skim milk
- ¹/₂ cup fat-free cholesterol-free egg product
- 1 cup Bisquick® Reduced Fat baking mix
- ¹/₂ teaspoon onion powder

Heat oven to 425°. Spray square pan, 8 × 8 × 2 inches, with cooking spray. Sprinkle ¹/₂ cup of the Cheddar cheese, the mozzarella cheese and chilies in pan.

Place remaining ingredients except ¹/₄ cup Cheddar in blender or food processor. Cover and blend on high speed about 30 seconds or until smooth. Pour into pan.

Bake uncovered about 25 minutes or until toothpick inserted in center comes out clean. Sprinkle with remaining ¹/₄ cup Cheddar cheese. Cut into squares. Serve warm.

1 Serving: Calories 235 (Calories from Fat 65); Fat 7g (Saturated 4g); Cholesterol 15mg; Sodium 700mg; Carbohydrate 26g (Dietary Fiber 1g); Protein 18g
% Daily Value: Vitamin A 10%; Vitamin C 16%; Calcium 36%; Iron 10%
Diet Exchanges: 1¹/₂ starch, 2 lean meat

Tomato-Corn Quiche

LO CAL / LO FAT / LO CHOL

PREP: 10 MIN; BAKE: 45 MIN; STAND: 10 MIN

6 SERVINGS

Evaporated skimmed milk is a healthy alternative to half-and-half or whipping (heavy) cream.

- 1 cup evaporated skimmed milk
- ¹/₂ cup fat-free cholesterol-free egg product
- 2 tablespoons all-purpose flour
- 1 tablespoon chopped fresh cilantro
- ¹/₂ teaspoon chili powder
- ¹/₄ teaspoon onion powder
- ¹/₄ teaspoon salt
- ¹/₄ teaspoon pepper
- 1 cup frozen (thawed) whole kernel corn
- ³/₄ cup shredded reduced-fat Cheddar cheese (3 ounces)
- 1 medium tomato, seeded and chopped (³/₄ cup)

Heat oven to 350°. Spray pie plate, 9 × 1¹/₄ inches, with cooking spray. Mix all ingredients except corn, cheese and tomato in medium bowl until blended. Stir in remaining ingredients; pour into pie plate.

Bake 35 to 45 minutes or until knife inserted in center comes out clean. Let stand 10 minutes before cutting.

1 Serving: Calories 95 (Calories from Fat 10); Fat 1g (Saturated 1g); Cholesterol 5mg; Sodium 270mg; Carbohydrate 14g (Dietary Fiber 1g); Protein 9g
% Daily Value: Vitamin A 10%; Vitamin C 4%; Calcium 18%; Iron 4%
Diet Exchanges: 1 starch, 1 very lean meat

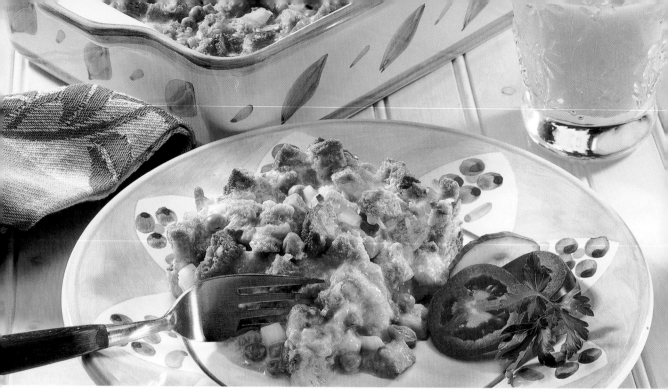

Vegetable-Cheese Bake

Vegetable-Cheese Bake

LO CAL / HI FIB

PREP: 10 MIN; BAKE: 30 MIN

6 SERVINGS

If you're a fan of pumpernickel or light rye bread, use one of them instead of the whole wheat.

8	slices soft whole wheat bread, cut into $^{1}/_{2}$-inch cubes
2	cups shredded reduced-fat mozzarella cheese (8 ounces)
$1^{1}/_{2}$	cups frozen green peas or whole kernel corn
1	small onion, finely chopped ($^{1}/_{4}$ cup)
$1^{1}/_{2}$	cups fat-free cholesterol-free egg product
1	can (12 ounces) evaporated skimmed milk
$^{1}/_{2}$	cup plain fat-free yogurt
1	tablespoon mustard

Heat oven to 350°. Spray square baking dish, 8 × 8 × 2 inches, with cooking spray.

Mix bread cubes, cheese, peas and onion in large bowl. Mix remaining ingredients; pour over bread mixture and stir to coat. Pour into baking dish.

Bake uncovered about 30 minutes or until golden brown and center is set.

1 Serving: Calories 295 (Calories from Fat 80); Fat 9g (Saturated 5g); Cholesterol 25mg; Sodium 610mg; Carbohydrate 33g (Dietary Fiber 6g); Protein 26g
% Daily Value: Vitamin A 14%; Vitamin C 4%; Calcium 50%; Iron 18%
Diet Exchanges: 2 starch, 3 lean meat

Savory Mushroom Strata

LO CAL / LO FAT / LO CHOL / HI FIB

PREP: 20 MIN; CHILL: 2 HR; BAKE: 50 MIN;

STAND: 10 MIN

6 SERVINGS

Don't throw away that day-old bread! Slightly dried-out bread slices are perfect for soaking up all the wonderful flavors in this dish.

3	cups chopped mushrooms (12 ounces)
1	cup fat-free small-curd cottage cheese
2	medium green onions, chopped (2 tablespoons)
1	teaspoon chopped fresh or $1/2$ teaspoon dried rosemary leaves
1	clove garlic, finely chopped
12	slices whole-grain or white bread
$1^1/_2$	cups skim milk
1	cup fat-free cholesterol-free egg product
$1/4$	cup shredded reduced-fat Monterey Jack cheese (1 ounce)

Spray square baking pan, 9 × 9 × 2 inches, with cooking spray. Mix mushrooms, cottage cheese, onions, rosemary and garlic. Place 4 of the bread slices in pan. Spread with half of the mushroom mixture.

Beat milk and egg product until blended; pour one-third of the milk mixture over bread slices in pan. Spread 4 of the bread slices with remaining mushroom mixture. Place bread, mushroom sides up, in pan. Top with remaining 4 slices bread; press down gently if bread is higher than edge of dish. Pour remaining milk mixture over bread. Sprinkle with cheese. Cover and refrigerate at least 2 hours but no longer than 24 hours.

Heat oven to 325°. Bake uncovered 45 to 50 minutes or until set and top is golden brown. Let stand 10 minutes before serving.

1 Serving: Calories 215 (Calories from Fat 35); Fat 4g (Saturated 2g); Cholesterol 5mg; Sodium 550mg; Carbohydrate 33g (Dietary Fiber 5g); Protein 17g
% Daily Value: Vitamin A 8%; Vitamin C 2%; Calcium 20%; Iron 18%
Diet Exchanges: 1 starch, 1 lean meat, 2 vegetable, $1/2$ skim milk

Tortilla Casserole

LO CAL / LO FAT / LO CHOL / HI FIB

PREP: 25 MIN; BAKE: 35 MIN

6 SERVINGS

The Spicy Fresh Chili Sauce also makes a great condiment for other Mexican favorites, such as tacos, burritos and enchiladas.

1	can (15 to 16 ounces) kidney beans, drained
1/2	cup skim milk
1/4	cup fat-free cholesterol-free egg product or 2 egg whites
1/4	cup chopped fresh cilantro
1/2	cup ready-to-serve vegetable broth
1	large onion, chopped (1 cup)
1	medium green bell pepper, chopped (1 cup)
2	cloves garlic, finely chopped
2	cans (4 ounces each) chopped mild green chilies, drained
4	cups Baked Tortilla Chips (page 62) or reduced-fat tortilla chips
1	cup shredded reduced-fat Cheddar cheese (4 ounces)
	Spicy Fresh Chili Sauce (right) or 3/4 cup salsa
	Reduced-fat sour cream, if desired

Heat oven to 375°. Spray 2-quart casserole with cooking spray. Mash beans and milk in medium bowl until smooth. Stir in egg product and 2 table-spoons of the cilantro; reserve. (Or place beans, milk, egg product and 2 tablespoons of the cilantro in blender or food processor; cover and blend until smooth.)

Cook broth, onion, bell pepper, garlic and chilies in 10-inch nonstick skillet over medium heat about 5 minutes, stirring occasionally, until onion is tender. Stir in remaining 2 tablespoons cilantro.

Coarsely chop half of the tortilla chips. Place 1 cup of the chopped chips in bottom of casserole. Spread reserved bean mixture over chips. Spread vegetable mixture over bean mixture. Sprinkle with 1/2 cup of the cheese. Top with remaining chopped chips. Sprinkle with remaining 1/2 cup cheese.

Bake uncovered 30 to 35 minutes or until hot and cheese is golden brown. Serve with Spicy Fresh Chili Sauce, the remaining chips and sour cream.

Spicy Fresh Chili Sauce

1	medium tomato, finely chopped (3/4 cup)
3	medium green onions, sliced (3 tablespoons)
1	medium jalapeño chili, seeded and finely chopped
1	clove garlic, finely chopped
1	tablespoon chopped fresh cilantro
1/4	teaspoon ground cumin

Mix all ingredients. Serve immediately, or refrigerate until serving.

1 Serving: Calories 180 (Calories from Fat 20); Fat 2g (Saturated 1g); Cholesterol 5mg; Sodium 460mg; Carbohydrate 33g (Dietary Fiber 6g); Protein 13g
% Daily Value: Vitamin A 16%; Vitamin C 50%; Calcium 14%; Iron 18%
Diet Exchanges: 2 starch, 1 very lean meat

Cheddar, Egg and Rice Bake

LO CAL / LO FAT / LO CHOL

PREP: 40 MIN; BAKE: 55 MIN; STAND: 5 MIN

6 SERVINGS

Eggs are a nutritional bargain. Because they are one of the food proteins that best match human protein needs, scientists call eggs "reference proteins" and compare the quality of other proteins, such as meat, fish and legumes, to them.

1	package (8 ounces) sliced mushrooms (3 cups)
1	medium onion, chopped ($^1/_2$ cup)
$^2/_3$	cup uncooked regular long grain rice
$1^1/_3$	cups water
1	cup frozen chopped broccoli
1	cup fat-free small-curd cottage cheese
1	cup shredded reduced-fat Cheddar cheese (4 ounces)
2	tablespoons dry bread crumbs
1	tablespoon chopped fresh or 1 teaspoon dried basil leaves
$^1/_4$	teaspoon salt
$^1/_4$	teaspoon pepper
$^1/_2$	cup fat-free cholesterol-free egg product

Spray quiche dish, 9 × $1^1/_2$ inches, or pie plate, 9 × $1^1/_4$ inches, with cooking spray. Mix mushrooms, onion, rice and water in 3-quart saucepan. Heat to boiling; reduce heat. Cover and simmer about 20 minutes, stirring occasionally, until rice is tender.

Heat oven to 325°. Stir broccoli and cottage cheese into mushroom mixture. Stir in $^3/_4$ cup of the Cheddar cheese and the remaining ingredients. Spoon into dish.

Bake 40 minutes. Sprinkle with remaining $^1/_4$ cup Cheddar cheese. Bake 10 to 15 minutes or until center is hot. Let stand 5 minutes before cutting.

1 Serving: Calories 170 (Calories from Fat 20); Fat 2g (Saturated 2g); Cholesterol 50mg; Sodium 400mg; Carbohydrate 26g (Dietary Fiber 2g); Protein 14g
% Daily Value: Vitamin A 8%; Vitamin C 12%; Calcium 14%; Iron 12%
Diet Exchanges: 1 starch, 1 lean meat, 2 vegetable

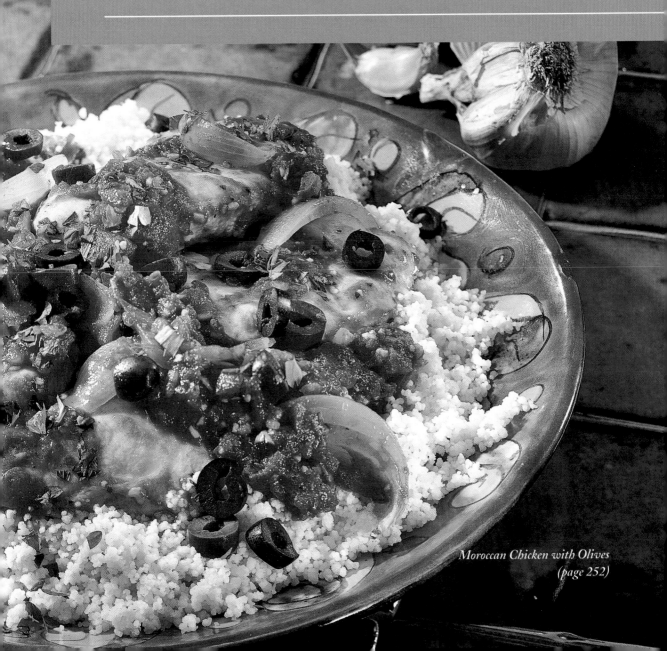

CHICKEN AND TURKEY

Moroccan Chicken with Olives
(page 252)

Country-Style Chicken

LO CAL / HI FIB

PREP: 25 MIN; BAKE: 2 HR; COOK: 5 MIN

6 SERVINGS

Leaving the skin on the chicken during the baking time helps lock in flavorful juices and keeps the meat both tender and moist.

3 to 3½   pound whole broiler-fryer chicken

1   tablespoon margarine

1   can (10½ ounces) condensed chicken broth

¾   teaspoon chopped fresh or ¼ teaspoon dried thyme leaves

¼   teaspoon pepper

8   medium carrots, cut into fourths

8   whole small white onions

4   medium turnips, cut into fourths

½   cup dry white wine or chicken broth

2   tablespoons cold water

1   tablespoon cornstarch

Chopped fresh thyme, if desired

Fold wings of chicken across back with tips touching. Tie or skewer drumsticks to tail. Melt margarine in ovenproof nonstick Dutch oven over medium heat. Cook chicken in margarine until brown on all sides; drain.

Heat oven to 375°. Pour broth over chicken in Dutch oven. Sprinkle with thyme and pepper. Insert meat thermometer in chicken so tip is in thickest part of inside thigh muscle and does not touch bone. Cover and bake 45 minutes.

Arrange carrots, onions and turnips around chicken. Cover and bake 1 to 1¼ hours or until thermometer reads 180° and juice of chicken is no longer pink when center of thigh is cut. Remove chicken and vegetables from Dutch oven; keep warm.

Skim fat from pan drippings in Dutch oven. Stir wine into juices. Heat to boiling. Mix cold water and cornstarch; stir into wine mixture. Heat to boiling, stirring constantly. Boil and stir 1 minute. Remove and discard chicken skin. Serve chicken and vegetables with sauce. Sprinkle with thyme.

1 Serving: Calories 330 (Calories from Fat 145); Fat 16g (Saturated 5g); Cholesterol 85mg; Sodium 480mg; Carbohydrate 22g (Dietary Fiber 6g); Protein 31g
% Daily Value: Vitamin A 100%; Vitamin C 18%; Calcium 8%; Iron 12%
Diet Exchanges: 1 starch, 3 medium-fat meat, 1 vegetable

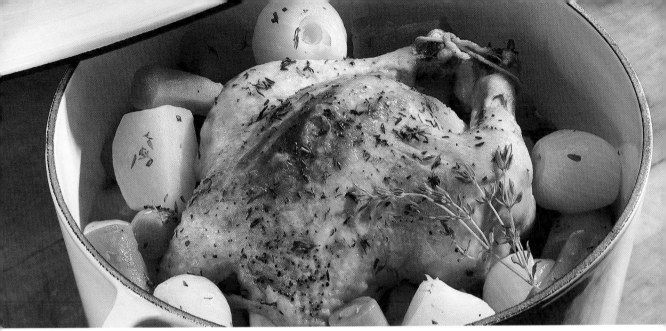

Country-Style Chicken

Rosemary-Lemon Chicken

LOW CALORIE

PREP: 20 MIN; ROAST: 1½ HR; STAND: 10 MIN

6 SERVINGS

2 large shallots or 1 small onion, finely chopped (¼ cup)

1 garlic clove, finely chopped

1 teaspoon grated lemon peel

½ teaspoon dried rosemary leaves, crumbled

½ teaspoon salt

¼ teaspoon pepper

3 to 3½ pound whole broiler-fryer chicken

1 medium lemon, cut in half

½ teaspoon paprika

Heat oven to 350°. Mix all ingredients except chicken, lemon and paprika. Gently loosen breast skin from chicken with fingers, reaching as far back as possible without tearing skin. Spread herb mixture over breast meat; cover with skin. Squeeze lemon halves over outside of chicken and inside body cavity; place lemon halves in cavity.

Fold wings of chicken across back with tips touching. Tie or skewer drumsticks to tail. Sprinkle paprika over chicken. Place chicken, breast side up, on rack in shallow roasting pan. Insert meat thermometer in chicken so tip is in thickest part of inside thigh muscle and does not touch bone.

Roast uncovered about 1½ hours or until thermometer reads 180° and juice of chicken is no longer pink when center of thigh is cut. Let stand 10 minutes before carving. Remove and discard chicken skin and lemon.

1 Serving: Calories 230 (Calories from Fat 115); Fat 13g (Saturated 4g); Cholesterol 85mg; Sodium 280mg; Carbohydrate 1g (Dietary Fiber 0g); Protein 27g
% Daily Value: Vitamin A 6%; Vitamin C 0%; Calcium 2%; Iron 8%
Diet Exchanges: 3 medium-fat meat

Wine-Sauced Chicken

LOW CALORIE

PREP: 10 MIN; ROAST: 1¼ HR; STAND: 10 MIN

6 SERVINGS

3 to 3½	pound whole broiler-fryer chicken
1	cup dry red wine or grape juice
1	tablespoon chopped fresh or 1 teaspoon dried basil leaves
½	teaspoon salt
1	medium onion, finely chopped (½ cup)
2	large cloves garlic, finely chopped
1	can (8 ounces) tomato sauce

Heat oven to 375°. Fold wings of chicken across back with tips touching. Tie or skewer drumsticks to tail. Place chicken, breast side up, on rack in shallow roasting pan. Insert meat thermometer in chicken so tip is in thickest part of inside thigh muscle and does not touch bone.

Roast uncovered 1 to 1¼ hours or until thermometer reads 180° and juice of chicken is no longer pink when center of thigh is cut. Let stand 10 minutes before carving. Remove and discard chicken skin.

While chicken is roasting, mix remaining ingredients in 1½-quart saucepan. Heat to boiling, stirring occasionally; reduce heat to low. Cover and simmer 30 minutes. Serve with chicken.

1 Serving: Calories 250 (Calories from Fat 115); Fat 13g (Saturated 4g); Cholesterol 85mg; Sodium 510mg; Carbohydrate 5g (Dietary Fiber 1g); Protein 27g
% Daily Value: Vitamin A 8%; Vitamin C 4%; Calcium 2%; Iron 10%
Diet Exchanges: 3 medium-fat meat, 1 vegetable

Honey-Mustard Chicken

LOW CALORIE

PREP: 10 MIN; BAKE: 1 HR

6 SERVINGS

3 to 3½	pound cut-up broiler-fryer chicken
⅓	cup country-style Dijon mustard
3	tablespoons honey
1	tablespoon mustard seed
½	teaspoon pepper

Heat oven to 375°. Place chicken, skin sides down, in ungreased rectangular pan, 13 × 9 × 2 inches. Mix remaining ingredients; brush over chicken.

Cover and bake 30 minutes. Turn chicken; brush with mustard mixture. Bake uncovered about 30 minutes longer or until juice of chicken is no longer pink when centers of thickest pieces are cut. (If chicken begins to brown too quickly, cover with aluminum foil.) Discard any remaining mustard mixture.

To Grill: Heat coals or gas grill. Place chicken, skin sides up, on grill. Brush with mustard mixture. Cover and grill 5 to 6 inches from medium heat 15 minutes. Turn chicken; brush with mustard mixture. Cover and grill 20 to 40 minutes longer, turning and brushing with mustard mixture, until juice of chicken is no longer pink when centers of thickest pieces are cut. Discard any remaining mustard mixture.

1 Serving: Calories 285 (Calories from Fat 135); Fat 15g (Saturated 4g); Cholesterol 85mg; Sodium 250mg; Carbohydrate 10g (Dietary Fiber 0g); Protein 28g
% Daily Value: Vitamin A 4%; Vitamin C 0%; Calcium 2%; Iron 10%
Diet Exchanges: 4 lean meat, ½ fruit, 1 fat

Chicken-Potato Roast

LOW CALORIE

PREP: 20 MIN; ROAST: 1$\frac{1}{4}$ HR; STAND: 10 MIN

6 SERVINGS

For a savory, herb flavor, add dried rosemary or sage to the margarine mixture before brushing it on the chicken.

3 to 3$\frac{1}{2}$	pound whole broiler-fryer chicken
1	medium apple, cut into fourths
1	medium onion, cut into fourths
2	cloves garlic, cut into fourths
3	unpeeled medium baking potatoes, cut into fourths
2	tablespoons margarine, melted
1	teaspoon dried thyme leaves
1	teaspoon paprika
$\frac{1}{2}$	teaspoon salt

Heat oven to 375°. Fold wings of chicken across back with tips touching. Place apple, onion and garlic in body cavity. Tie or skewer drumsticks to tail. Place chicken, breast side up, on rack in shallow roasting pan.

Cut potatoes crosswise about three-fourths of the way through into $\frac{1}{4}$-inch slices. Place on rack around chicken. Mix remaining ingredients; brush over chicken and potatoes. Insert meat thermometer in chicken so tip is in thickest part of inside thigh muscle and does not touch bone.

Roast uncovered 1 to 1$\frac{1}{4}$ hours, brushing chicken and potatoes with margarine mixture every 30 minutes, until thermometer reads 180° and juice of chicken is no longer pink when center of thigh is cut. Let chicken stand 10 minutes before carving; keep potatoes warm. Discard apple, onion and garlic. Remove and discard chicken skin.

1 Serving: Calories 340 (Calories from Fat 155); Fat 17g (Saturated 5g); Cholesterol 85mg; Sodium 330mg; Carbohydrate 21g (Dietary Fiber 2g); Protein 28g
% Daily Value: Vitamin A 12%; Vitamin C 18%; Calcium 2%; Iron 12%
Diet Exchanges: 2 starch, 3 medium-fat meat, 1 vegetable

Chinese Pepper Chicken

LOW CALORIE

PREP: 15 MIN; MARINATE: 1 HR; COOK: 45 MIN

6 SERVINGS

The mild, sweet flavor of rice vinegar really lets the delicate flavors of this dish shine. If it is not available, substitute half cider vinegar and half water.

2	tablespoons reduced-sodium soy sauce
2	tablespoons rice vinegar
1	teaspoon sugar
2	teaspoons sesame or vegetable oil
1/2	teaspoon red pepper sauce
3 to 3 1/2	pound cut-up broiler-fryer chicken
2	tablespoons vegetable oil
1	teaspoon finely chopped gingerroot
2	cloves garlic, finely chopped
3	medium green onions, sliced (3 tablespoons)
1 1/2	cups sliced mushrooms (4 ounces)
3	medium bell peppers, cut into 1-inch pieces

Mix soy sauce, vinegar, sugar, sesame oil and pepper sauce in shallow glass or plastic dish or heavy resealable plastic food-storage bag. Add chicken; turn to coat with marinade. Cover dish or seal bag and refrigerate, turning chicken occasionally, at least 1 hour but no longer than 24 hours. Remove chicken from marinade; reserve marinade.

Heat vegetable oil in 12-inch nonstick skillet or Dutch oven over medium heat. Cook chicken in oil about 15 minutes, turning occasionally, until brown on all sides. Cover and cook over low heat about 20 minutes or until juice is no longer pink when centers of thickest pieces are cut. Remove chicken from skillet, using tongs; keep warm.

Drain all but 1 teaspoon drippings from skillet. Heat 1 teaspoon drippings and the marinade in skillet over medium-high heat. Stir in gingerroot, garlic and onions. Cook and stir about 30 seconds or until garlic is light golden brown. Stir in mushrooms and bell peppers. Cook about 5 minutes, stirring occasionally, until bell peppers are crisp-tender. Serve with chicken.

1 Serving: Calories 305 (Calories from Fat 170); Fat 19g (Saturated 5g); Cholesterol 85mg; Sodium 260mg; Carbohydrate 7g (Dietary Fiber 1g); Protein 28g
% Daily Value: Vitamin A 8%; Vitamin C 46%; Calcium 2%; Iron 10%
Diet Exchanges: 4 medium-fat meat, 1 vegetable

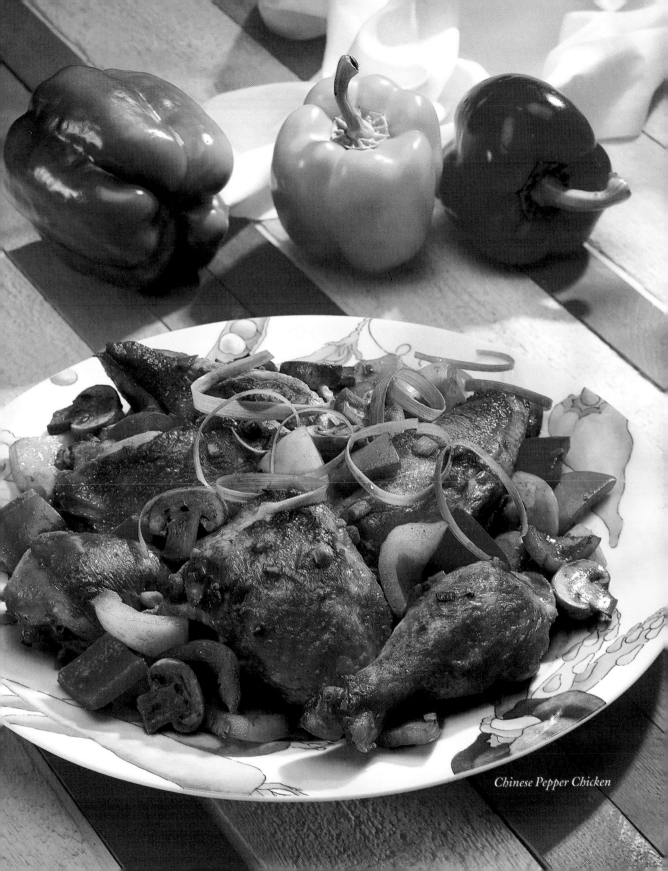

Chinese Pepper Chicken

Herbed Chicken and Vegetables

HIGH FIBER

PREP: 30 MIN; COOK: 1 HR

6 SERVINGS

Because potatoes are root vegetables, they contain many trace minerals that come from the surrounding soil, even after a good cleaning. Potatoes can be a particularly good source of chromium, manganese, molybdenum and copper.

3 to 3½   pound cut-up broiler-fryer chicken

¼   cup all-purpose flour

1   tablespoon chopped fresh or 1 teaspoon dried basil leaves

1½   teaspoons chopped fresh or ½ teaspoon dried oregano leaves

1   teaspoon paprika

¾   teaspoon chopped fresh or ¼ teaspoon dried marjoram leaves

¼   teaspoon pepper

2   tablespoons vegetable oil

1   cup dry white wine or chicken broth

12   small pitted ripe olives

8   medium carrots, cut into fourths

8   whole small onions

4   medium baking potatoes, cut into fourths

1   tablespoon cornstarch

1   tablespoon cold water

Remove skin and fat from chicken pieces. Mix flour, basil, oregano, paprika, marjoram and pepper. Coat chicken with flour mixture. Heat oil in nonstick Dutch oven or 12-inch nonstick skillet over medium-high heat. Cook chicken in oil about 15 minutes or until light brown on all sides; remove chicken and drain.

Stir wine, olives, carrots, onions and potatoes into Dutch oven; add chicken. Heat to boiling; reduce heat. Cover and simmer 35 to 40 minutes or until juice of chicken is no longer pink when centers of thickest pieces are cut. Remove chicken and vegetables; keep warm.

Mix cornstarch and cold water; stir into liquid in Dutch oven. Heat to boiling, stirring constantly. Boil and stir 1 minute. Serve with chicken and vegetables.

1 Serving: Calories 445 (Calories from Fat 170); Fat 19g (Saturated 5g); Cholesterol 85mg; Sodium 350mg; Carbohydrate 43g (Dietary Fiber 7g); Protein 32g
% Daily Value: Vitamin A 100%; Vitamin C 20%; Calcium 8%; Iron 20%
Diet Exchanges: 2 starch, 3 medium-fat meat, 2 vegetable

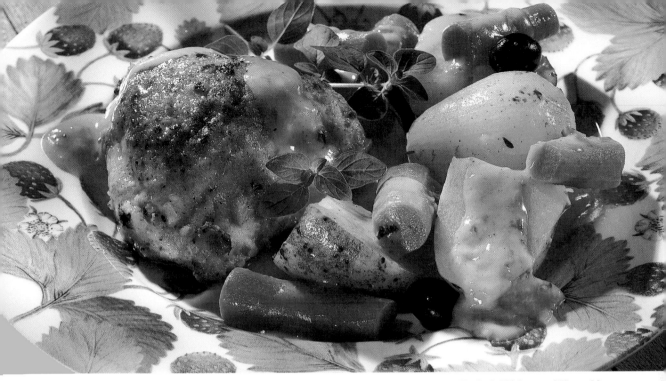

Herbed Chicken and Vegetables

Oriental Barbecued Chicken

LOW CALORIE

PREP: 10 MIN; BROIL: 14 MIN

4 SERVINGS

Hoisin sauce, a key ingredient in Chinese cooking, is a thick paste-like blend of soy sauce, garlic, chili peppers and various spices.

4	skinless, boneless chicken breast halves (about 1 pound)
$^1/_2$	cup hoisin sauce
1	tablespoon sesame or vegetable oil
1	tablespoon tomato paste
$^1/_2$	teaspoon ground ginger
2	cloves garlic, finely chopped

Set oven control to broil. Remove fat from chicken. Spray broiler or pan rack with cooking spray. Place chicken on rack in broiler pan. Mix remaining ingredients; brush some of the sauce over chicken.

Broil chicken with tops 5 to 7 inches from heat 7 minutes, turn, brush with sauce. Broil 7 minutes longer or until juice of chicken is no longer pink when centers of thickest pieces are cut.

While chicken is broiling, heat remaining sauce to boiling; boil 1 minute. Serve with chicken.

1 Serving: Calories 240 (Calories from Fat 80); Fat 9g (Saturated 2g); Cholesterol 70mg; Sodium 610mg; Carbohydrate 14g (Dietary Fiber 1g); Protein 27g
% Daily Value: Vitamin A 6%; Vitamin C 4%; Calcium 4%; Iron 10%
Diet Exchanges: $3^1/_2$ lean meat, 1 fruit

Lemon-Pistachio Chicken

LOW CALORIE

PREP: 10 MIN; COOK: 20 MIN

4 SERVINGS

Generally, unshelled nuts will keep their freshness twice as long as shelled ones. If you purchase unshelled pistachios, look for those with partially open shells. A closed shell means that the nutmeat is immature. Plus removing the nut is much easier when the shell is slightly open.

- 4 skinless, boneless chicken breast halves (about 1 pound)
- 1 teaspoon lemon pepper
- 1 tablespoon vegetable oil
- 3 tablespoons lemon juice
- 1 teaspoon grated lemon peel
- ¼ cup chopped pistachio nuts, toasted*

  Lemon slices, if desired

Remove fat from chicken. Flatten chicken breast halves to ¼-inch thickness between sheets of plastic wrap or waxed paper. Sprinkle both sides of chicken with lemon pepper.

Heat oil in 10-inch nonstick skillet over medium-high heat. Cook chicken, lemon juice and lemon peel in oil 15 to 20 minutes, turning chicken once and stirring juice mixture occasionally, until juice of chicken is no longer pink when centers of thickest pieces are cut. Serve chicken topped with juice mixture, nuts and lemon slices.

*To toast nuts, bake uncovered in ungreased shallow pan in 350° oven about 10 minutes, stirring occasionally, until golden brown. Or cook in ungreased skillet over medium-low heat 5 to 7 minutes, stirring frequently until browning begins, then stirring constantly until golden brown.

1 Serving: Calories 210 (Calories from Fat 100); Fat 11g (Saturated 2g); Cholesterol 70mg; Sodium 150mg; Carbohydrate 3g (Dietary Fiber 1g); Protein 26g
% Daily Value: Vitamin A 0%; Vitamin C 2%; Calcium 2%; Iron 8%
Diet Exchanges: 4 lean meat

Jamaican Jerk Chicken

LO CAL / LO FAT

PREP: 10 MIN; BAKE: 25 MIN

6 SERVINGS

This easy-to-fix recipe relies on the Jamaican cooking technique of "jerking"—rubbing a food with a dry mixture of herbs and spices—to boost flavor without adding fat and calories.

6   skinless, boneless chicken breast halves (about 1¹/₂ pounds)

2   tablespoons freeze-dried chives

1   tablespoon instant minced onion

1   tablespoon instant minced garlic

1   teaspoon crushed red pepper

1   teaspoon ground coriander

1   teaspoon ground ginger

1   medium pineapple (3 pounds), peeled and cut into 6 slices

Hot cooked rice, if desired

Heat oven to 425°. Spray rectangular pan, 13 × 9 × 2 inches, with cooking spray. Remove fat from chicken.

Place chives, onion flakes, garlic flakes, red pepper, coriander and ginger in blender or food processor. Cover and blend on high speed about 30 seconds or until blended. Rub both sides of chicken breast halves with chive mixture.

Place pineapple slices in pan. Place 1 chicken breast half on each pineapple slice. Bake uncovered about 25 minutes or until juice of chicken is no longer pink when centers of thickest pieces are cut. Serve chicken and pineapple over rice.

1 Serving: Calories 190 (Calories from Fat 35); Fat 4g (Saturated 1g); Cholesterol 70mg; Sodium 65mg; Carbohydrate 16g (Dietary Fiber 2g); Protein 25g
% Daily Value: Vitamin A 2%; Vitamin C 16%; Calcium 2%; Iron 8%
Diet Exchanges: 4 very lean meat, 1 fruit

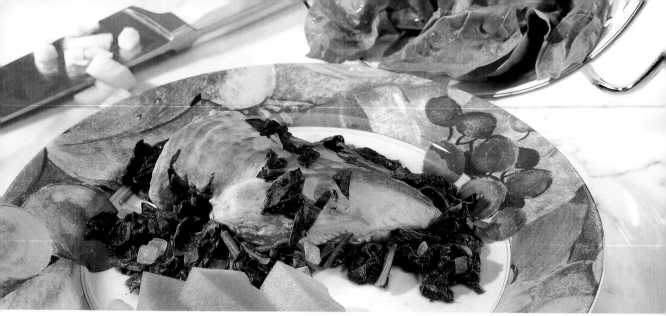

Spinach and Chicken Sauté

Spinach and Chicken Sauté

LO CAL / LO FAT

PREP: 10 MIN; COOK: 15 MIN

6 SERVINGS

Milk, a key player in our diets, supplies much of the calcium and vitamin D we need for healthy bones and teeth. Adequate amounts of calcium can also help prevent osteoporosis.

- 6   skinless, boneless chicken breast halves (about 1¹/₂ pounds)
- 1   cup skim milk
- ¹/₂ cup chicken broth
- 1   medium onion, chopped (¹/₂ cup)
- 1   bag (10 ounces) washed fresh spinach, chopped
- ¹/₄ teaspoon salt
- ¹/₄ teaspoon pepper
- ¹/₄ teaspoon ground nutmeg

Remove fat from chicken. Spray 12-inch nonstick skillet with cooking spray; heat skillet over medium heat. Cook chicken in skillet 2 minutes on each side; reduce heat to medium-low. Stir in milk, broth and onion. Cook about 5 minutes, turning chicken occasionally, until onion is tender.

Stir in spinach. Cook 3 to 4 minutes, stirring occasionally, until spinach is completely wilted and juice of chicken is no longer pink when centers of thickest pieces are cut. Remove chicken from skillet; keep warm.

Increase heat to medium. Cook spinach mixture about 3 minutes or until liquid has almost evaporated. Stir in salt, pepper and nutmeg. Serve chicken on spinach.

1 Serving: Calories 165 (Calories from Fat 35); Fat 4g (Saturated 2g); Cholesterol 70mg; Sodium 300mg; Carbohydrate 5g (Dietary Fiber 1g); Protein 28g
% Daily Value: Vitamin A 26%; Vitamin C 4%; Calcium 10%; Iron 8%
Diet Exchanges: 4 very lean meat, 1 vegetable

Broiled Sage Chicken

LO CAL / LO FAT

PREP: 10 MIN; MARINATE: 3 HR; BROIL: 14 MIN

6 SERVINGS

Prepare a flavorful sauce for this dish by adding mustard to reduced-fat sour cream. Begin with 2 to 3 teaspoons mustard per 1/2 cup of sour cream, and adjust to suit your taste. Just before serving, spoon the sauce over the chicken and sprinkle with sage leaves.

6	skinless, boneless chicken breast halves (about 1¹/₂ pounds)
2	tablespoons chopped fresh or 2 teaspoons dried sage leaves
2	tablespoons chopped onion
2	tablespoons reduced-fat sour cream
2	tablespoons lime juice
2	teaspoons Dijon mustard
¹/₂	teaspoon salt
¹/₄	teaspoon pepper

Remove fat from chicken. Mix remaining ingredients in shallow glass or plastic dish. Add chicken; turn to coat with marinade. Cover and refrigerate at least 3 hours but no longer than 24 hours.

Set oven control to broil. Spray broiler pan rack with cooking spray. Place chicken on rack in pan. Broil chicken with tops 5 to 7 inches from heat 7 minutes; turn. Broil about 7 minutes longer or until juice of chicken is no longer pink when centers of thickest pieces are cut.

1 Serving: Calories 145 (Calories from Fat 35); Fat 4g (Saturated 2g); Cholesterol 70mg; Sodium 290mg; Carbohydrate 2g (Dietary Fiber 0g); Protein 25g
% Daily Value: Vitamin A 2%; Vitamin C 0%; Calcium 2%; Iron 4%
Diet Exchanges: 3 lean meat

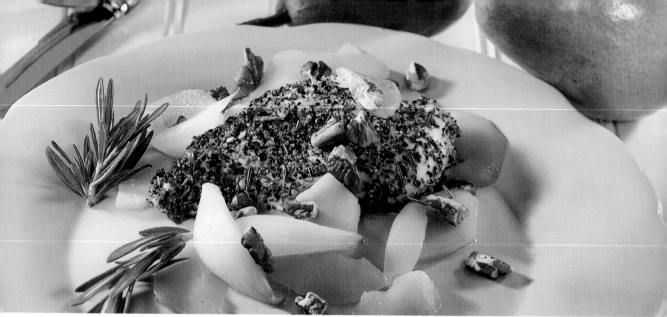

Peppery Chicken with Pears

Peppery Chicken with Pears

LO CAL / LO FAT / HI FIB

PREP: 15 MIN; BAKE: 25 MIN

4 SERVINGS

Cracked black pepper adds a slightly hot flavor and crunchy texture to this dish. If you prefer a less peppery bite, decrease the black pepper to 2 teaspoons.

4   skinless, boneless chicken breast halves (about 1 pound)

3   teaspoons cracked black pepper

1   teaspoon dried rosemary leaves, crumbled

¼   teaspoon crushed red pepper

2   medium pears (1 pound), peeled and cored, cut lengthwise in half, then cut crosswise into thin slices

1   medium onion, cut into 8 wedges and separated

2   tablespoons honey

2   tablespoons white wine vinegar

Coarsely chopped pecans or walnuts, toasted (page 242), if desired

Heat oven to 425°. Spray square pan, 9 × 9 × 2 inches, with cooking spray. Remove fat from chicken.

Mix black pepper, rosemary and red pepper. Sprinkle on both sides of chicken breast halves; press in gently. Place in pan. Bake uncovered about 25 minutes or until juice of chicken is no longer pink when centers of thickest pieces are cut.

While chicken is baking, spray 10-inch nonstick skillet with cooking spray; heat over medium heat. Cook pears and onion in skillet about 3 minutes, stirring frequently, until pears are almost tender. Stir in honey and vinegar; reduce heat to low. Cover and simmer 2 minutes longer. Serve pear mixture with chicken. Sprinkle with pecans.

1 Serving: Calories 225 (Calories from Fat 35); Fat 4g (Saturated 1g); Cholesterol 70mg; Sodium 65mg; Carbohydrate 25g (Dietary Fiber 3g); Protein 25g
% Daily Value: Vitamin A 0%; Vitamin C 4%; Calcium 2%; Iron 8%
Diet Exchanges: 3 very lean meat, 2 vegetable, 1 fruit

Lemon-Dill Chicken

LO CAL / LO FAT

PREP: 10 MIN; MARINATE: 3 HR; BROIL: 14 MIN

6 SERVINGS

When marinating chicken, you should always place it in a nonmetal container. Lemon juice, which is very acidic, can react with metal and cause undesirable and off-flavors to develop.

6	skinless, boneless chicken breast halves (about 1½ pounds)
½	cup chicken broth
¼	cup lemon juice
2	teaspoons dried dill weed
¼	teaspoon salt
¼	teaspoon pepper
1	medium onion, chopped (½ cup)
2	cloves garlic, finely chopped

Remove fat from chicken. Mix remaining ingredients in shallow glass or plastic dish. Add chicken; turn to coat with marinade. Cover and refrigerate at least 3 hours but no longer than 24 hours.

Set oven control to broil. Spray broiler pan rack with cooking spray. Remove chicken from marinade; reserve marinade. Place chicken on rack in pan. Broil chicken with tops 5 to 7 inches from heat 7 minutes. Turn chicken; brush with marinade. Broil about 7 minutes longer or until juice of chicken is no longer pink when centers of thickest pieces are cut. Discard any remaining marinade.

1 Serving: Calories 150 (Calories from Fat 35); Fat 4g (Saturated 1g); Cholesterol 70mg; Sodium 250mg; Carbohydrate 3g (Dietary Fiber 0g); Protein 25g
% Daily Value: Vitamin A 0%; Vitamin C 2%; Calcium 2%; Iron 6%
Diet Exchanges: 4 very lean meat

Thai Chicken with Cucumber-Red Onion Relish

LO CAL / LO FAT

PREP: 10 MIN; MARINATE: 15 MIN; BROIL: 14 MIN

6 SERVINGS

Refreshingly light and simple with a hint of hotness, this Thai-influenced cucumber relish, made without oil, is a sensational serve-along for broiled fish, pork chops and burgers, as well as chicken.

$1/4$ **cup water**

$1/2$ **cup lime juice**

$1/2$ **cup reduced-sodium soy sauce**

2 **serrano or jalapeño chilies, seeded and finely chopped**

2 **tablespoons sugar**

2 **cups chopped peeled cucumber**

1 **small red onion, cut lengthwise in half, then cut crosswise into thin slices**

6 **skinless, boneless chicken breast halves (about 1$1/2$ pounds)**

Place water, $1/4$ cup of the lime juice, $1/4$ cup of the soy sauce, the chilies and sugar in blender or food processor. Cover and blend on high speed about 1 minute or until blended. Place cucumber and onion in shallow dish; add blended mixture. Cover and refrigerate until serving.

Remove fat from chicken. Mix remaining $1/4$ cup lime juice and remaining $1/4$ cup soy sauce in shallow glass or plastic dish or resealable plastic bag. Add chicken; turn to coat with marinade. Cover dish or seal bag and refrigerate 15 minutes.

Set oven control to broil. Spray broiler pan rack with cooking spray. Remove chicken from marinade; reserve marinade. Place chicken on rack in broiler pan. Brush chicken with marinade. Broil chicken with tops 5 to 7 inches from heat 7 minutes. Turn chicken; brush with marinade. Broil about 7 minutes longer or until juice of chicken is no longer pink when centers of thickest pieces are cut. Discard any remaining marinade. Serve cucumber relish with chicken.

1 Serving: Calories 185 (Calories from Fat 35); Fat 4g (Saturated 1g); Cholesterol 70mg; Sodium 780mg; Carbohydrate 11g (Dietary Fiber 1g); Protein 27g
% Daily Value: Vitamin A 16%; Vitamin C 40%; Calcium 2%; Iron 8%
Diet Exchanges: 4 very lean meat, 2 vegetable

Golden Potato-Coated Baked Chicken

LO CAL / LO FAT / LO SODIUM

PREP: 10 MIN; BAKE: 25 MIN

4 SERVINGS

For a fresh-tasting accompaniment to this crispy chicken, sprinkle chopped fresh basil leaves over sliced roma (plum) tomatoes. Then drizzle on reduced-calorie or fat-free Italian dressing.

- 4   skinless, boneless chicken breast halves (about 1 pound)
- 1   egg white
- 2   tablespoons water
- ¼   cup mashed potato mix (dry)
- 1   tablespoon cornstarch
- 2   teaspoons Italian seasoning
- ¼   teaspoon ground red pepper (cayenne)
-     Butter-flavored cooking spray

Heat oven to 425°. Spray 12-inch pizza pan or jelly roll pan, 15½ × 10½ × 1 inch, with cooking spray. Remove fat from chicken.

Mix egg white and water. Mix potato mix, cornstarch, Italian seasoning and red pepper in a second bowl. Dip chicken into egg white mixture, then coat with potato mixture. Place in pan so pieces don't touch. Spray chicken lightly with cooking spray.

Bake uncovered about 25 minutes or until juice of chicken is no longer pink when centers of thickest pieces are cut (do not turn chicken while baking).

1 Serving: Calories 160 (Calories from Fat 35); Fat 4g (Saturated 1g); Cholesterol 70mg; Sodium 80mg; Carbohydrate 5g (Dietary Fiber 0g); Protein 26g
% Daily Value: Vitamin A 0%; Vitamin C 0%; Calcium 2%; Iron 6%
Diet Exchanges: 4 very lean meat, 1 vegetable

Honey-Spiced Chicken with Carrots and Grapes

LO CAL / LO FAT / LO SODIUM

PREP: 10 MIN; COOK: 16 MIN

4 SERVINGS

If your family prefers dark chicken meat, make this recipe with boneless thighs. Just keep in mind, however, that dark meat is higher in fat than white meat. A 3-ounce portion of dark meat has about 25 more calories and 1 gram more fat than the same-size portion of white meat.

4	skinless, boneless chicken breast halves (about 1 pound)
3	medium carrots, cut into julienne strips (2 cups)
2	cups seedless red grapes, cut in half
$1/3$	cup orange juice
1	tablespoon honey
1	tablespoon balsamic or red wine vinegar
$1/4$	teaspoon ground cinnamon
$1/4$	teaspoon ground nutmeg
	Hot cooked rice, if desired
	Chopped fresh parsley, if desired

Remove fat from chicken. Place chicken and remaining ingredients except rice and parsley in 10-inch nonstick skillet. Heat to boiling; reduce heat. Cover and simmer about 10 minutes, stirring occasionally, until juice of chicken is no longer pink when centers of thickest pieces are cut.

Remove chicken; keep warm. Heat sauce in skillet to boiling; reduce heat. Simmer uncovered 2 minutes, stirring occasionally. Serve chicken on rice; pour sauce over chicken. Sprinkle with parsley.

1 Serving: Calories 235 (Calories from Fat 35); Fat 4g (Saturated 2g); Cholesterol 70mg; Sodium 80mg; Carbohydrate 26g (Dietary Fiber 2g); Protein 26g
% Daily Value: Vitamin A 72%; Vitamin C 16%; Calcium 4%; Iron 8%
Diet Exchanges: $3^1/_2$ lean meat, 2 vegetable, 1 fruit

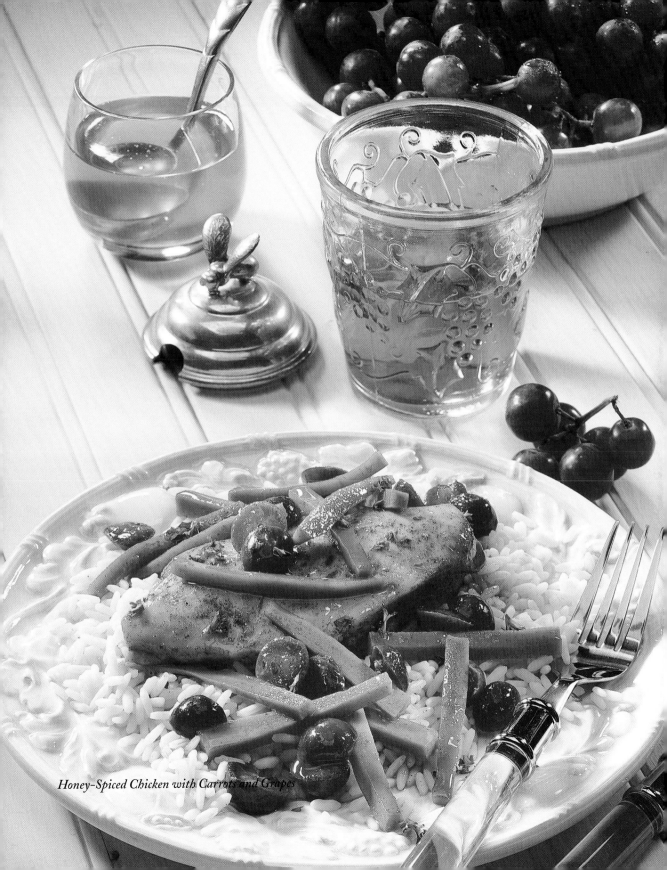

Honey-Spiced Chicken with Carrots and Grapes

Moroccan Chicken with Olives

LO CAL / LO FAT

PREP: 10 MIN; COOK: 20 MIN

4 SERVINGS

The seasonings in the sauce have their roots in Moroccan cooking, but the home-style flavor of this dish makes it all-American. This dish is especially enticing served over hot cooked couscous or rice (photo, page 233).

4	skinless, boneless chicken breast halves (about 1 pound)
1	can ($14^{1}/_{2}$ ounces) Italian-style stewed tomatoes
1	medium onion, cut into 8 wedges and separated
3	cloves garlic, finely chopped
$^{1}/_{2}$	cup dry white wine or chicken broth
$^{1}/_{2}$	teaspoon ground cumin
$^{1}/_{2}$	teaspoon ground ginger
$^{1}/_{2}$	teaspoon crushed red pepper
	Hot cooked couscous, if desired
	Chopped fresh parsley, if desired
	Imported Greek or Italian black olives, pitted and sliced, if desired

Remove fat from chicken. Drain tomatoes, reserving liquid. Cut up tomatoes.

Heat chicken, tomatoes, tomato liquid, onion, garlic, wine, cumin, ginger and red pepper to boiling in 12-inch nonstick skillet; reduce heat. Cover and simmer about 10 minutes or until juice of chicken is no longer pink when centers of thickest pieces are cut. Remove chicken; keep warm.

Heat sauce to boiling; reduce heat. Simmer uncovered 2 minutes. Serve chicken over couscous. Pour sauce over chicken. Sprinkle with parsley and olives.

1 Serving: Calories 180 (Calories from Fat 35); Fat 4g (Saturated 1g); Cholesterol 70mg; Sodium 350mg; Carbohydrate 11g (Dietary Fiber 1g); Protein 26g
% Daily Value: Vitamin A 6%; Vitamin C 12%; Calcium 4%; Iron 8%
Diet Exchanges: $3^{1}/_{2}$ lean meat, 2 vegetable

Wild Mushroom Herbed Chicken

LO CAL / LO FAT

PREP: 10 MIN; COOK: 20 MIN

6 SERVINGS

Wild mushrooms have a fuller and more robust flavor than the white cultivated mushrooms you find most often in the store. Look for varieties such as oyster, shiitake or chanterelle.

6	skinless, boneless chicken breast halves (about 1$\frac{1}{2}$ pounds)
$\frac{3}{4}$	pound assorted wild mushrooms (such as oyster, shiitake, chanterelle), coarsely chopped (5 cups)
1	medium leek, sliced (2 cups)
3	cloves garlic, finely chopped
1	can (14$\frac{1}{2}$ ounces) ready-to-serve chicken broth
$\frac{1}{2}$	cup dry white wine or chicken broth
2	tablespoons cornstarch
$\frac{1}{2}$	teaspoon dried thyme leaves
	Hot cooked couscous, if desired

Remove fat from chicken. Spray 12-inch nonstick skillet with cooking spray; heat over medium heat. Cook chicken in skillet about 12 minutes, turning once, until juice is no longer pink when centers of thickest pieces are cut. Remove chicken from skillet; keep warm.

Cook mushrooms, leek and garlic in same skillet about 3 minutes, stirring frequently, until leek is tender. Mix remaining ingredients except couscous; stir into mushroom mixture. Heat to boiling, stirring occasionally. Boil and stir about 1 minute or until slightly thickened. Add chicken; heat through. Serve chicken on couscous.

1 Serving: Calories 170 (Calories from Fat 35); Fat 4g (Saturated 1g); Cholesterol 70mg; Sodium 360mg; Carbohydrate 7g (Dietary Fiber 1g); Protein 28g
% Daily Value: Vitamin A 0%; Vitamin C 4%; Calcium 2%; Iron 12%
Diet Exchanges: 4 very lean meat, 1 vegetable

Curried Chicken Kabobs

LO CAL / LO FAT / LO SODIUM / HI FIB

PREP: 10 MIN; MARINATE: 30 MIN; BROIL: 15 MIN

4 SERVINGS

Curry powder is a blend of several spices, including cumin, turmeric and pepper just to name a few. In addition to the standard curry powder, there is also a style termed madras, which is much hotter than the basic variety.

- 4 skinless, boneless chicken breast halves (about 1 pound)

  Curry Marinade (right)
- 2 cups cubed pineapple
- 2 cups cubed papaya
- 2 medium green bell peppers, cut into 1-inch pieces

Remove fat from chicken. Cut chicken into 1-inch cubes. Place chicken in shallow glass or plastic dish. Prepare Curry Marinade; pour over chicken. Cover and refrigerate 30 minutes.

Set oven control to broil. Remove chicken from marinade; reserve marinade. Thread chicken, pineapple, papaya and bell pepper pieces alternately on each of four 15-inch metal skewers,* leaving space between each piece. Place on rack in broiler pan.

Broil with tops 5 to 6 inches from heat 10 to 15 minutes, turning and brushing frequently with marinade, until chicken is no longer pink in center. Discard any remaining marinade.

Curry Marinade

- 3 tablespoons lime juice
- 2 tablespoons honey
- 1 tablespoon vegetable oil
- 2 teaspoons curry powder

Beat all ingredients, using wire whisk.

To Grill: Heat coals or gas grill. Cover and grill kabobs 4 to 6 inches from medium heat 10 to 15 minutes, turning and brushing frequently with marinade, until chicken is no longer pink in center. Discard any remaining marinade.

*If using bamboo skewers, soak in water at least 30 minutes before using to prevent burning.

1 Serving: Calories 240 (Calories from Fat 55); Fat 6g (Saturated 2g); Cholesterol 70mg; Sodium 65mg; Carbohydrate 24g (Dietary Fiber 3g); Protein 26g
% Daily Value: Vitamin A 6%; Vitamin C 80%; Calcium 4%; Iron 8%
Diet Exchanges: 3 lean meat, 1½ fruit

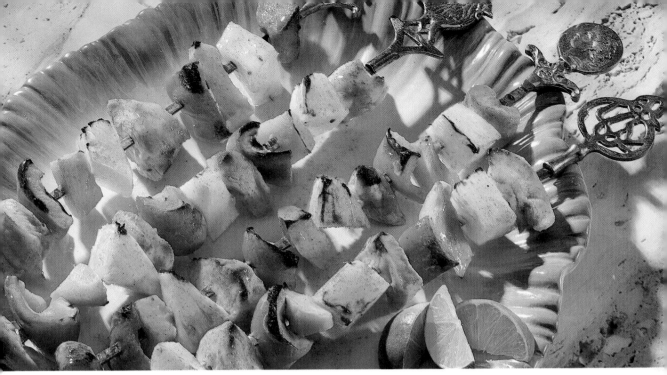

Curried Chicken Kabobs

Crunchy Garlic Chicken

LOW CALORIE

PREP: 15 MIN; BAKE: 25 MIN

6 SERVINGS

To boost the fiber in this dish, try wheat or bran flakes in place of the cornflakes. If you want variety, use a combination of all three!

6	skinless, boneless chicken breast halves (about 1¹/₂ pounds)
3	tablespoons margarine, melted
1	tablespoon skim milk
1	tablespoon chopped fresh chives or parsley
¹/₂	teaspoon salt
¹/₂	teaspoon garlic powder
2	cups cornflakes, crushed (1 cup)
3	tablespoons chopped fresh parsley
¹/₂	teaspoon paprika
	Cooking spray

Heat oven to 425°. Spray rectangular pan, 13 × 9 × 2 inches, with cooking spray. Remove fat from chicken. Mix margarine, milk, chives, salt and garlic powder. Mix cornflakes, parsley and paprika.

Dip chicken into margarine mixture, then coat lightly and evenly with cornflakes mixture. Place in pan. Spray chicken with cooking spray. Bake uncovered 20 to 25 minutes or until juice of chicken is no longer pink when centers of thickest pieces are cut.

1 Serving: Calories 220 (Calories from Fat 80); Fat 9g (Saturated 3g); Cholesterol 70mg; Sodium 430mg; Carbohydrate 9g (Dietary Fiber 0g); Protein 26g
% Daily Value: Vitamin A 18%; Vitamin C 6%; Calcium 2%; Iron 22%
Diet Exchanges: ¹/₂ starch, 3 lean meat

Chicken Breasts with Sun-Dried Tomato Sauce

LO CAL / LO FAT

PREP: 30 MIN; COOK: 25 MIN

4 SERVINGS

Use kitchen scissors to snip the sun-dried tomatoes into small pieces before soaking them in the chicken broth.

1/4 cup coarsely chopped sun-dried tomatoes (not oil-packed)

1/2 cup chicken broth

4 skinless, boneless chicken breast halves (about 1 pound)

1/2 cup sliced mushrooms

2 medium green onions, chopped (2 tablespoons)

2 cloves garlic, finely chopped

2 tablespoons dry red wine or chicken broth

1 teaspoon vegetable oil

1/2 cup skim milk

2 teaspoons cornstarch

2 teaspoons chopped fresh or 1/2 teaspoon dried basil leaves

2 cups hot cooked fettuccine, if desired

Mix tomatoes and broth. Let stand 30 minutes. Remove fat from chicken.

Cook mushrooms, onions and garlic in wine in 10-inch nonstick skillet over medium heat about 3 minutes, stirring occasionally, until mushrooms are tender; remove mixture from skillet.

Add oil to skillet. Cook chicken in oil over medium heat until brown on both sides. Add tomato mixture. Heat to boiling; reduce heat. Cover and simmer about 10 minutes, stirring occasionally, until juice of chicken is no longer pink when centers of thickest pieces are cut. Remove chicken from skillet; keep warm.

Mix milk, cornstarch and basil; stir into tomato mixture. Heat to boiling, stirring constantly. Boil and stir 1 minute. Stir in mushroom mixture; heat through. Serve over chicken and fettuccine.

1 Serving: Calories 275 (Calories from Fat 55); Fat 6g (Saturated 2g); Cholesterol 90mg; Sodium 250mg; Carbohydrate 26g (Dietary Fiber 2g); Protein 31g
% Daily Value: Vitamin A 2%; Vitamin C 2%; Calcium 6%; Iron 14%
Diet Exchanges: 1 starch, 3 lean meat, 2 vegetable

Chicken Picadillo

LO CAL / LO FAT

PREP: 15 MIN; COOK: 18 MIN

4 SERVINGS

Traditional Mexican picadillo is a ground beef hash that's made with a chili-spiced sauce and sweetened with raisins. This first-rate adaptation combines that same sauce with chicken, apple and a hint of orange.

4	skinless, boneless chicken breast halves (about 1 pound)
1	can (14$^1/_2$ ounces) Mexican-style stewed tomatoes
1	medium unpeeled tart cooking apple, coarsely chopped (1 cup)
$^1/_3$	cup orange juice
1 to 2	jalapeño chilies, seeded and finely chopped
2	tablespoons raisins
2	tablespoons white vinegar
3	tablespoons orange juice
2	teaspoons cornstarch
	Hot cooked rice, if desired
	Slivered almonds, toasted, if desired (page 242)

Remove fat from chicken. Cut chicken into 2-inch pieces. Drain tomatoes, reserving liquid. Cut up tomatoes.

Heat tomatoes, tomato liquid, apple, $^1/_3$ cup orange juice, the chilies, raisins and vinegar to boiling in 12-inch nonstick skillet; reduce heat. Stir in chicken. Cover and simmer about 10 minutes or until juice of chicken is no longer pink when centers of thickest pieces are cut.

Mix 3 tablespoons orange juice and the cornstarch; stir into chicken mixture. Heat to boiling, stirring constantly. Boil and stir 1 minute. Serve chicken mixture on rice. Sprinkle with almonds.

1 Serving: Calories 220 (Calories from Fat 35); Fat 4g (Saturated 1g); Cholesterol 70mg; Sodium 350mg; Carbohydrate 22g (Dietary Fiber 2g); Protein 26g
% Daily Value: Vitamin A 16%; Vitamin C 38%; Calcium 4%; Iron 10%
Diet Exchanges: 4 very lean meat, 1$^1/_2$ fruit

Savory Chicken and Rice

LOW CALORIE

PREP: 10 MIN; COOK: 25 MIN

4 SERVINGS

Skinless chicken breast, loaded with vitamin B6, niacin and zinc, is the leanest cut of chicken. Serving to serving, chicken breast has less fat than dark meat, but the amount of cholesterol is the same.

4	skinless, boneless chicken breast halves (about 1 pound)
1¹⁄₂	cups sliced mushrooms (4 ounces)
1	cup baby-cut carrots
1¹⁄₂	cups water
1	package (4.1 ounces) long grain and wild rice mix with chicken and herbs

Remove fat from chicken. Cut chicken into 1-inch pieces. Spray 10-inch nonstick skillet with cooking spray; heat over medium heat. Cook chicken in skillet about 5 minutes, stirring occasionally, until no longer pink in center.

Stir in remaining ingredients. Heat to boiling; reduce heat to low. Cover and simmer 15 minutes, stirring occasionally. Uncover and simmer about 3 minutes longer, stirring occasionally, until carrots are tender and liquid is absorbed.

1 Serving: Calories 220 (Calories from Fat 65); Fat 7g (Saturated 2g); Cholesterol 70mg; Sodium 200mg; Carbohydrate 13g (Dietary Fiber 2g); Protein 27g
% Daily Value: Vitamin A 96%; Vitamin C 0%; Calcium 2%; Iron 10%
Diet Exchanges: 1 starch, 3 lean meat

Wine-Poached Chicken Breasts

LO CAL / LO FAT

PREP: 5 MIN; COOK: 15 MIN

4 SERVINGS

Complement this entrée with a side of steamed broccoli spears, high in vitamins A and C. Squirt a little lemon juice over the veggies, and you have a healthy and elegant meal.

4	skinless, boneless chicken breast halves (about 1 pound)
¹⁄₂	cup dry white wine or chicken broth
1	tablespoon lemon juice
¹⁄₄	teaspoon salt

Remove fat from chicken. Place chicken and remaining ingredients in 10-inch nonstick skillet. Heat to boiling; reduce heat. Cover and simmer about 10 minutes or until juice of chicken is no longer pink when centers of thickest pieces are cut.

1 Serving: Calories 140 (Calories from Fat 35); Fat 4g (Saturated 1g); Cholesterol 70mg; Sodium 210mg; Carbohydrate 1g (Dietary Fiber 0g); Protein 25g
% Daily Value: Vitamin A 0%; Vitamin C 0%; Calcium 0%; Iron 4%
Diet Exchanges: 4 very lean meat

Balsamic Chicken

LOW CALORIE

PREP: 10 MIN; MARINATE: 2 HR; COOK: 30 MIN

6 SERVINGS

Balsamic vinegar has a sweet, rich, oak-like flavor.

12   skinless, boneless chicken thighs (about
      1¹/₂ pounds)

¹/₂   cup white wine or apple juice

¹/₂   cup chicken broth

2   tablespoons lemon juice

2   tablespoons balsamic or red wine vinegar

1   tablespoon chopped fresh or ¹/₂ teaspoon
      dried thyme leaves

2   teaspoons grated lemon peel

1   teaspoon paprika

¹/₂   teaspoon salt

¹/₄   teaspoon pepper

Remove fat from chicken. Mix remaining ingredients in shallow glass or plastic dish. Add chicken; turn to coat with marinade. Cover and refrigerate at least 2 hours but no longer than 24 hours.

Place chicken and marinade in 12-inch nonstick skillet. Heat to boiling; reduce heat. Cover and simmer 15 to 20 minutes or until juice of chicken is no longer pink when centers of thickest pieces are cut. Remove chicken; keep warm.

Heat marinade to boiling. Boil about 6 minutes or until liquid is reduced by half. Pour over chicken.

1 Serving: Calories 180 (Calories from Fat 80); Fat 9g (Saturated 3g); Cholesterol 70mg; Sodium 350mg; Carbohydrate 1g (Dietary Fiber 0g); Protein 24g
% Daily Value: Vitamin A 2%; Vitamin C 2%; Calcium 2%; Iron 12%
Diet Exchanges: 3 lean meat

Tequila Chicken

LOW CALORIE

PREP: 10 MIN; COOK: 23 MIN

4 SERVINGS

If you like, serve this Tex-Mex-style barbecued chicken over cooked brown rice or whole wheat fettuccine.

8   skinless, boneless chicken thighs (about
      1¹/₃ pounds)

1   medium onion, cut into 8 wedges and
      separated

1   can (15 ounces) tomato sauce

¹/₄   cup tequila or chicken broth

2   tablespoons molasses

1   tablespoon lime juice

1   teaspoon crushed red pepper

¹/₂   teaspoon ground cumin
      Hot cooked brown rice, if desired
      Lime wedges, if desired

Remove fat from chicken. Spray 12-inch nonstick skillet with cooking spray; heat over medium heat. Cook chicken in skillet about 5 minutes, turning once, until brown. Remove chicken from skillet.

Add remaining ingredients except rice and lime wedges to skillet. Heat to boiling; reduce heat. Return chicken to skillet. Cover and simmer about 10 minutes or until juice of chicken is no longer pink when centers of thickest pieces are cut. Uncover and simmer 3 minutes longer.

Serve chicken on rice; pour sauce over chicken. Serve with lime wedges.

1 Serving: Calories 305 (Calories from Fat 110); Fat 12g (Saturated 4g); Cholesterol 95mg; Sodium 730mg; Carbohydrate 18g (Dietary Fiber 2g); Protein 33g
% Daily Value: Vitamin A 12%; Vitamin C 14%; Calcium 8%; Iron 22%
Diet Exchanges: 1 starch, 3¹/₂ lean meat, 1 vegetable

Chicken Fricassee with Apples and Sour Cream Sauce

LO CAL / HI FIB

PREP: 10 MIN; COOK: 30 MIN

4 SERVINGS

The tart flavor and red color of Jonathan, McIntosh, Rome Beauty and York Imperial apples make them top picks for this creamy chicken dish simmered in a skillet.

- 4 skinless, boneless chicken thighs (about $^3/_4$ pound)
- $^1/_2$ cup all-purpose flour
- 2 teaspoons dried marjoram leaves
- $^1/_3$ cup buttermilk or skim milk
- 3 medium unpeeled tart red cooking apples, cut into 8 wedges
- 1 bag (16 ounces) frozen small whole onions, thawed
- 1 can (14$^1/_2$ ounces) ready-to-serve chicken broth
- $^2/_3$ cup reduced-fat sour cream

    Hot cooked mashed potatoes or noodles, if desired

Remove fat from chicken. Mix flour and marjoram in shallow dish or resealable plastic bag. Dip chicken into buttermilk, then coat with flour mixture.

Spray 12-inch nonstick skillet with cooking spray; heat over medium heat. Cook chicken in skillet about 5 minutes, turning once, until brown. Add apples, onions and broth. Heat to boiling; reduce heat. Cover and simmer about 10 minutes or until juice of chicken is no longer pink when centers of thickest pieces are cut. Remove chicken and onion mixture from skillet, using slotted spoon; keep warm.

Skim fat from liquid in skillet. Heat liquid to boiling; reduce heat. Simmer uncovered about 6 minutes or until liquid is reduced to $^1/_3$ cup. Stir sour cream into liquid in skillet. Heat over medium heat just until heated through. Serve chicken and onion mixture on mashed potatoes; pour sauce over chicken.

1 Serving: Calories 340 (Calories from Fat 90); Fat 10g (Saturated 4g); Cholesterol 55mg; Sodium 570mg; Carbohydrate 44g (Dietary Fiber 5g); Protein 23g
% Daily Value: Vitamin A 8%; Vitamin C 10%; Calcium 14%; Iron 16%
Diet Exchanges: 2 starch, 2$^1/_2$ lean meat, 1 fruit

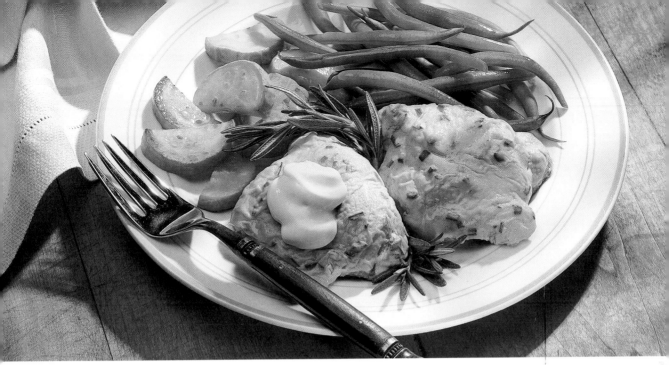

Rosemary-Mustard Chicken

LOW CALORIE

PREP: 10 MIN; MARINATE: 3 HR; BAKE: 20 MIN

6 SERVINGS

The name rosemary comes from the Latin word ros marinum, *meaning "dew of the sea." Traditionally, brides have carried rosemary at their weddings as a symbol of fidelity and remembrance.*

- 12 skinless, boneless chicken thighs (about 1½ pounds)
- 1 tablespoon chopped fresh or 1 teaspoon dried rosemary leaves, crumbled
- 3 tablespoons reduced-fat sour cream
- 3 tablespoons Dijon mustard
- ¼ teaspoon white pepper

Additional reduced-fat sour cream, if desired

Chopped fresh or dried rosemary leaves, crumbled, if desired

Remove fat from chicken. Mix 1 tablespoon rosemary, 3 tablespoons sour cream, the mustard and white pepper in shallow glass or plastic dish. Add chicken; turn to coat with marinade. Cover and refrigerate at least 3 hours but no longer than 24 hours.

Heat oven to 400°. Spray rectangular pan, 13 × 9 × 2 inches, with cooking spray. Place chicken in pan. Bake uncovered about 20 minutes or until juice of chicken is no longer pink when centers of thickest pieces are cut. Serve with sour cream and rosemary.

1 Serving: Calories 320 (Calories from Fat 180); Fat 20g (Saturated 6g); Cholesterol 120mg; Sodium 210mg; Carbohydrate 2g (Dietary Fiber 0g); Protein 33g
% Daily Value: Vitamin A 8%; Vitamin C 0%; Calcium 4%; Iron 10%
Diet Exchanges: 4½ medium-fat meat

Chicken with Basil-Seasoned Vegetables

LO CAL / HI FIB

PREP: 10 MIN; COOK: 27 MIN

4 SERVINGS

To make this mouthwatering chicken even healthier, serve it over cholesterol-free noodles.

   2   pounds chicken drumsticks

   1   can (14$^1\!/_2$ ounces) ready-to-serve chicken broth

   1   can (5$^1\!/_2$ ounces) spicy eight-vegetable juice

1$^1\!/_2$ teaspoons dried basil leaves

   $^1\!/_2$ teaspoon cracked black pepper

   1   bag (16 ounces) frozen green beans, potatoes, onions and red peppers, thawed

   2   tablespoons cornstarch

       Hot cooked noodles, if desired

Spray 12-inch nonstick skillet with cooking spray; heat over medium heat. Cook chicken in skillet about 10 minutes, turning occasionally, until brown on all sides. Remove chicken from skillet; keep warm.

Reserve 2 tablespoons of the broth. Add remaining broth, the vegetable juice, basil and pepper to skillet. Heat to boiling; reduce heat. Arrange chicken in broth mixture. Add vegetables. Cover and simmer about 15 minutes, stirring occasionally, until juice of chicken is no longer pink when centers of thickest pieces are cut. Remove chicken; keep warm.

Mix reserved 2 tablespoons broth and the cornstarch; stir into vegetable mixture. Heat to boiling, stirring constantly. Boil and stir 1 minute. Serve over chicken and noodles.

1 Serving: Calories 300 (Calories from Fat 110); Fat 12g (Saturated 4g); Cholesterol 90mg; Sodium 630mg; Carbohydrate 17g (Dietary Fiber 3g); Protein 34g
% Daily Value: Vitamin A 22%; Vitamin C 58%; Calcium 6%; Iron 20%
Diet Exchanges: 1 starch, 4 lean meat

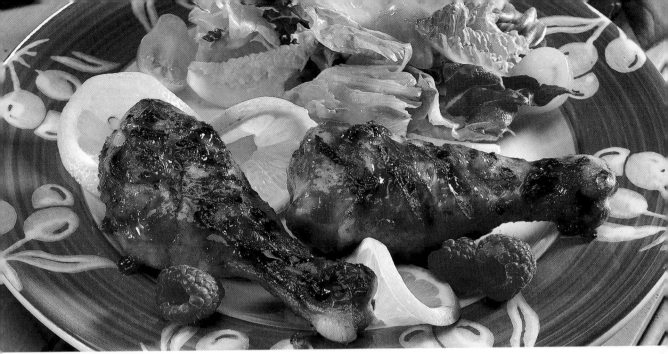

Grilled Raspberry- and Sage-Glazed Chicken Drumsticks

Grilled Raspberry- and Sage-Glazed Chicken Drumsticks

LO CAL / LO SODIUM

PREP: 10 MIN; GRILL: 25 MIN

4 SERVINGS

The fruity accents of raspberry and lemon fuse with the bite of brown mustard and sage to make these roasted drumsticks high in taste appeal and low in fat and calories. For a different twist, use strawberry or apricot spreadable fruit.

¹/₄   **cup seedless raspberry spreadable fruit**

1   **tablespoon lemon juice**

1   **tablespoon spicy brown mustard**

¹/₄   **teaspoon ground sage**

2   **pounds chicken drumsticks**

Brush grill rack with vegetable oil. Heat coals or gas grill for direct heat. Mix spreadable fruit, lemon juice, mustard and sage; brush over chicken.

Cover and grill chicken 4 to 6 inches from medium heat 20 to 25 minutes, turning once, until juice of chicken is no longer pink when centers of thickest pieces are cut.

To Broil: Set oven control to broil. Place chicken, skin sides down, on broiler pan. Brush with fruit mixture. Broil chicken with tips 7 to 9 inches from heat 20 minutes; turn. Brush with fruit mixture. Broil 10 to 15 minutes longer or until juice of chicken is no longer pink when centers of thickest pieces are cut.

1 Serving: Calories 270 (Calories from Fat 110); Fat 12g (Saturated 4g); Cholesterol 90mg; Sodium 130mg; Carbohydrate 10g (Dietary Fiber 0g); Protein 30g
% Daily Value: Vitamin A 0%; Vitamin C 0%; Calcium 4%; Iron 14%
Diet Exchanges: 4¹/₂ lean meat, ¹/₂ fruit

Southwestern Drumsticks

LO CAL / LO FAT

PREP: 20 MIN; BAKE: 45 MIN

4 SERVINGS

For a little extra fiber, toss in ¼ cup of oat bran with the cornmeal mixture.

2 **pounds chicken drumsticks**

⅔ **cup yellow cornmeal**

1 **teaspoon ground cumin**

1 **teaspoon chili powder**

¼ **teaspoon salt**

⅓ **cup buttermilk**

¼ **teaspoon red pepper sauce**

Cooking spray

1 **cup thick-and-chunky salsa, if desired**

Heat oven to 400°. Spray rectangular pan, 13 × 9 × 2 inches, with cooking spray. Remove skin and fat from chicken.

Mix cornmeal, cumin, chili powder and salt in heavy resealable plastic food-storage bag. Mix buttermilk and pepper sauce in medium bowl. Dip chicken into buttermilk mixture, then shake in bag to coat with cornmeal mixture. Place in pan. Spray chicken lightly with cooking spray.

Bake uncovered 40 to 45 minutes or until juice of chicken is no longer pink when centers of thickest pieces are cut. Serve with salsa.

1 Serving: Calories 220 (Calories from Fat 55); Fat 6g (Saturated 2g); Cholesterol 90mg; Sodium 240mg; Carbohydrate 19g (Dietary Fiber 2g); Protein 25g
% Daily Value: Vitamin A 2%; Vitamin C 0%; Calcium 4%; Iron 18%
Diet Exchanges: 1 starch, 2 lean meat, 1 vegetable

Creamy Chicken and Corn with Fettuccine

HIGH FIBER

PREP: 10 MIN; COOK: 5 MIN

4 SERVINGS

If you'd like to reduce the fat in this recipe even more, substitute fat-free cream cheese with garden vegetables for the roasted-garlic version.

8	ounces uncooked fettuccine or linguine
1	package (10 ounces) frozen whole kernel corn, thawed
6	medium green onions, sliced (6 tablespoons)
1	tub (8 ounces) roasted-garlic reduced-fat cream cheese
$1/3$	cup skim milk
$1^1/2$	cups cut-up cooked chicken or turkey
1	jar (2 ounces) diced pimientos, drained
$1/4$	teaspoon pepper
	Chopped fresh parsley, if desired

Cook fettuccine as directed on package. While fettuccine is cooking, spray 12-inch nonstick skillet with cooking spray; heat over medium heat. Cook corn and onions in skillet about 4 minutes, stirring frequently, until corn is crisp-tender.

Stir cream cheese and milk into corn mixture until blended. Stir in chicken, pimientos and pepper; heat through.

Drain fettuccine. Stir fettuccine into cheese sauce mixture; heat through. Sprinkle with parsley.

1 Serving: Calories 465 (Calories from Fat 135); Fat 15g (Saturated 8g); Cholesterol 120mg; Sodium 340mg; Carbohydrate 57g (Dietary Fiber 4g); Protein 30g
% Daily Value: Vitamin A 26%; Vitamin C 12%; Calcium 14%; Iron 22%
Diet Exchanges: 3 starch, 2 medium-fat meat, 2 vegetable, $1/2$ fat

Chicken Enchiladas

LO CAL / LO FAT

PREP: 20 MIN; BAKE: 25 MIN

6 SERVINGS

Fresh cilantro and parsley will keep up to a week in the refrigerator if they are wrapped in a slightly damp towel and placed in a sealed plastic bag. Just before using, wash the fresh herbs, and dry them with a paper towel.

1   cup bottled mild green sauce or salsa

1/4   cup cilantro sprigs

1/4   cup parsley sprigs

1   tablespoon lime juice

2   cloves garlic

2   cups chopped cooked chicken or turkey

3/4   cup shredded reduced-fat mozzarella cheese (3 ounces)

6   fat-free flour tortillas (6 to 8 inches in diameter)

1   medium lime, cut into wedges

Heat oven to 350°. Spray rectangular baking dish, 11 × 7 × 1½ inches, with cooking spray. Place green sauce, cilantro, parsley, lime juice and garlic in blender or food processor. Cover and blend on high speed about 30 seconds or until smooth. Reserve half of mixture.

Mix remaining sauce mixture, the chicken and 1/4 cup of the cheese. Spoon about 1/4 cup chicken mixture onto each tortilla. Roll tortilla around filling; place seam side down in baking dish.

Pour reserved sauce mixture over enchiladas. Sprinkle with remaining 1/2 cup cheese. Bake uncovered 20 to 25 minutes or until hot. Serve with lime wedges.

1 Serving: Calories 235 (Calories from Fat 55); Fat 6g (Saturated 3g); Cholesterol 50mg; Sodium 570mg; Carbohydrate 27g (Dietary Fiber 2g); Protein 20g
% Daily Value: Vitamin A 6%; Vitamin C 10%; Calcium 14%; Iron 12%
Diet Exchanges: 1 starch, 2 lean meat, 2 vegetable

Creamy Chicken and Vegetables with Noodles

LO CAL / LO FAT / HI FIB

PREP: 10 MIN; COOK: 5 MIN

4 SERVINGS

Using chicken or turkey breast in this colorful meal-in-a-skillet helps keep it lower in fat and calories than if you made it with dark meat.

5   cups uncooked medium noodles
     (10 ounces)

2   cups frozen mixed vegetables, thawed

6   medium green onions, sliced
     (6 tablespoons)

1   tub (8 ounces) garden vegetable fat-free
     cream cheese

1¼   cups skim milk

1½   cups cut-up cooked chicken or turkey

½   teaspoon garlic salt

¼   teaspoon pepper

     Chopped fresh parsley, if desired

Cook noodles as directed on package. While noodles are cooking, spray 12-inch nonstick skillet with cooking spray; heat over medium heat. Cook vegetables and onions in skillet about 4 minutes, stirring frequently, until vegetables are crisp-tender.

Stir cream cheese and milk into vegetable mixture until blended. Stir in chicken, garlic salt and pepper; heat through.

Drain noodles. Stir noodles into cheese sauce mixture; heat through. Sprinkle with parsley.

1 Serving: Calories 280 (Calories from Fat 45); Fat 5g (Saturated 1g); Cholesterol 70mg; Sodium 340mg; Carbohydrate 38g (Dietary Fiber 3g); Protein 24g
% Daily Value: Vitamin A 34%; Vitamin C 12%; Calcium 20%; Iron 16%
Diet Exchanges: 2 starch, 2 lean meat, 1½ vegetable

Chicken Paprika

LOW CALORIE

PREP: 10 MIN; COOK: 12 MIN

4 SERVINGS

This updated version of Chicken Paprikash allows you to enjoy the traditional spicy flavor of the dish with less fat and sodium and fewer calories than old-time recipes. For a touch of authenticity, use fiery Hungarian paprika, but use only 1 tablespoon to start and then add more to taste.

 2 medium onions, cut lengthwise in half, then cut crosswise into very thin slices

 2 medium stalks celery, sliced (1 cup)

 4 cloves garlic, finely chopped

 2 tablespoons paprika

 1/4 teaspoon pepper

 1 1/2 cups cut-up cooked chicken or turkey

 1/2 cup chicken broth

 1 cup reduced-fat sour cream

   Hot cooked wide egg noodles, if desired

   Chopped fresh parsley, if desired

Spray 10-inch nonstick skillet with cooking spray; heat over medium heat. Cook onions, celery and garlic in skillet about 5 minutes, stirring frequently, until onions are tender. Stir in paprika and pepper. Cook 1 minute, stirring constantly.

Stir in chicken and broth. Heat to boiling; reduce heat to medium. Stir sour cream into liquid in skillet. Heat over medium heat just until heated through. Serve over noodles. Sprinkle with parsley.

1 Serving: Calories 225 (Calories from Fat 80); Fat 9g (Saturated 4g); Cholesterol 65mg; Sodium 250mg; Carbohydrate 17g (Dietary Fiber 2g); Protein 21g
% Daily Value: Vitamin A 32%; Vitamin C 6%; Calcium 12%; Iron 10%
Diet Exchanges: 1 starch, 2 1/2 lean meat

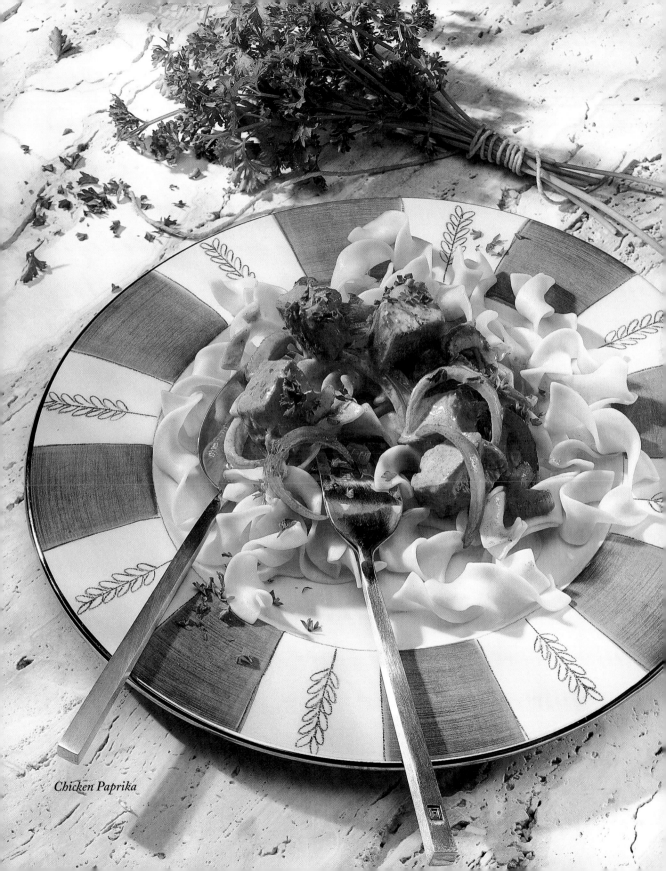

Chicken Paprika

Chicken Thermidor

LO CAL / LO FAT

PREP: 10 MIN; COOK: 15 MIN

4 SERVINGS

By using chicken instead of lobster, fat-free half-and-half in place of rich cream and no butter for sautéing, classic Lobster Thermidor is transformed into this exquisite, good-for-you entrée.

1½ cups sliced mushrooms (4 ounces)

2 large shallots or 1 small onion, finely chopped (¼ cup)

2 tablespoons all-purpose flour

1 teaspoon chicken bouillon granules

1¼ cups fat-free half-and-half or refrigerated fat-free nondairy creamer

1½ cups cut-up cooked chicken or turkey

2 tablespoons dry white wine or chicken broth

½ teaspoon dried tarragon leaves

4 slices white or whole wheat bread, toasted and cut into fourths, or 2 English muffins, split, toasted and cut into fourths

Grated Parmesan cheese, if desired

Spray 2-quart saucepan with cooking spray; heat over medium heat. Cook mushrooms and shallots in saucepan about 5 minutes, stirring frequently, until mushrooms are tender. Stir in flour and bouillon granules. Cook over medium heat, stirring constantly, until mixture is bubbly; remove from heat.

Gradually stir in half-and-half. Heat to boiling, stirring constantly. Boil and stir 1 minute. Stir in chicken, wine and tarragon; reduce heat to low. Cook about 5 minutes, stirring occasionally, until heated through. Spoon over toast. Sprinkle with cheese.

1 Serving: Calories 220 (Calories from Fat 45); Fat 5g (Saturated 2g); Cholesterol 45mg; Sodium 580mg; Carbohydrate 25g (Dietary Fiber 1g); Protein 20g
% Daily Value: Vitamin A 10%; Vitamin C 2%; Calcium 14%; Iron 12%
Diet Exchanges: 1 starch, 2 lean meat, 2 vegetable

Asian Turkey

LO CAL / LO FAT

PREP: 20 MIN; MARINATE: 2 HR; BAKE: 35 MIN

6 SERVINGS

If you have time, make the salsa the day before, so the flavors have a chance to develop and blend.

- 1/4 cup lemon juice
- 1 tablespoon grated lemon peel
- 2 tablespoons red wine vinegar
- 2 tablespoons reduced-sodium soy sauce
- 1 tablespoon olive or vegetable oil
- 1 clove garlic, finely chopped
- 1 1/2 pounds turkey breast tenderloins
- Red Onion Salsa (right)

Mix all ingredients except turkey and Red Onion Salsa in shallow glass or plastic dish. Add turkey; turn to coat with marinade. Cover and refrigerate, turning once, at least 2 hours but no longer than 24 hours. Prepare Red Onion Salsa.

Heat oven to 350°. Spray rectangular pan, 13 × 9 × 2 inches, with cooking spray. Remove turkey from marinade; discard marinade. Place turkey in pan. Bake uncovered about 35 minutes, brushing with pan drippings after 10 minutes, until juice of turkey is no longer pink when centers of thickest pieces are cut. Serve with salsa.

Red Onion Salsa

- 2 medium red onions, finely chopped (1 1/2 cups)
- 1 medium tomato, finely chopped (3/4 cup)
- 4 medium green onions, chopped (1/4 cup)
- 4 cloves garlic, finely chopped
- 1/4 cup lemon juice
- 2 tablespoons chopped fresh cilantro
- 2 tablespoons balsamic or red wine vinegar
- 1 tablespoon olive or vegetable oil
- 1 teaspoon reduced-sodium soy sauce
- 1/4 teaspoon ground red pepper (cayenne)

Mix all ingredients in glass or plastic bowl. Cover and refrigerate at least 2 hours.

1 Serving: Calories 190 (Calories from Fat 55); Fat 6g (Saturated 1g); Cholesterol 75mg; Sodium 260mg; Carbohydrate 8g (Dietary Fiber 1g); Protein 27g
% Daily Value: Vitamin A 2%; Vitamin C 10%; Calcium 2%; Iron 10%
Diet Exchanges: 3 lean meat, 1 vegetable

Turkey Tenderloins and Mixed Sweet Peppers

LO CAL / LO FAT

PREP: 10 MIN; COOK: 20 MIN

4 SERVINGS

Turkey tenderloins, unlike turkey breast slices, are pieces of whole muscle taken from the inside of the turkey breast. They are narrow pieces that are roughly triangular in shape with one pointed end.

1   **pound turkey breast tenderloins**

3   **medium red, yellow, orange or green bell peppers, cut into $1/4$-inch strips**

$2/3$ **cup chicken broth**

1   **teaspoon dried basil leaves**

$1/4$ **teaspoon salt**

$1/4$ **teaspoon ground red pepper (cayenne)**

3   **tablespoons white wine vinegar**

1   **tablespoon cornstarch**

Spray 10-inch nonstick skillet with cooking spray; heat over medium heat. Cook turkey in skillet about 5 minutes, turning once, until brown. Remove turkey from skillet.

Add bell peppers to skillet. Cook over medium heat about 3 minutes, stirring frequently, until crisp-tender. Stir in broth, basil, salt and red pepper. Heat to boiling; reduce heat. Return turkey to skillet. Cover and simmer about 10 minutes, stirring occasionally, until juice of turkey is no longer pink when centers of thickest pieces are cut.

Remove turkey from skillet; keep warm. Push bell peppers from center of skillet. Mix vinegar and cornstarch; stir into liquid in skillet. Heat to boiling, stirring constantly. Boil and stir 1 minute. Stir peppers into sauce to coat. Cut turkey into thin slices. Serve sauce with turkey.

1 Serving: Calories 155 (Calories from Fat 10); Fat 1g (Saturated 0g); Cholesterol 75mg; Sodium 370mg; Carbohydrate 9g (Dietary Fiber 1g); Protein 28g
% Daily Value: Vitamin A 20%; Vitamin C 100%; Calcium 2%; Iron 10%
Diet Exchanges: 3 very lean meat, 2 vegetable

Turkey Smothered with Maple Sweet Potatoes

LO CAL / LO FAT / HI FIB

PREP: 10 MIN; COOK: 20 MIN

4 SERVINGS

All the wonderful flavors of Thanksgiving dinner are wrapped up in this quick-as-a-wink entrée. Top it off with Streusel Pumpkin Pie (page 405) for dessert.

1   pound turkey breast tenderloins

⅓   cup dried cranberries, dried cherries or currants

¼   cup orange juice

⅓   cup reduced-calorie maple-flavored syrup

1   tablespoon margarine

¼   teaspoon ground cinnamon

1   can (23 ounces) sweet potatoes in light syrup, drained

Spray 10-inch nonstick skillet with cooking spray; heat over medium heat. Cook turkey in skillet about 5 minutes, turning once, until brown.

While turkey is cooking, heat cranberries, orange juice, maple syrup, margarine and cinnamon to boiling in 1-quart saucepan. Arrange sweet potatoes around turkey. Pour orange juice mixture over turkey and potatoes.

Cover and cook over low heat 10 minutes. Uncover and cook about 5 minutes longer or until juice of turkey is no longer pink when centers of thickest pieces are cut and sauce is slightly thickened.

1 Serving: Calories 290 (Calories from Fat 35); Fat 4g (Saturated 1g); Cholesterol 75mg; Sodium 170mg; Carbohydrate 42g (Dietary Fiber 7g); Protein 28g
% Daily Value: Vitamin A 80%; Vitamin C 22%; Calcium 4%; Iron 14%
Diet Exchanges: 2 starch, 2 very lean meat, 1 fruit

Turkey Smothered with Maple Sweet Potatoes

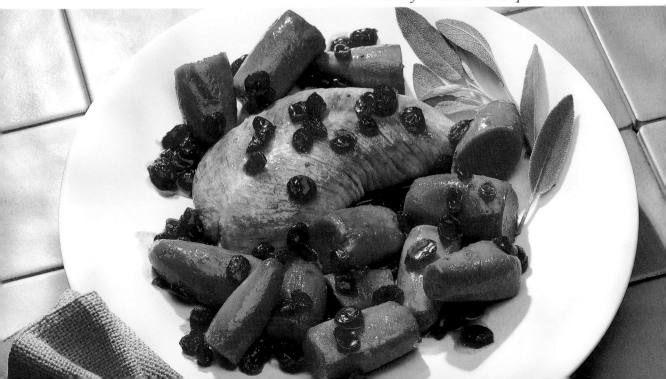

Roast Spiced Turkey with Cherry Sauce

LO CAL / LO FAT

PREP: 10 MIN; BAKE: 25 MIN

6 SERVINGS

For a no-fuss menu, serve this delectable fruit-sauced turkey with a tossed salad made from packaged mixed greens and steamed asparagus spears seasoned with a squirt of lemon juice.

- 1 tablespoon olive or vegetable oil
- 1 teaspoon ground allspice
- 1/2 teaspoon cracked black pepper
- 1/2 teaspoon salt
- 1 1/2 pounds turkey breast tenderloins
- 2/3 cup orange juice
- 1 tablespoon cornstarch
- 1 tablespoon packed brown sugar
- 1 bag (16 ounces) frozen dark sweet cherries, partially thawed and drained

  Hot cooked couscous, if desired

Heat oven to 350°. Spray rectangular pan, 13 × 9 × 2 inches, with cooking spray. Mix oil, allspice, pepper and salt. Rub top of turkey tenderloins with oil mixture. Place in pan.

Bake uncovered about 25 minutes or until juice is no longer pink when centers of thickest pieces are cut.

While turkey is baking, mix orange juice, cornstarch and brown sugar. Mix orange juice mixture and cherries in 2-quart saucepan. Heat to boiling, stirring constantly. Boil and stir 1 minute. Cut turkey into thin slices. Serve turkey with couscous; pour sauce over turkey.

1 Serving: Calories 220 (Calories from Fat 35); Fat 4g (Saturated 1g); Cholesterol 75mg; Sodium 250mg; Carbohydrate 23g (Dietary Fiber 2g); Protein 27g
% Daily Value: Vitamin A 2%; Vitamin C 12%; Calcium 2%; Iron 10%
Diet Exchanges: 4 very lean meat, 1 1/2 fruit

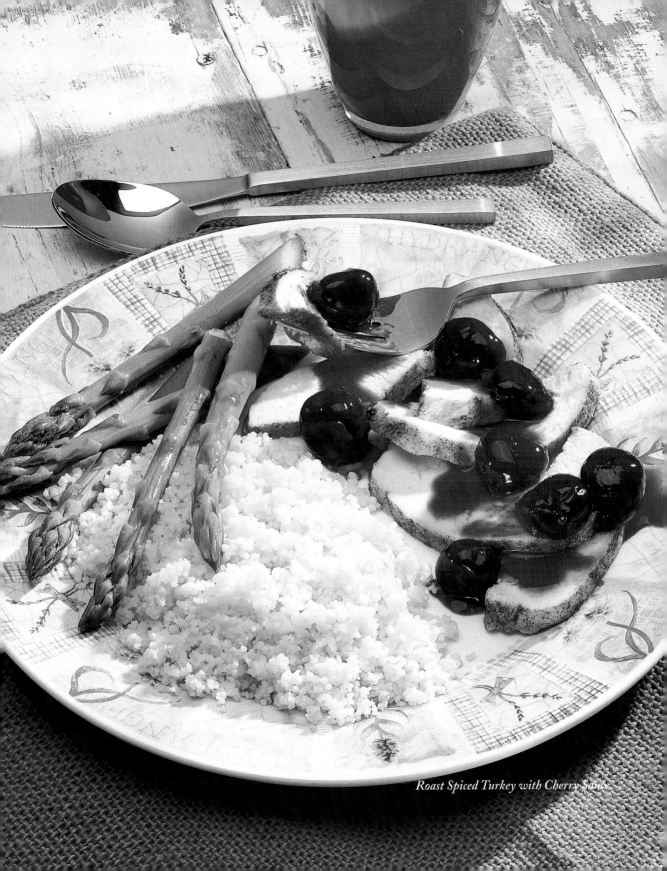

Roast Spiced Turkey with Cherry Sauce

Glazed Turkey Tenderloins

LO CAL / LO FAT / LO SODIUM

PREP: 5 MIN; COOK: 20 MIN

4 SERVINGS

For an impressive presentation, place turkey tenderloins, overlapping slightly, around the edge of a serving platter. Serve with hot cooked whole wheat spaghetti, and garnish with thin twists or curls of orange peel or thin slices of orange.

1 pound turkey breast tenderloins

1/3 cup orange marmalade spreadable fruit

1 teaspoon finely chopped gingerroot or 1/2 teaspoon ground ginger

1 teaspoon Worcestershire sauce

Spray 10-inch nonstick skillet with cooking spray. Cook turkey in skillet over medium heat about 5 minutes or until brown on one side; turn. Stir in remaining ingredients; reduce heat.

Cover and simmer about 15 minutes, stirring sauce occasionally, until sauce is thickened and juice of turkey is no longer pink when centers of thickest pieces are cut. Cut turkey into thin slices. Spoon sauce over turkey.

1 Serving: Calories 175 (Calories from Fat 10); Fat 1g (Saturated 0g); Cholesterol 75mg; Sodium 65mg; Carbohydrate 16g (Dietary Fiber 1g); Protein 27g
% Daily Value: Vitamin A 0%; Vitamin C 2%; Calcium 2%; Iron 8%
Diet Exchanges: 4 very lean meat, 1 fruit

Turkey Medallions with Cranberry and Orange

LO FAT / LO SODIUM / HI FIB

PREP: 10 MIN; MARINATE: 30 MIN; COOK: 20 MIN

4 SERVINGS

For a touch of the tropics, use pineapple chunks or mandarin orange segments in place of the cranberries.

1/4 cup dry white wine or chicken broth

2 tablespoons orange juice

1 1/2 pounds turkey breast tenderloins, cut into 1/2-inch slices

1 cup orange marmalade spreadable fruit

1/2 cup dried or fresh cranberries

1/4 cup orange juice

Mix wine and 2 tablespoons orange juice in shallow glass or plastic dish. Add turkey; stir to coat with marinade. Cover and refrigerate 30 minutes.

Place turkey and marinade in 10-inch nonstick skillet. Cook over medium heat 15 to 20 minutes, stirring occasionally, until turkey is no longer pink in center.

Mix spreadable fruit, cranberries and 1/4 cup orange juice in 1-quart saucepan. Cook over low heat 5 minutes, stirring occasionally. Place turkey on serving platter. Top with fruit mixture.

1 Serving: Calories 460 (Calories from Fat 20); Fat 2g (Saturated 1g); Cholesterol 115mg; Sodium 110mg; Carbohydrate 70g (Dietary Fiber 6g); Protein 41g
% Daily Value: Vitamin A 0%; Vitamin C 26%; Calcium 4%; Iron 16%
Diet Exchanges: 5 1/2 very lean meat, 4 1/2 fruit

Eggplant-Turkey Parmigiana

LOW CALORIE

PREP: 25 MIN; BAKE: 20 MIN

6 SERVINGS

1/2 cup dry bread crumbs

2 teaspoons chopped fresh or 1/2 teaspoon dried oregano leaves

1 1/2 pounds uncooked turkey breast slices, about 1/4 inch thick

2 egg whites, slightly beaten

2 cups cubed peeled eggplant

1 1/2 cups spaghetti sauce

1/2 cup shredded reduced-fat mozzarella cheese (2 ounces)

1/2 cup grated Parmesan cheese

Heat oven to 375°. Spray 10-inch nonstick skillet with cooking spray. Mix bread crumbs and oregano. Dip turkey into egg whites, then coat with bread crumb mixture.

Heat skillet about 30 seconds. Cook half of the turkey in skillet 3 to 4 minutes, turning once, until light brown. Repeat with remaining turkey.

Spray rectangular baking dish, 13 × 9 × 2 inches, with cooking spray. Place turkey in single layer in baking dish. Top with eggplant, spaghetti sauce and cheeses. Bake uncovered about 20 minutes or until cheese is bubbly and mixture is heated through.

1 Serving: Calories 280 (Calories from Fat 65); Fat 7g (Saturated 3g); Cholesterol 85mg; Sodium 630mg; Carbohydrate 21g (Dietary Fiber 2g); Protein 35g
% Daily Value: Vitamin A 6%; Vitamin C 8%; Calcium 20%; Iron 6%
Diet Exchanges: 1 starch, 4 very lean meat, 1 vegetable, 1 fat

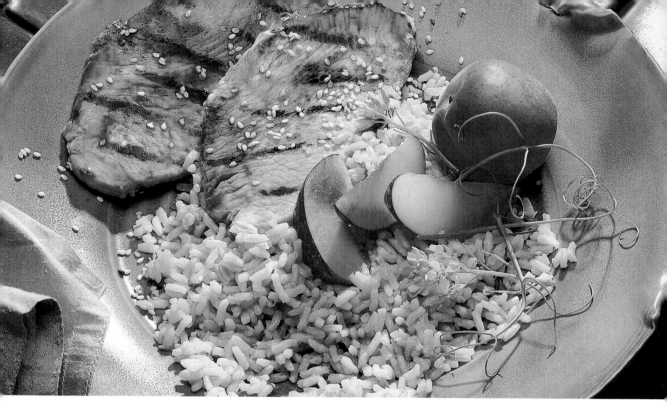

Grilled Sesame-Ginger Turkey Slices

Grilled Sesame-Ginger Turkey Slices

LO CAL / LO FAT

PREP: 5 MIN; GRILL: 20 MIN

4 SERVINGS

If you can't find turkey breast slices in your supermarket, use boneless, skinless breast halves pounded to ¼-inch thickness.

2 tablespoons teriyaki sauce

1 tablespoon sesame seed, toasted (page 124)

1 teaspoon ground ginger

1 pound uncooked turkey breast slices, about ¼ inch thick

4 cups hot cooked rice, if desired

Heat coals or gas grill. Mix teriyaki sauce, sesame seed and ginger.

Cover and grill turkey 4 to 6 inches from medium heat 15 to 20 minutes, brushing frequently with sauce mixture and turning after 10 minutes, until turkey is no longer pink in center. Discard any remaining sauce mixture. Serve turkey with rice.

1 Serving: Calories 135 (Calories from Fat 20); Fat 2g (Saturated 1g); Cholesterol 75mg; Sodium 390mg; Carbohydrate 2g (Dietary Fiber 0g); Protein 27g
% Daily Value: Vitamin A 0%; Vitamin C 0%; Calcium 2%; Iron 10%
Diet Exchanges: 4 very lean meat

Turkey with Herb-and-Garlic Sour Cream Sauce

LO CAL / LO FAT / HI FIB

PREP: 10 MIN; COOK: 16 MIN

4 SERVINGS

Turkey breast slices are crosswise cutlets that are cut from the breast. They are normally between ¹/₄ and ³/₈ inch thick. Look for packages of the slices in your supermarket's poultry case.

1   pound uncooked turkey breast slices, about ¹/₄ inch thick

1   bag (16 ounces) baby-cut carrots

3   medium stalks celery, sliced (1¹/₂ cups)

1   can (14¹/₂ ounces) ready-to-serve chicken broth

1   envelope (1.2 ounces) herb-and-garlic soup mix

³/₄   cup reduced-fat sour cream

2   tablespoons all-purpose flour

2   tablespoons Dijon mustard

Hot cooked noodles, if desired

Spray 12-inch nonstick skillet with cooking spray; heat over medium heat. Cook turkey in skillet about 5 minutes, turning once, until brown. Remove turkey from skillet.

Add carrots and celery to skillet. Stir in broth and soup mix (dry). Heat to boiling; reduce heat. Add turkey. Cover and simmer about 6 minutes, stirring occasionally, until turkey is no longer pink in center. Remove turkey and vegetables from skillet, using slotted spoon; keep warm.

Mix sour cream, flour and mustard until blended. Beat sour cream mixture into liquid in skillet with wire whisk. Heat over medium heat about 1 minute, beating constantly with whisk, just until heated through. Serve turkey and vegetables on noodles; pour sauce over turkey.

1 Serving: Calories 275 (Calories from Fat 45); Fat 5g (Saturated 3g); Cholesterol 90mg; Sodium 1430mg; Carbohydrate 28g (Dietary Fiber 5g); Protein 34g
% Daily Value: Vitamin A 100%; Vitamin C 12%; Calcium 14%; Iron 16%
Diet Exchanges: 1 starch, 3 very lean meat, 3 vegetable

Country French Turkey and Red Potatoes

LO FAT / LO SODIUM / HI FIB

PREP: 10 MIN; COOK: 18 MIN

4 SERVINGS

¼ cup all-purpose flour

⅛ teaspoon pepper

1 pound uncooked turkey breast slices, about ¼ inch thick

1 pound mushrooms, cut in half

8 large shallots, cut into fourths

8 small red potatoes (about ¾ pound), cut into 6 wedges

⅓ cup dry white wine or chicken broth

½ teaspoon dried rosemary leaves

Mix flour and pepper in shallow dish or resealable plastic bag. Coat turkey with flour mixture. Spray 12-inch nonstick skillet with cooking spray; heat over medium heat. Cook turkey in skillet about 5 minutes, turning once, until brown. Remove turkey from skillet; keep warm.

Add mushrooms and shallots to skillet. Cook about 3 minutes, stirring frequently, until shallots are tender. Stir in remaining ingredients. Heat to boiling, stirring constantly. Boil and stir 2 minutes. Add turkey; reduce heat to low. Cover and simmer about 6 minutes, stirring occasionally, until turkey is no longer pink in center.

1 Serving: Calories 370 (Calories from Fat 20); Fat 2g (Saturated 1g); Cholesterol 75mg; Sodium 75mg; Carbohydrate 61g (Dietary Fiber 7g); Protein 34g
% Daily Value: Vitamin A 2%; Vitamin C 28%; Calcium 6%; Iron 34%
Diet Exchanges: 4 starch, 2 very lean meat

Baked Turkey Roll-Ups

LO CAL / LO FAT

PREP: 15 MIN; BAKE: 25 MIN

6 SERVINGS

Let's talk turkey! Turkey breast is heralded as a top meat choice. It's loaded with phosphorus, a mineral important in building strong bones and helping muscles function properly.

½ cup fat-free ricotta cheese

½ cup frozen chopped spinach, thawed and squeezed to drain

¼ cup dry bread crumbs

2 tablespoons chopped fresh or 2 teaspoons dried basil leaves

1½ pounds uncooked turkey breast slices, about ¼ inch thick

¼ teaspoon salt

¼ teaspoon pepper

½ cup chicken broth

Heat oven to 350°. Spray square pan, 9 × 9 × 2 inches, with cooking spray. Mix ricotta cheese, spinach, bread crumbs and basil. Sprinkle turkey with salt and pepper.

Spread spinach mixture evenly over turkey slices; roll up. Place seam sides down in pan. Pour broth over rolls. Cover and bake about 25 minutes or until turkey is no longer pink in center.

1 Serving: Calories 160 (Calories from Fat 20); Fat 2g (Saturated 1g); Cholesterol 75mg; Sodium 300mg; Carbohydrate 6g (Dietary Fiber 1g); Protein 30g
% Daily Value: Vitamin A 16%; Vitamin C 2%; Calcium 8%; Iron 12%
Diet Exchanges: 4 very lean meat, 1 vegetable

Texas-Style Turkey and Taters

LO CAL / LO FAT / HI FIB

PREP: 10 MIN; COOK: 8 MIN

4 SERVINGS

Tailor this hearty spud supper to your family's taste by using the variety of barbecue sauce everyone likes best. Western-style and mesquite-flavored sauces are especially tasty.

1   pound ground turkey breast

1   medium onion, chopped (½ cup)

1   medium stalk celery, sliced (½ cup)

2   cloves garlic, finely chopped

1   cup barbecue sauce

1   can (4 ounces) chopped green chilies, drained

4   hot baked potatoes

Cook turkey, onion, celery and garlic in 10-inch nonstick skillet over medium-high heat about 5 minutes, stirring occasionally, until turkey is no longer pink and vegetables are tender.

Stir in barbecue sauce and chilies. Cook uncovered about 3 minutes, stirring frequently, until heated through. Spoon turkey mixture over baked potatoes.

1 Serving: Calories 300 (Calories from Fat 20); Fat 2g (Saturated 1g); Cholesterol 75mg; Sodium 620mg; Carbohydrate 43g (Dietary Fiber 4g); Protein 31g
% Daily Value: Vitamin A 6%; Vitamin C 30%; Calcium 4%; Iron 20%
Diet Exchanges: 3 starch, 2 very lean meat

California-Style Turkey Patties with Corn and Tomato Relish

LO CAL / LO FAT

PREP: 10 MIN; BROIL: 12 MIN

6 SERVINGS

Another time, use this tangy, multicolored relish to top off grilled or broiled fish or chicken breasts.

1½   pounds ground turkey breast

1   medium onion, chopped (½ cup)

1   cup soft bread crumbs (about 1½ slices bread)

½   teaspoon salt

¼   teaspoon pepper

⅓   cup chicken broth

    Corn and Tomato Relish (right)

Mix turkey, onion, bread crumbs, salt, pepper and broth. Shape mixture into 6 patties, each about ½ inch thick.

Set oven control to broil. Spray broiler pan rack with cooking spray. Place patties on rack in broiler pan. Broil with tops 4 inches from heat about 12 minutes, turning once, until no longer pink in center. Serve patties with Corn and Tomato Relish.

Corn and Tomato Relish

1   can (11 ounces) whole kernel corn with red and green peppers, drained

2   medium stalks celery, sliced (1 cup)

12   cherry tomatoes, cut into fourths

2   tablespoons lemon juice

Mix all ingredients.

1 Serving: Calories 220 (Calories from Fat 20); Fat 2g (Saturated 1g); Cholesterol 100mg; Sodium 470mg; Carbohydrate 16g (Dietary Fiber 2g); Protein 37g
% Daily Value: Vitamin A 2%; Vitamin C 10%; Calcium 4%; Iron 14%
Diet Exchanges: 4 very lean meat, 3 vegetable

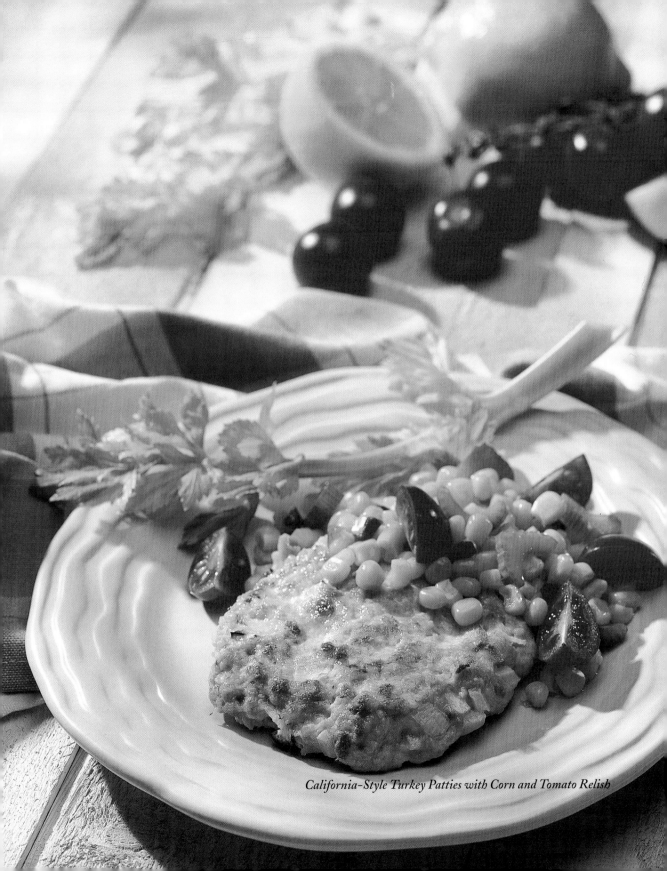

California-Style Turkey Patties with Corn and Tomato Relish

Wild Rice and Turkey Casserole

LOW CALORIE

PREP: 10 MIN; BAKE: 1 HR 5 MIN

6 SERVINGS

This dish is a great way to use up those Thanksgiving leftovers. If you like, toss in chopped vegetables, such as carrots or celery, for a healthy and hearty one-dish meal.

2	cups cut-up cooked turkey
2¼	cups boiling water
⅓	cup skim milk
1	small onion, chopped (¼ cup)
1	can (10¾ ounces) condensed cream of mushroom soup
1	package (6.2 ounces) fast-cooking long grain and wild rice mix

Heat oven to 350°. Mix all ingredients, including contents of seasoning packet from rice mix, in ungreased 2-quart casserole.

Cover and bake 45 to 50 minutes or until rice is tender. Uncover and bake 10 to 15 minutes longer or until liquid is absorbed.

1 Serving: Calories 170 (Calories from Fat 65); Fat 7g (Saturated 2g); Cholesterol 40mg; Sodium 500mg; Carbohydrate 12g (Dietary Fiber 0g); Protein 15g
% Daily Value: Vitamin A 2%; Vitamin C 0%; Calcium 4%; Iron 6%
Diet Exchanges: 1 starch, 2 lean meat

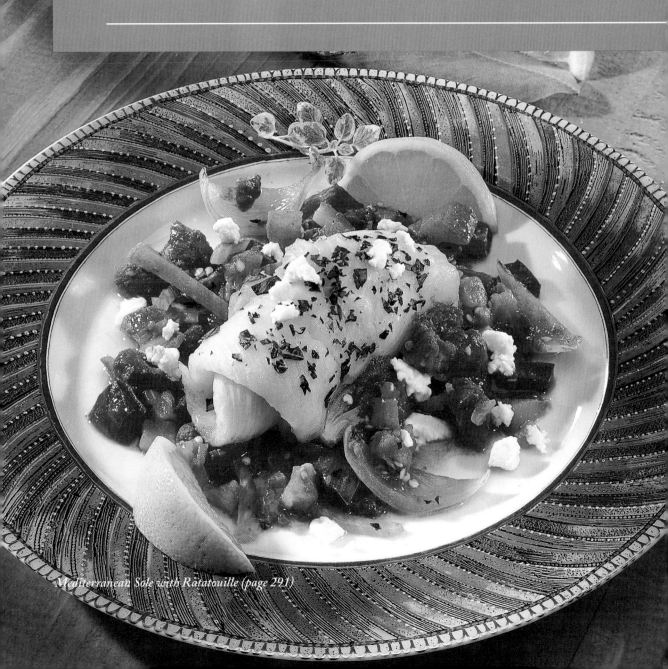

FISH
AND SEAFOOD

Mediterranean Sole with Ratatouille (page 291)

Walleye with Dill and Lemon Pepper Vegetables

LO CAL / LO FAT / HI FIB

PREP: 10 MIN; COOK: 15 MIN

4 SERVINGS

Impressive enough for company, this simple-to-fix fish recipe is low in fat and calories. Who could ask for more? Serve it with fresh fruit or sherbet for dessert.

1   pound walleye pike, haddock or other lean fish fillets, $1/2$ inch thick

1   can ($14^{1}/_{2}$ ounces) ready-to-serve chicken broth

1   small red onion, cut lengthwise in half, then cut crosswise into thin slices

2   teaspoons lemon pepper

$1/2$ teaspoon dried dill weed

1   bag (16 ounces) frozen baby peas, carrots, snow peas and baby corn cob, thawed

2   tablespoons cornstarch

Hot cooked fettuccine, if desired

Cut fish into 4 serving pieces. Reserve 2 tablespoons of the broth.

Heat remaining broth, the onion, lemon pepper and dill weed to boiling in 12-inch nonstick skillet; reduce heat. Cover and simmer about 3 minutes or until onion is tender.

Stir in vegetables. Arrange fish in vegetable mixture. Heat to boiling; reduce heat to medium. Cover and cook about 4 minutes or until fish flakes easily with fork.

Carefully remove fish from skillet, using wide slotted spatula. Mix reserved 2 tablespoons broth and the cornstarch; stir into vegetable mixture. Heat to boiling, stirring constantly. Boil and stir 1 minute. Serve fish and vegetables over fettuccine.

1 Serving: Calories 190 (Calories from Fat 20); Fat 2g (Saturated 0g); Cholesterol 65mg; Sodium 510mg; Carbohydrate 21g (Dietary Fiber 5g); Protein 27g
% Daily Value: Vitamin A 48%; Vitamin C 4%; Calcium 4%; Iron 8%
Diet Exchanges: 1 starch, 3 very lean meat, 1 vegetable

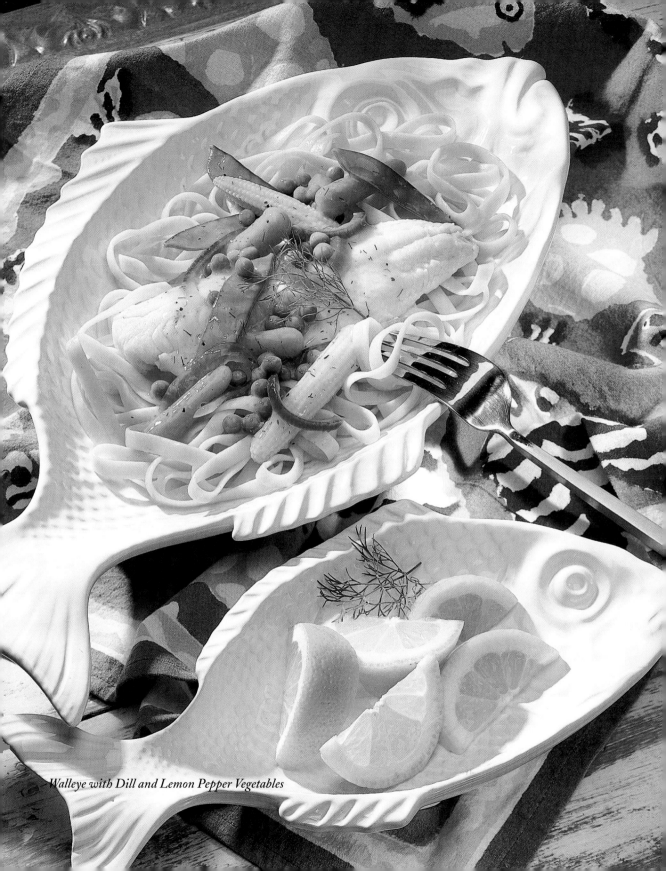

Walleye with Dill and Lemon Pepper Vegetables

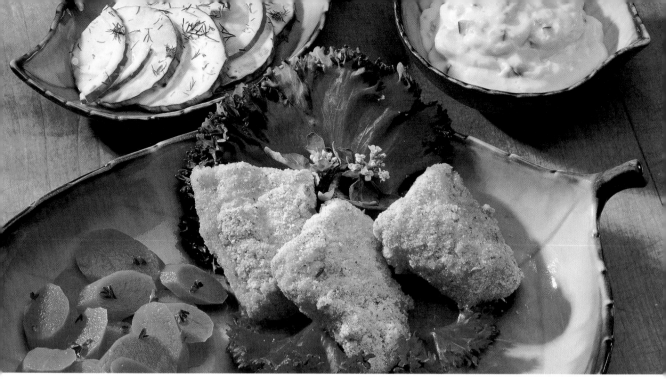

Cajun Oven-Fried Catfish

Cajun Oven-Fried Catfish

LO CAL / LO FAT

PREP: 10 MIN; BAKE: 10 MIN

4 SERVINGS

Cajun seasoning, a blend of spices and flavorings that's traditionally used to prepare foods such as gumbo and jambalaya, adds an inviting bite to this catfish.

1 **pound catfish, trout or other medium-fat fish fillets, about $^3/_4$ inch thick**

$^1/_4$ **cup buttermilk or skim milk**

1 **egg white, slightly beaten**

$^1/_3$ **cup yellow cornmeal**

$^1/_3$ **cup dry bread crumbs**

1 **teaspoon Cajun Creole seasoning**

Butter-flavored cooking spray

Lemon wedges, if desired

Move oven rack to position slightly above middle of oven. Heat oven to 500°. Remove and discard skin from fish. Cut fish into 2 × $1^1/_2$-inch pieces.

Mix buttermilk and egg white with fork. Mix cornmeal, bread crumbs and Cajun Creole seasoning. Dip fish into buttermilk mixture, then coat with cornmeal mixture. Place in ungreased rectangular pan, 13 × 9 × 2 inches. Lightly spray cooking spray on fish.

Bake uncovered about 10 minutes or until fish flakes easily with fork. Serve with lemon wedges.

1 Serving: Calories 190 (Calories from Fat 20); Fat 2g (Saturated 1g); Cholesterol 70mg; Sodium 220mg; Carbohydrate 16g (Dietary Fiber 1g); Protein 28g
% Daily Value: Vitamin A 2%; Vitamin C 0%; Calcium 6%; Iron 8%
Diet Exchanges: 1 starch, 3 very lean meat

Creole Mustard-Broiled Whitefish

LOW CALORIE

PREP: 10 MIN; BROIL: 8 MIN

6 SERVINGS

One of the favorite seasonings of Louisiana's German-Creole cooks, Creole mustard is spicy-hot with a whisper of horseradish. Look for it in food specialty shops or the mustard aisle of your supermarket.

6	whitefish, swordfish or other medium-fat fish steaks, about $3/4$ inch thick (about $1^1/4$ pounds)
$2/3$	cup reduced-fat mayonnaise or salad dressing
1	tablespoon chopped fresh chives
1	tablespoon Creole mustard or spicy brown mustard
$1/2$	teaspoon reduced-sodium Worcestershire sauce
$1/8$	teaspoon pepper

Set oven control to broil. Spray broiler pan rack with cooking spray. Place fish on rack in broiler pan. Broil with tops about 4 inches from heat 5 minutes.

While fish is broiling, mix remaining ingredients. Carefully turn fish, using wide slotted spatula. Spread mayonnaise mixture over tops of fish. Broil about 3 minutes or until fish flakes easily with fork.

Creole Mustard-Broiled Walleye Fillets: Substitute $1^1/2$ pounds walleye pike or other lean fish fillets, cut into 4 serving pieces, for the whitefish steaks. Broil with tops about 4 inches from heat about 5 minutes or until fish flakes easily with fork (do not turn). Spread mayonnaise mixture over fish during last 2 minutes of broiling.

1 Serving: Calories 305 (Calories from Fat 170); Fat 19g (Saturated 3g); Cholesterol 95mg; Sodium 300mg; Carbohydrate 2g (Dietary Fiber 0g); Protein 31g
% Daily Value: Vitamin A 2%; Vitamin C 0%; Calcium 2%; Iron 8%
Diet Exchanges: $4^1/2$ lean meat, 1 fat

Poached Tilapia with Raspberry Vinegar Sauce

LO CAL / LO FAT

PREP: 10 MIN; COOK: 6 MIN

6 SERVINGS

Tilapia, sometimes called St. Peter's fish, is a white fish that's raised primarily on fish farms. It has a delicate flavor and slightly firm texture.

1/2 cup reduced-fat sour cream

1/2 cup plain low-fat or fat-free yogurt

1 tablespoon raspberry vinegar or white wine vinegar

1/2 teaspoon chopped fresh or 1/4 teaspoon dried thyme leaves

2 cups dry white wine or vegetable broth

1 small onion, sliced

3 bay leaves

6 tilapia, red snapper or other lean fish fillets, 1/4 to 1/2 inch thick (about 1 1/2 pounds)

Mix sour cream, yogurt, vinegar and thyme. Cover and refrigerate until serving.

Heat wine, onion and bay leaves to boiling in 12-inch nonstick skillet; reduce heat. Cover and simmer 5 minutes. Add fish. Heat to boiling; reduce heat. Simmer uncovered about 6 minutes or until fish flakes easily with fork. Carefully remove fish from skillet, using wide slotted spatula. Serve fish with raspberry vinegar sauce.

1 Serving: Calories 145 (Calories from Fat 25); Fat 3g (Saturated 2g); Cholesterol 70mg; Sodium 130mg; Carbohydrate 6g (Dietary Fiber 0g); Protein 24g
% Daily Value: Vitamin A 4%; Vitamin C 0%; Calcium 8%; Iron 2%
Diet Exchanges: 3 very lean meat, 1 vegetable

Parmesan-Basil Perch

LO CAL / LO FAT

PREP: 10 MIN; BAKE: 10 MIN

4 SERVINGS

A perch is a perch by so many names! There are yellow perch, common or river perch and the pike perch, including the walleye and sauger or sand pike. Perch has a mild, delicate flavor and firm yet tender flesh.

2 tablespoons dry bread crumbs

2 tablespoons grated Parmesan cheese

1 tablespoon chopped fresh or 1 teaspoon dried basil leaves

1/2 teaspoon paprika

Dash of pepper

1 pound ocean perch or other lean fish fillets, cut into 4 serving pieces

1 tablespoon margarine, melted

1 tablespoon chopped fresh parsley

Move oven rack to position slightly above middle of oven. Heat oven to 375°. Spray rectangular pan, 13 × 9 × 2 inches, with cooking spray.

Mix all ingredients except fish, margarine and parsley. Brush one side of fish with margarine; dip into crumb mixture. Place fish, coated sides up, in pan. Bake uncovered 15 to 20 minutes or until fish flakes easily with fork. Sprinkle with parsley.

1 Serving: Calories 145 (Calories from Fat 45); Fat 5g (Saturated 1g); Cholesterol 60mg; Sodium 180mg; Carbohydrate 3g (Dietary Fiber 0g); Protein 22g
% Daily Value: Vitamin A 8%; Vitamin C 2%; Calcium 4%; Iron 4%
Diet Exchanges: 3 very lean meat, 1 fat

Mediterranean Sole with Ratatouille

LO CAL / LO FAT / HI FIB

PREP: 10 MIN; COOK: 28 MIN

4 SERVINGS

Fennel, with a celery-like bulb, is eaten as a vegetable. It has a very subtle anise flavor and is rich in vitamin A (photo, page 285).

1   medium red or green bell pepper, chopped (1 cup)

1   medium onion, cut into 8 wedges and separated

1   small bulb fennel, thinly sliced

1   small eggplant (1 pound), peeled and cut into $1/2$-inch cubes

1   can ($14^1/2$ ounces) diced tomatoes with garlic and onion, undrained

2   teaspoons chopped fresh or 1 teaspoon dried oregano leaves

4   sole, orange roughy or other lean fish fillets, about $1/4$ inch thick (about $3/4$ pound)

2   teaspoons chopped fresh or 1 teaspoon dried oregano leaves

Feta cheese, if desired

Spray 12-inch nonstick skillet with cooking spray; heat over medium heat. Cook bell pepper, onion and fennel in skillet about 5 minutes, stirring frequently, until vegetables are crisp-tender.

Stir in eggplant, tomatoes and 2 teaspoons oregano; reduce heat to medium-low. Cover and cook 15 minutes, stirring frequently.

Beginning from narrow end, roll up each fillet and secure with toothpicks; sprinkle with remaining oregano. Place fish rolls, seam sides down, in eggplant mixture. Cover and cook about 8 minutes or until fish flakes easily with fork.

Remove fish to serving platter, using slotted spoon. Remove toothpicks from fish. Serve eggplant mixture with fish. Sprinkle with cheese.

1 Serving: Calories 175 (Calories from Fat 20); Fat 2g (Saturated 1g); Cholesterol 55mg; Sodium 400mg; Carbohydrate 23g (Dietary Fiber 6g); Protein 22g
% Daily Value: Vitamin A 24%; Vitamin C 66%; Calcium 8%; Iron 10%
Diet Exchanges: $1/2$ starch, 2 very lean meat, 3 vegetable

Garlic- and Herb-Broiled Rainbow Trout

LOW CALORIE

PREP: 10 MIN; BROIL: 4 MIN

4 SERVINGS

Spooning the bread crumb mixture on only one side of the fish saves time and helps keep the coating crisp.

4   rainbow trout, lake perch or other medium-fat fish fillets, $1/4$ to $1/2$ inch thick (about 1 pound)

2   tablespoons lime or lemon juice

$2/3$ cup soft bread crumbs (about 1 slice bread)

1   teaspoon Italian seasoning

2   teaspoons olive or vegetable oil

$1/2$ teaspoon garlic powder

$1/4$ teaspoon pepper

Set oven control to broil. Spray broiler pan rack with cooking spray. Place fish on rack in broiler pan. Brush with lime juice. Broil with tops about 4 inches from heat 3 minutes.

While fish is broiling, mix remaining ingredients. Spoon bread crumb mixture on top of fish. Broil about 1 minute or until fish flakes easily with fork.

1 Serving: Calories 195 (Calories from Fat 80); Fat 9g (Saturated 3g); Cholesterol 75mg; Sodium 105mg; Carbohydrate 4g (Dietary Fiber 0g); Protein 25g
% Daily Value: Vitamin A 4%; Vitamin C 2%; Calcium 2%; Iron 6%
Diet Exchanges: 3 lean meat, 1 vegetable

Ginger Baked Flounder

LO CAL / LO FAT / LO SODIUM

PREP: 10 MIN; MARINATE: 1 HR; BAKE: 20 MIN

6 SERVINGS

Flounder is a fine-textured fish with a very mild flavor.

6   small flounder or sole fillets (about $1^1/2$ pounds)

$1/3$ cup dry sherry or apple juice

3   tablespoons lemon juice

2   teaspoons finely chopped gingerroot

1   teaspoon vegetable oil

2   teaspoons honey

$1/4$ teaspoon pepper

2   medium green onions, chopped (2 tablespoons)

2   cloves garlic, finely chopped

Spray rectangular pan, 13 × 9 × 2 inches, with cooking spray. Place fish in pan. Mix remaining ingredients; spoon over fish. Cover and refrigerate 1 hour.

Heat oven to 375°. Bake covered 15 to 20 minutes or until fish flakes easily with fork.

1 Serving: Calories 120 (Calories from Fat 20); Fat 2g (Saturated 0g); Cholesterol 55mg; Sodium 90mg; Carbohydrate 5g (Dietary Fiber 0g); Protein 20g
% Daily Value: Vitamin A 0%; Vitamin C 2%; Calcium 2%; Iron 2%
Diet Exchanges: 3 very lean meat

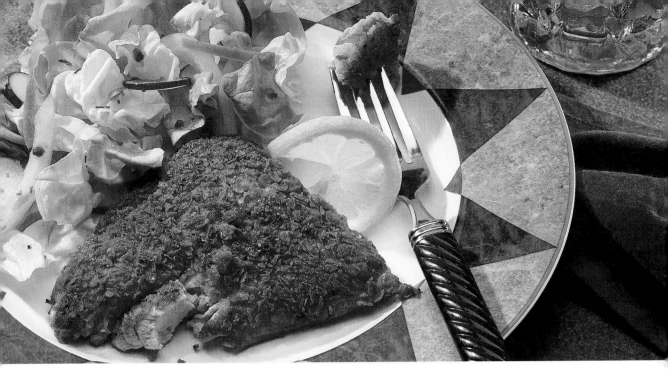

Potato-Crusted Salmon

Potato-Crusted Salmon

LOW CALORIE

PREP: 10 MIN; COOK: 6 MIN

4 SERVINGS

This crispy-coated fish tastes like it's deep-fried, but only uses 1 tablespoon of oil for cooking.

1 pound salmon, artic char or other medium-fat fish fillets, about ³/₄ inch thick

1 egg white, slightly beaten

2 tablespoons water

¹/₃ cup mashed potato mix (dry)

2 teaspoons cornstarch

1 teaspoon paprika

1 teaspoon lemon pepper

1 tablespoon olive or vegetable oil

Remove and discard skin from fish. Cut fish into 4 serving pieces. Mix egg white and water with fork. Mix potato mix, cornstarch, paprika and lemon pepper. Dip just the top sides of fish into egg white mixture, then press into potato mixture.

Spray 12-inch nonstick skillet with cooking spray. Heat oil in skillet over high heat. Cook fish, potato sides down, in oil 3 minutes. Carefully turn fish, using wide slotted spatula. Reduce heat to medium. Cook about 3 minutes longer or until fish flakes easily with fork.

1 Serving: Calories 220 (Calories from Fat 100); Fat 11g (Saturated 2g); Cholesterol 65mg; Sodium 160mg; Carbohydrate 5g (Dietary Fiber 0g); Protein 25g
% Daily Value: Vitamin A 4%; Vitamin C 2%; Calcium 4%; Iron 10%
Diet Exchanges: 3¹/₂ lean meat, 1 vegetable

Halibut-Asparagus Stir-Fry

LO CAL / LO FAT / HI FIB

PREP: 15 MIN; COOK: 10 MIN

4 SERVINGS

Halibut is one of the "big fish" in the pond, in this case the Atlantic or Pacific Ocean. Although it can weigh as much as 1 ton, it usually tips the scales between 50 and 100 pounds.

1	pound halibut, swordfish or tuna fillets, cut into 1-inch pieces
1	medium onion, thinly sliced
3	cloves garlic, finely chopped
1	teaspoon finely chopped gingerroot
1	package (10 ounces) frozen asparagus cuts, thawed and drained
1	package (8 ounces) sliced mushrooms (3 cups)
1	medium tomato, cut into thin wedges
2	tablespoons reduced-sodium soy sauce
1	tablespoon lemon juice

Spray 10-inch nonstick skillet with cooking spray; heat over medium-high heat. Add fish, onion, garlic, gingerroot and asparagus; stir-fry 2 to 3 minutes or until fish almost flakes with fork.

Carefully stir in remaining ingredients. Cook until heated through and fish flakes easily with fork. Serve with additional reduced-sodium soy sauce if desired.

1 Serving: Calories 180 (Calories from Fat 20); Fat 2g (Saturated 1g); Cholesterol 75mg; Sodium 390mg; Carbohydrate 11g (Dietary Fiber 3g); Protein 32g
% Daily Value: Vitamin A 8%; Vitamin C 22%; Calcium 4%; Iron 10%
Diet Exchanges: 4 very lean meat, 2 vegetable

Oven-Poached Halibut

LO CAL / LO FAT

PREP: 5 MIN; BAKE: 25 MIN

4 SERVINGS

Like most varieties of fish, halibut is naturally low in fat. Halibut has a firm eating texture and is mild flavored.

4	halibut, swordfish or tuna fillets, about 1 inch thick (about 1 1/2 pounds)
1/4	teaspoon salt
4	sprigs dill weed
4	slices lemon
4	black peppercorns
1/4	cup dry white wine or chicken broth

Heat oven to 450°. Place fish in ungreased rectangular baking dish, 11 × 7 × 1 1/2 inches. Sprinkle with salt. Place dill weed sprig and lemon slice on each. Top with peppercorns. Pour wine over fish. Bake uncovered 20 to 25 minutes or until fish flakes easily with fork.

1 Serving: Calories 140 (Calories from Fat 20); Fat 2g (Saturated 0g); Cholesterol 90mg; Sodium 290mg; Carbohydrate 1g (Dietary Fiber 0g); Protein 30g
% Daily Value: Vitamin A 2%; Vitamin C 2%; Calcium 2%; Iron 4%
Diet Exchanges: 4 very lean meat

Flounder Florentine

LO CAL / LO FAT / HI FIB

PREP: 15 MIN; BAKE: 30 MIN

4 SERVINGS

If you'd like a spicier flavor, increase the red pepper sauce to ¼ teaspoon.

2   packages (10 ounces each) frozen chopped spinach, thawed and squeezed to drain

1   pound flounder, sole or orange roughy fillets, about ½ inch thick

¼   teaspoon salt

½   cup roasted red bell peppers (from 7-ounce jar)

¼   cup chopped fresh or 2 teaspoons dried basil leaves

1   tablespoon skim milk

⅛   teaspoon red pepper sauce

Heat oven to 400°. Spread spinach evenly in ungreased rectangular pan, 11 × 7 × 1½ inches. Arrange fish on spinach. Sprinkle with salt.

Place bell peppers, basil, milk and pepper sauce in blender or food processor. Cover and blend on high speed about 15 seconds or until smooth; pour over fish. Cover and bake 25 to 30 minutes or until fish flakes easily with fork.

1 Serving: Calories 105 (Calories from Fat 10); Fat 1g (Saturated 0g); Cholesterol 50mg; Sodium 310mg; Carbohydrate 6g (Dietary Fiber 3g); Protein 21g
% Daily Value: Vitamin A 80%; Vitamin C 34%; Calcium 16%; Iron 10%
Diet Exchanges: 2 very lean meat, 1 vegetable

Snapper with Sautéed Tomato-Pepper Sauce

LO CAL / LO FAT

PREP: 10 MIN; COOK: 10 MIN

4 SERVINGS

For a bit of sweeter-tasting salsa, select a red, yellow or orange bell pepper.

1   pound red snapper, cod or flounder fillets

1   large tomato, chopped (1 cup)

1   small green bell pepper, chopped (½ cup)

1   small onion, sliced

2   tablespoons finely chopped fresh cilantro or parsley

¼   teaspoon salt

¼   cup dry white wine or chicken broth

If fish fillets are large, cut into 4 serving pieces. Spray 10-inch nonstick skillet with cooking spray; heat over medium heat. Arrange fish in single layer in skillet. Cook uncovered 4 to 6 minutes, turning once, until fish flakes easily with fork. Remove fish to warm platter; keep warm.

Cook remaining ingredients except wine in same skillet over medium heat 3 to 5 minutes, stirring frequently, until bell pepper and onion are crisp-tender. Stir in wine, cook until hot. Spoon tomato mixture over fish.

1 Serving: Calories 120 (Calories from Fat 20); Fat 2g (Saturated 0); Cholesterol 60mg; Sodium 250mg; Carbohydrate 5g (Dietary Fiber 1g); Protein 22g
% Daily Value: Vitamin A 4%; Vitamin C 22%; Calcium 2%; Iron 4%
Diet Exchanges: 3 very lean meat, 1 vegetable

Caribbean Swordfish with Papaya Salsa

LOW CALORIE

PREP: 10 MIN; MARINATE: 2 HR; BROIL: 15 MIN

4 SERVINGS

Papayas are ripe when their skin is golden yellow and they give slightly to gentle pressure when pressed; slightly green papayas will ripen more quickly if placed in a paper bag. Papaya is a good source of vitamin C.

- 4 swordfish or shark steaks, 1 inch thick (about 1¹/₂ pounds)
- 1 tablespoon grated lime peel
- ¹/₄ cup lime juice
- ¹/₄ cup grapefruit juice
- ¹/₂ teaspoon salt
- 1 clove garlic, finely chopped

  Papaya Salsa (right)

Place fish in ungreased square baking dish, 8 × 8 × 2 inches. Mix remaining ingredients except Papaya Salsa; pour over fish. Cover and refrigerate 2 hours. Prepare Papaya Salsa.

Set oven control to broil. Spray broiler pan rack with cooking spray. Remove fish from marinade; reserve marinade. Place fish on rack in broiler pan. Broil with tops about 4 inches from heat about 16 minutes, turning and brushing with marinade after 8 minutes, until fish flakes easily with fork. Discard any remaining marinade. Serve fish with salsa.

Papaya Salsa

- 1 large papaya, peeled, seeded and chopped (2 cups)
- ¹/₄ cup finely chopped red bell pepper
- 1 medium green onion, finely chopped (1 tablespoon)
- 1 tablespoon chopped fresh cilantro
- 2 to 3 tablespoons grapefruit juice
- ¹/₈ teaspoon salt

Mix all ingredients in glass or plastic bowl. Cover and refrigerate 1 hour.

1 Serving: Calories 220 (Calories from Fat 60); Fat 7g (Saturated 2g); Cholesterol 80mg; Sodium 450mg; Carbohydrate 14g (Dietary Fiber 2g); Protein 27g
% Daily Value: Vitamin A 12%; Vitamin C 74%; Calcium 4%; Iron 6%
Diet Exchanges: 4 very lean meat, 1¹/₂ fruit

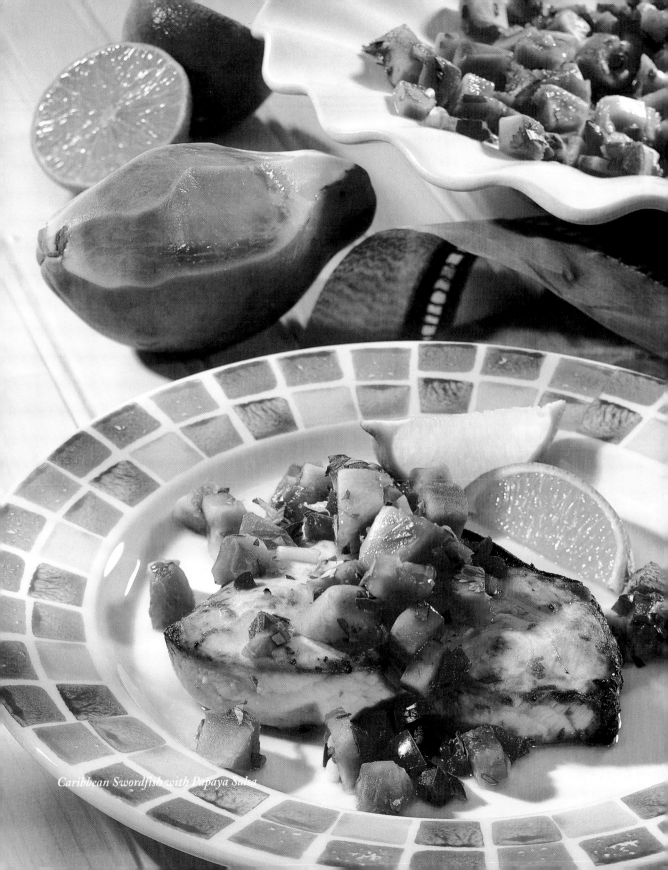

Caribbean Swordfish with Papaya Salsa

Teriyaki Swordfish Kabobs

LO CAL / LO FAT

PREP: 15 MIN; BROIL: 10 MIN

4 SERVINGS

Teriyaki marinade and sauce looks like soy sauce, and you'll find it in the Asian foods section of the grocery store.

- ¹⁄₂   cup teriyaki marinade and sauce
- ¹⁄₄   cup orange marmalade
- 2   teaspoons grated gingerroot
- 1   large unpeeled orange, cut into 8 wedges
- 1   pound swordfish or tuna fillets, cut into 24 one-inch pieces
- 1   large red bell pepper, cut into 24 pieces

Mix teriyaki sauce, marmalade and gingerroot in small bowl.

Set oven control to broil. Thread 1 orange wedge on each of four 15-inch metal skewers*. On each skewer, alternate a total of 6 fish pieces and 6 red pepper pieces, leaving a space between each piece. Thread another orange wedge on each skewer. Place on rack in broiler pan. (For easy cleanup, line broiler pan with aluminum foil before placing kabobs on rack.) Brush kabobs with sauce.

Broil kabobs with tops about 4 inches from heat 5 minutes, brushing frequently with sauce. Turn kabobs; brush with sauce. Broil 4 to 6 minutes longer or until fish flakes easily with fork. Discard any remaining sauce.

*If using bamboo skewers, soak in water at least 30 minutes before using to prevent burning.

1 Serving: Calories 230 (Calories from Fat 45); Fat 5g (Saturated 2g); Cholesterol 60mg; Sodium 1440mg; Carbohydrate 27g; (Dietary Fiber 2g); Protein 22g
% Daily Value: Vitamin A 26%; Vitamin C 86%; Calcium 4%; Iron 8%
Diet Exchanges: 3 very lean meat, 2 fruit

Summer Swordfish with Citrus and Basil

LO CAL / LO FAT

PREP: 15 MIN; MARINATE: 30 MIN; BAKE: 15 MIN

6 SERVINGS

Swordfish are found in warm ocean waters; they are large, generally weighing from 200 to 600 pounds. Swordfish has a meatlike texture and mild flavor.

6	small swordfish, redfish or salmon steaks, about 1 inch thick (about 1½ pounds)
1	cup orange juice
¼	cup chopped fresh basil leaves
1	teaspoon grated lemon peel
1	teaspoon grated lime peel
2	tablespoons lemon juice
2	tablespoons lime juice
1	teaspoon olive or vegetable oil
½	teaspoon salt
¼	teaspoon pepper
	Lemon wedges

Place fish in shallow glass or plastic dish. Mix remaining ingredients except lemon wedges; pour over fish. Cover and refrigerate at least 30 minutes.

Heat oven to 375°. Place fish with marinade in ungreased rectangular pan, 13 × 9 × 2 inches. Cover and bake 10 to 15 minutes or until fish flakes easily with fork. Serve with lemon wedges.

1 Serving: Calories 155 (Calories from Fat 55); Fat 6g (Saturated 2g); Cholesterol 60mg; Sodium 255mg; Carbohydrate 5g (Dietary Fiber 0g); Protein 20g
% Daily Value: Vitamin A 4%; Vitamin C 14%; Calcium 2%; Iron 4%
Diet Exchanges: 3 very lean meat, ½ fruit, ½ fat

Sautéed Tuna with Creamy Tarragon Sauce

LO CAL / LO FAT / LO SODIUM

PREP: 5 MIN; COOK: 15 MIN

6 SERVINGS

Tuna is moderately high in fat, firm in texture and stronger in flavor than many other types of fish. The fresh variety is head and shoulders above the canned variety—give it a try.

6	small yellowfin tuna, grouper or sea bass steaks, about 1 inch thick (about 1½ pounds)
¾	cup apple juice
3	tablespoons reduced-fat sour cream
2	tablespoons chopped fresh or 2 teaspoons dried tarragon leaves
¼	teaspoon ground mustard (dry)

Spray 10-inch nonstick skillet with cooking spray; heat over medium-high heat. Cook fish in skillet 5 minutes; turn. Cover and cook 5 to 6 minutes longer or until fish flakes easily with fork. Mix remaining ingredients.

Remove fish from skillet; keep warm. Add apple juice mixture to skillet; heat to boiling. Boil 5 to 6 minutes or until reduced to ½ cup. Serve over fish.

1 Serving: Calories 130 (Calories from Fat 20); Fat 2g (Saturated 1g); Cholesterol 65mg; Sodium 110mg; Carbohydrate 5g (Dietary Fiber 0g); Protein 23g
% Daily Value: Vitamin A 2%; Vitamin C 0%; Calcium 2%; Iron 2%
Diet Exchanges: 2 very lean meat, ½ fruit

Soft Fish Tacos

HIGH FIBER

PREP: 20 MIN; BROIL: 10 MIN

4 SERVINGS

Regular flour tortillas are often made with lard or shortening, with just one tortilla often having at least 4 grams of fat. Fortunately for all tortilla lovers, you can now buy a fat-free version!

Spicy Fresh Chili Sauce (right)

2 tablespoons lime juice

1 teaspoon vegetable oil

1 pound yellowfin tuna, halibut or red snapper fillets, about 1 inch thick

8 fat-free flour tortillas (6 to 8 inches in diameter), warmed

3/4 cup shredded lettuce

1 small red bell pepper, chopped (1/2 cup)

1 medium onion, chopped (1/2 cup)

Prepare Spicy Fresh Chili Sauce. Set oven control to broil. Spray broiler pan rack with cooking spray. Mix lime juice and oil; brush over fish. Place fish on rack in broiler pan. Broil with tops about 4 inches from heat 5 minutes; turn. Broil 5 to 8 minutes longer or until fish flakes easily with fork.

Break fish into large flakes, or cut into 1-inch cubes. Spoon scant 1/2 cup fish onto center of each tortilla. Top with lettuce, bell pepper and onion. Roll up tortillas. Serve with sauce.

Spicy Fresh Chili Sauce

1 medium tomato, chopped (3/4 cup)

5 medium green onions, sliced (1/3 cup)

1 clove garlic, finely chopped

1 tablespoon finely chopped hot green chili (1 small)

1 tablespoon chopped fresh cilantro

1/4 teaspoon ground cumin

Mix all ingredients.

1 Serving: Calories 405 (Calories from Fat 80); Fat 9g (Saturated 1g); Cholesterol 60mg; Sodium 520mg; Carbohydrate 55g (Dietary Fiber 5g); Protein 31g
% Daily Value: Vitamin A 22%; Vitamin C 58%; Calcium 14%; Iron 20%
Diet Exchanges: 3 starch, 4 very lean meat, 1 vegetable

Yellowfin Tuna with Pear Salsa

LO CAL / LO FAT

PREP: 15 MIN; CHILL: 1 HR; BROIL: 5 MIN

6 SERVINGS

Fresh peaches or nectarines can be used instead of a fresh pear in this refreshing salsa.

Pear Salsa (below)

6 small yellowfin tuna, mahimahi or scrod fish fillets (about 1½ pounds)

Prepare Pear Salsa. Set oven control to broil. Spray broiler pan rack with cooking spray. Place fish on rack in broiler pan. Broil with tops about 4 inches from heat about 5 minutes or until fish flakes easily with fork. Top with salsa.

Pear Salsa

1 large unpeeled pear, chopped (1½ cups)

2 medium green onions, chopped (2 tablespoons)

1 medium hot yellow chili, chopped (2 tablespoons)

2 tablespoons chopped fresh cilantro

2 tablespoons lemon juice

2 teaspoons grated lemon peel

½ teaspoon salt

Mix all ingredients in small glass or plastic bowl. Cover and refrigerate 1 hour.

1 Serving: Calories 130 (Calories from Fat 20); Fat 2g (Saturated 0g); Cholesterol 60mg; Sodium 290mg; Carbohydrate 7g (Dietary Fiber 1g); Protein 22g
% Daily Value: Vitamin A 4%; Vitamin C 16%; Calcium 2%; Iron 2%
Diet Exchanges: 3 very lean meat, ½ fruit

Shrimp Creole

LO CAL / LO FAT

PREP: 10 MIN; COOK: 15 MIN

4 SERVINGS

Many new flavored tomato products are appearing on grocery store shelves. If you can't find the flavor called for in this recipe, choose another one that sounds good to you; it will work just fine.

2 cups frozen stir-fry bell peppers and onions (from 16-ounce bag)

1 can (14½ ounces) chunky tomatoes with crushed red pepper, undrained

1 pound uncooked peeled deveined medium shrimp, thawed if frozen

1 teaspoon chopped fresh or ¼ teaspoon dried thyme leaves

⅛ teaspoon garlic powder

Hot cooked rice, if desired

Spray 12-inch nonstick skillet with cooking spray; heat over medium-high heat. Cook stir-fry vegetables in skillet about 3 minutes, stirring occasionally, until crisp-tender.

Stir in remaining ingredients except rice. Heat to boiling; reduce heat. Cover and simmer 8 to 10 minutes, stirring occasionally, until shrimp are pink and firm. Serve with rice.

1 Serving: Calories 110 (Calories from Fat 10); Fat 1g (Saturated 0g); Cholesterol 160mg; Sodium 330mg; Carbohydrate 8g (Dietary Fiber 2g); Protein 19g
% Daily Value: Vitamin A 12%; Vitamin C 3%; Calcium 6%; Iron 18%
Diet Exchanges: 2 very lean meat, 2 vegetable

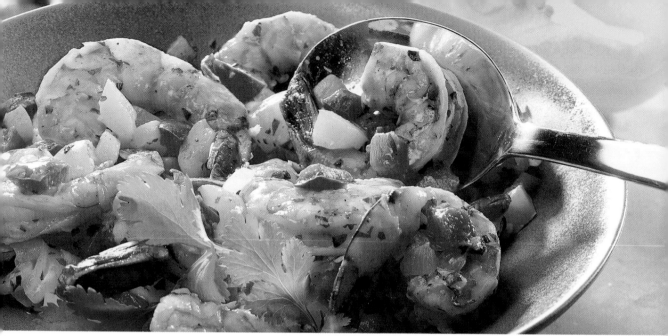

Southwestern Stir-Fried Shrimp

Southwestern Stir-Fried Shrimp

LO CAL / LO FAT

PREP: 15 MIN; MARINATE: 1 HR; COOK: 5 MIN

6 SERVINGS

Cumin is a frequent dinner guest in southwestern cuisine. It has a warm, earthy flavor and pungent aroma. You are probably most familiar with its flavor from eating chili.

2	tablespoons lime juice
2	teaspoons cornstarch
$1/2$	teaspoon ground cumin
$1/4$	teaspoon salt
$1/4$	teaspoon pepper
$1^1/2$	pounds uncooked peeled deveined large shrimp (about 24), thawed if frozen
1	large yellow bell pepper, chopped ($1^1/2$ cups)
1	large red bell pepper, chopped ($1^1/2$ cups)
1	medium onion, chopped ($1/2$ cup)
$1/3$	cup chicken broth
2	cloves garlic, finely chopped
$1/8$	teaspoon ground red pepper (cayenne)
2	tablespoons chopped fresh cilantro

Mix lime juice, cornstarch, cumin, salt and pepper in medium glass or plastic bowl. Stir in shrimp. Cover and refrigerate 1 hour.

Spray 12-inch nonstick skillet with cooking spray; heat over medium heat. Add bell peppers, onion, broth, garlic, red pepper and cilantro; stir-fry 2 minutes. Add shrimp mixture; stir-fry 3 to 4 minutes or until shrimp are pink and firm.

1 Serving: Calories 65 (Calories from Fat 10) Fat 1g (Saturated 0g); Cholesterol 55g; Sodium 220g; Carbohydrate 9g (Dietary Fiber 2g); Protein 7g
% Daily Value: Vitamin A 24%; Vitamin C 100%; Calcium 2%; Iron 8%
Diet Exchanges: 1 very lean meat, $1/2$ vegetable

Shrimp Florentine Stir-Fry

LO CAL / LO FAT / HI FIB

PREP: 10 MIN; COOK: 8 MIN

4 SERVINGS

Serve this elegant stir-fry with rice, rolls and fresh fruit.

- 1 tablespoon olive or vegetable oil
- 1 pound uncooked peeled deveined medium shrimp, thawed if frozen
- 4 cups lightly packed spinach leaves
- 1 can (14 ounces) baby corn nuggets, drained
- 1/4 cup coarsely chopped roasted red bell peppers (from 7-ounce jar)
- 1 tablespoon chopped fresh or 1/2 teaspoon freeze-dried chives
- 1/2 teaspoon garlic salt
- Lemon wedges

Heat oil in 12-inch nonstick skillet over medium-high heat. Add shrimp; stir-fry 2 to 3 minutes or until shrimp are pink and firm.

Add spinach, corn, bell peppers, chives and garlic salt; stir-fry 2 to 4 minutes or until spinach is wilted. Serve with lemon wedges.

1 Serving: Calories 200 (Calories from Fat 45); Fat 5g (Saturated 1g); Cholesterol 160mg; Sodium 720mg; Carbohydrate 20g (Dietary Fiber 3g); Protein 21g
% Daily Value: Vitamin A 34%; Vitamin C 28%; Calcium 6%; Iron 24%
Diet Exchanges: 2 very lean meat, 4 vegetable, 1 fat

Summer Scallops with Melon Relish

LO CAL / LO FAT / LO CHOL

PREP: 15 MIN; MARINATE: 1 HR; BROIL: 6 MIN

4 SERVINGS

Chopped green onions can be substituted for the shallot.

½ medium cantaloupe, finely chopped
(1½ cups)

½ small honeydew melon, finely chopped
(1½ cups)

1 large shallot, finely chopped
(2 tablespoons)

3 tablespoons chopped fresh cilantro

2 tablespoons lemon juice

½ teaspoon salt

⅛ teaspoon pepper

⅛ teaspoon crushed pepper

1 pound sea scallops

Mix all ingredients except scallops; reserve 2 cups relish. Mix remaining relish and the scallops in glass or plastic bowl. Cover and refrigerate scallop mixture and 2 cups reserved relish separately at least 1 hour.

Set oven control to broil. Spray broiler pan rack with cooking spray. Remove scallops from melon mixture; discard melon mixture. Thread scallops on six 11-inch skewers.* Place on rack in broiler pan. Broil with tops about 4 inches from heat 3 minutes; turn. Broil about 3 minutes longer or until scallops are white. Serve reserved relish over scallops.

*If using bamboo skewers, soak in water at least 30 minutes before using to prevent burning.

1 Serving: Calories 120 (Calories from Fat 10); Fat 1g (Saturated 0g); Cholesterol 20mg; Sodium 460mg; Carbohydrate 14g (Dietary Fiber 1g); Protein 14g
% Daily Value: Vitamin A 20%; Vitamin C 72%; Calcium 8%; Iron 10%
Diet Exchanges: 2 very lean meat, 1 fruit

Scallops with Red Pepper Sauce

LO CAL / LO FAT / LO CHOL

PREP: 20 MIN; COOK: 5 MIN

4 SERVINGS

Red pepper sauce is a fiery little number made with peppers, vinegar and salt. Many brands are available, and the heat will vary greatly among them. Some are so hot that just a drop is enough; others are milder, allowing you to be more generous.

1   large red bell pepper, cut into fourths

¹/₈   teaspoon salt

10   drops red pepper sauce

1   clove garlic, finely chopped

¹/₄   cup plain fat-free yogurt

1   pound bay scallops

4   medium green onions, sliced (¹/₄ cup)

Fresh cilantro leaves

Hot cooked pasta or rice, if desired

Place steamer basket in ¹/₂ inch water in saucepan or skillet (water should not touch bottom of basket). Place bell pepper in basket. Cover tightly and heat to boiling; reduce heat. Steam 8 to 10 minutes or until tender.

Place bell pepper, salt, pepper sauce and garlic in blender or food processor. Cover and blend on medium speed until almost smooth. Heat bell pepper mixture in 1-quart saucepan over medium heat, stirring occasionally, until hot; remove from heat. Gradually stir in yogurt; keep warm.

Spray 10-inch nonstick skillet with cooking spray; heat over medium-high heat. Add scallops and onions; stir-fry 4 to 5 minutes or until scallops are white. Serve sauce with scallops. Garnish with cilantro. Serve with pasta or rice.

1 Serving: Calories 85 (Calories from Fat 10); Fat 1g (Saturated 0g); Cholesterol 20mg; Sodium 300mg; Carbohydrate 6g (Dietary Fiber 1g); Protein 14g
% Daily Value: Vitamin A 26%; Vitamin C 62%; Calcium 10%; Iron 10%
Diet Exchanges: 2 very lean meat, 1 vegetable

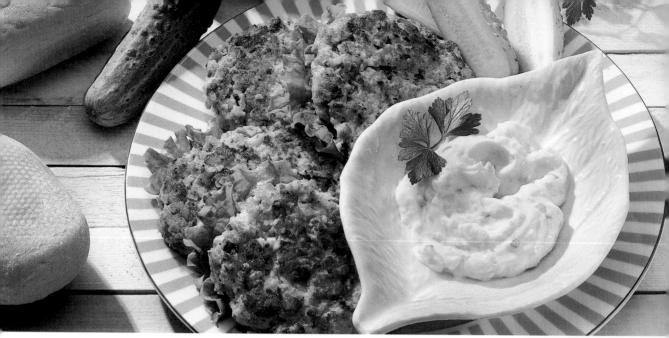

Whitefish and Shrimp Cakes

Whitefish and Shrimp Cakes

LO CAL / LO FAT

PREP: 20 MIN; COOK: 10 MIN

6 SERVINGS

This take on the classic crab cake can be eaten as is or served on buns with reduced-fat mayonnaise, tartar sauce or salsa.

$3/4$ **pound whitefish, trout or catfish fillets, cut up**

$1/2$ **pound uncooked peeled deveined medium shrimp, thawed if frozen**

4 **medium green onions, chopped ($1/4$ cup)**

2 **tablespoons fat-free cholesterol-free egg product or 1 egg white**

2 **tablespoons chopped fresh parsley**

1 **tablespoon all-purpose flour**

1 **tablespoon reduced-fat mayonnaise or salad dressing**

1 **teaspoon Dijon mustard**

$1/2$ **teaspoon salt**

$1/4$ **teaspoon pepper**

$1/8$ **teaspoon Worcestershire sauce**

Reduced-fat tartar sauce or salsa, if desired

Place all ingredients except tartar sauce in food processor. Cover and process, using quick on-and-off motions, until fish and shrimp are coarsely chopped.

Spray 12-inch nonstick skillet with cooking spray; heat over medium heat. Drop fish mixture by scant $1/3$ cupfuls into skillet; flatten with spatula. Cook 4 minutes; turn. Cook about 4 minutes longer or until patties are firm. Serve with tartar sauce.

1 Serving: Calories 125 (Calories from Fat 45); Fat 5g (Saturated 1g); Cholesterol 90mg; Sodium 230mg; Carbohydrate 2g (Dietary Fiber 0g); Protein 18g
% Daily Value: Vitamin A 4%; Vitamin C 2%; Calcium 2%; Iron 10%
Diet Exchanges: 3 very lean meat, $1/2$ fat

Garlic Shrimp

LO CAL / LO FAT

PREP: 15 MIN; COOK: 6 MIN

4 SERVINGS

Shrimp can be purchased already peeled and deveined, which can save about 10 minutes of preparation time.

- 1 tablespoon vegetable oil
- 3 large cloves garlic, finely chopped
- 1 pound uncooked peeled deveined medium shrimp, thawed if frozen
- 1 large carrot, cut into julienne strips (1 cup)
- 2 tablespoons chopped fresh parsley
- 2 cups hot cooked rice or noodles

Heat nonstick wok or 12-inch nonstick skillet over medium-high heat. Add oil; rotate wok to coat side.

Add garlic, stir-fry 1 minute. Add shrimp; stir-fry 1 minute. Add carrot; stir-fry about 3 minutes or until shrimp are pink and firm and carrot is crisp-tender. Stir in parsley. Serve over rice.

1 Serving: Calories 115 (Calories from Fat 35); Fat 4g (Saturated 1g); Cholesterol 160mg; Sodium 195mg; Carbohydrate 3g (Dietary Fiber 1g); Protein 18g
% Daily Value: Vitamin A 34%; Vitamin C 4%; Calcium 4%; Iron 16%
Diet Exchanges: 3 very lean meat, 1/2 vegetable

Savory Shrimp and Scallops

LOW CALORIE

PREP: 15 MIN; COOK: 10 MIN

4 SERVINGS

Sea scallops are the larger scallops, measuring up to 2 inches, versus the small bay scallops, which measure only 1/2 inch.

2 tablespoons olive or vegetable oil

1 clove garlic, finely chopped

2 medium green onions, sliced (2 tablespoons)

2 medium carrots, thinly sliced (1 cup)

1 tablespoon chopped fresh parsley or 1 teaspoon parsley flakes

1 pound uncooked peeled deveined medium shrimp, thawed if frozen

1 pound sea scallops, cut in half

1/2 cup dry white wine or chicken broth

1 tablespoon lemon juice

1/4 to 1/2 teaspoon crushed red pepper

Heat oil in 10-inch nonstick skillet over medium heat. Cook garlic, onions, carrots and parsley in oil about 5 minutes, stirring occasionally, until carrots are crisp-tender.

Stir in remaining ingredients. Cook 4 to 5 minutes, stirring frequently, until shrimp are pink and firm and scallops are white.

1 Serving: Calories 225 (Calories from Fat 80); Fat 9g (Saturated 1g); Cholesterol 180mg; Sodium 350mg; Carbohydrate 6g (Dietary Fiber 1g); Protein 31g
% Daily Value: Vitamin A 56%; Vitamin C 6%; Calcium 10%; Iron 26%
Diet Exchanges: 4 very lean meat, 1 vegetable, 1 fat

Thai Scallops and Noodles

LO CAL / LO CHOL / HI FIB

PREP: 10 MIN; COOK: 16 MIN

6 SERVINGS

If you can't find bay scallops at your supermarket or seafood shop, the larger sea scallops will work equally well—just cut them into fourths.

1 package (7 ounces) spaghetti, broken in half

5 cups broccoli pieces or 1 bag (16 ounces) frozen cut broccoli, thawed

3/4 pound bay scallops or quartered sea scallops or 1 package (12 ounces) frozen scallops, thawed

1/2 cup reduced-fat peanut butter spread

1/4 cup reduced-sodium soy sauce

1/4 cup rice vinegar

1 teaspoon red pepper sauce

2 tablespoons unsalted dry-roasted peanuts, finely chopped

Cook spaghetti as directed on package—except add broccoli and scallops during last 4 minutes of cooking. Scallops are done when they turn white.

While spaghetti, broccoli and scallops are cooking, beat peanut butter, soy sauce, vinegar and red pepper sauce with wire whisk until smooth.

Drain spaghetti mixture; return to saucepan. Add peanut butter mixture; toss gently to coat. Sprinkle with peanuts. Serve immediately.

1 Serving: Calories 320 (Calories from Fat 90); Fat 10g (Saturated 2g); Cholesterol 10mg; Sodium 600mg; Carbohydrate 41g (Dietary Fiber 4g); Protein 20g
% Daily Value: Vitamin A 8%; Vitamin C 46%; Calcium 8%; Iron 20%
Diet Exchanges: 2 starch, 1 1/2 lean meat, 2 vegetable, 1 fat

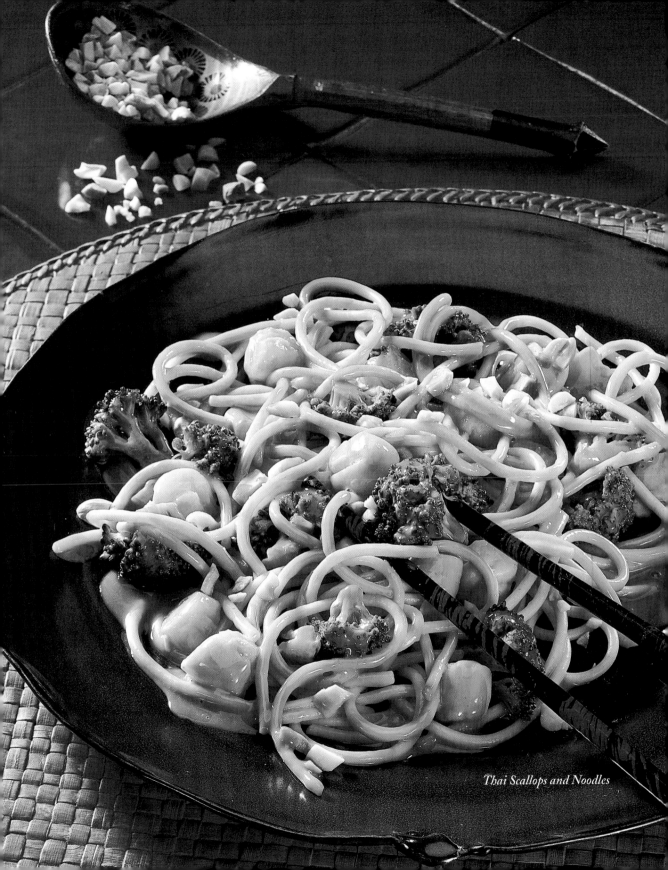

Thai Scallops and Noodles

Potato Frittata with Clams

LO CAL / LO FAT / LO CHOL / HI FIB

PREP: 10 MIN; COOK: 20 MIN

4 SERVINGS

You don't have to flip this fuss-free Italian frittata out of the pan. Simply bring it to the table right in the skillet, and cut it into wedges.

2	cups refrigerated shredded hash brown potatoes (from 1-pound 4-ounce bag)
4	medium green onions, sliced ($\frac{1}{4}$ cup)
$1\frac{1}{2}$	cups fat-free cholesterol-free egg product
$\frac{1}{4}$	cup skim milk
$\frac{1}{2}$	teaspoon garlic salt
$\frac{1}{4}$	teaspoon ground red pepper (cayenne)
1	can ($6\frac{1}{2}$ ounces) minced clams, drained
	Finely shredded or grated Parmesan cheese, if desired

Spray 10-inch nonstick skillet with cooking spray; heat over medium-low heat. Sprinkle potatoes and onions in skillet. Cook uncovered 10 minutes.

While potatoes are cooking, mix egg product, milk, garlic salt and red pepper with fork. Sprinkle clams over potato mixture. Pour egg mixture over clams. Cook uncovered over medium-low heat. As mixture begins to set on bottom and side, gently lift cooked portions with spatula so that thin, uncooked portion can flow to bottom. Cook about 5 minutes or until eggs are thickened throughout but still moist.

Sprinkle with cheese; reduce heat to low. Cover and cook about 10 minutes or until center is set. Loosen bottom of frittata with spatula. Cut into 4 wedges. Serve immediately.

1 Serving: Calories 150 (Calories from Fat 10); Fat 1g (Saturated 0g); Cholesterol 15mg; Sodium 220mg; Carbohydrate 23g (Dietary Fiber 3g); Protein 15g
% Daily Value: Vitamin A 8%; Vitamin C 12%; Calcium 8%; Iron 46%
Diet Exchanges: $1\frac{1}{2}$ starch, 1 very lean meat

Crab and Artichoke Bake

LO CAL / LO FAT / HI FIB

PREP: 10 MIN; BAKE: 25 MIN

4 SERVINGS

This classy casserole tastes delicious with a variety of vegetables. Besides the artichokes, you can make it with frozen (thawed) cut asparagus, cauliflower or Italian-style green beans.

2 cups skim milk

1/4 cup all-purpose flour

1 teaspoon chicken bouillon granules

1 teaspoon ground mustard (dry)

1/4 teaspoon pepper

1 cup shredded reduced-fat mozzarella cheese (4 ounces)

1 package (9 ounces) frozen artichoke hearts, thawed

1 package (8 ounces) refrigerated imitation crabmeat chunks

Heat oven to 425°. Gradually stir milk into flour in 2-quart saucepan. Stir in bouillon granules, mustard and pepper. Heat to boiling, stirring constantly. Boil and stir 1 minute; remove from heat. Stir in 1/2 cup of the cheese until melted. Stir in artichokes and crabmeat.

Pour mixture into ungreased 1 1/2-quart casserole. Sprinkle with remaining 1/2 cup cheese. Bake uncovered about 25 minutes or until hot and bubbly and cheese is golden brown.

1 Serving: Calories 235 (Calories from Fat 55); Fat 6g (Saturated 4g); Cholesterol 35mg; Sodium 1210mg; Carbohydrate 24g (Dietary Fiber 3g); Protein 24g
% Daily Value: Vitamin A 12%; Vitamin C 6%; Calcium 40%; Iron 8%
Diet Exchanges: 1 starch, 2 lean meat, 2 vegetable

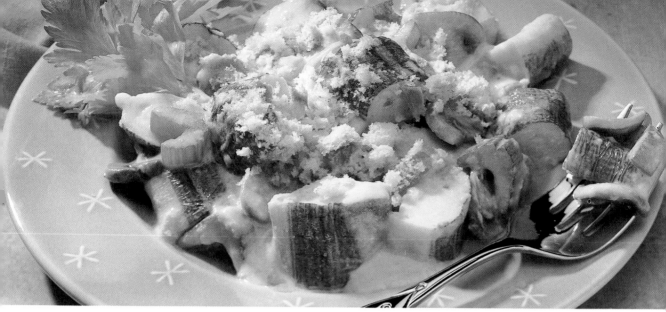

Creamy Crab au Gratin

Creamy Crab au Gratin

LO CAL / LO FAT

PREP: 15 MIN; BAKE: 15 MIN

4 SERVINGS

Forget ordinary tuna casserole, and try this enticing Crab au Gratin. Not only will you be pleased by its extraordinary flavor, you'll also applaud that it's low in fat. Steam some fresh pea pods to serve alongside.

1½ cups sliced mushrooms (4 ounces)

2 medium stalks celery, sliced (1 cup)

1 can (14½ ounces) ready-to-serve chicken broth

¾ cup fat-free half-and-half

3 tablespoons all-purpose flour

½ teaspoon red pepper sauce

2 packages (8 ounces each) refrigerated imitation crabmeat chunks or 2 cups chopped cooked crabmeat

1 cup soft bread crumbs (about 1½ slices bread)

Heat oven to 400°. Lightly spray rectangular baking dish, 11 × 7 × 1½ inches, with cooking spray.

Spray 3-quart saucepan with cooking spray; heat over medium heat. Cook mushrooms and celery in saucepan about 4 minutes, stirring constantly, until celery is tender. Stir in broth. Heat to boiling; reduce heat.

Beat half-and-half, flour and pepper sauce with wire whisk until smooth; stir into vegetable mixture. Heat to boiling, stirring constantly. Boil and stir 1 minute. Stir in crabmeat.

Spoon crabmeat mixture into baking dish. Top with bread crumbs. Bake uncovered about 15 minutes or until heated through.

1 Serving: Calories 200 (Calories from Fat 20); Fat 2g (Saturated 1g); Cholesterol 35mg; Sodium 1540mg; Carbohydrate 24g (Dietary Fiber 1g); Protein 23g
% Daily Value: Vitamin A 8%; Vitamin C 2%; Calcium 6%; Iron 8%
Diet Exchanges: ½ starch, 2 very lean meat, 2 vegetable, ½ skim milk

Lobster Newburg

LO CAL / LO FAT

PREP: 10 MIN; COOK: 6 MIN

4 SERVINGS

Classic Lobster Newburg uses butter, light cream and egg yolks. This health-conscious version skips the butter and egg yolks and uses fat-free half-and-half. The best part about this new Newburg is that it's still rich tasting, creamy and elegant.

1½   cups fat-free half-and-half or refrigerated fat-free nondairy creamer

2   tablespoons all-purpose flour

¼   teaspoon salt

⅛   teaspoon ground red pepper (cayenne)

⅛   teaspoon ground nutmeg

1   cup chopped cooked lobster or 1 package (8 ounces) refrigerated imitation lobster chunks

3   tablespoons dry sherry or apple juice

4   slices white or whole wheat bread, toasted and cut into fourths, or 4 English muffins, split and toasted

Gradually stir half-and-half into flour in 2-quart saucepan. Stir in salt, red pepper and nutmeg. Heat to boiling, stirring constantly. Boil and stir 1 minute. Stir in lobster and sherry; heat through. Serve over toast.

1 Serving: Calories 160 (Calories from Fat 10); Fat 1g (Saturated 0g); Cholesterol 25mg; Sodium 510mg; Carbohydrate 26g (Dietary Fiber 1g); Protein 13g
% Daily Value: Vitamin A 12%; Vitamin C 0%; Calcium 4%; Iron 6%
Diet Exchanges: 1 starch, 1 skim milk

Lobster Chow Mein Bake

LO CAL / HI FIB

PREP: 10 MIN; BAKE: 25 MIN

4 SERVINGS

Oriental vegetables and tender chunks of imitation lobster make a family-pleasing casserole that's easy on the cook and the budget. If you'd prefer, use refrigerated imitation crabmeat chunks in place of the lobster.

$^3/_4$	cup reduced-fat mayonnaise or salad dressing
1	tablespoon all-purpose flour
1	tablespoon reduced-sodium soy sauce
1	can (14 to 16 ounces) fancy mixed Chinese vegetables, drained
1	can (8 ounces) sliced water chestnuts, drained
1	package (8 ounces) refrigerated imitation lobster chunks
1	medium stalk celery, sliced ($^1/_2$ cup)
	Chow mein noodles, if desired

Heat oven to 350°. Mix mayonnaise, flour and soy sauce in $1^1/_2$-quart casserole. Stir in remaining ingredients except noodles.

Cover and bake about 25 minutes or until heated through. Sprinkle with noodles.

1 Serving: Calories 265 (Calories from Fat 145); Fat 16g (Saturated 3g); Cholesterol 30mg; Sodium 1000mg; Carbohydrate 22g (Dietary Fiber 4g); Protein 12g
% Daily Value: Vitamin A 28%; Vitamin C 100%; Calcium 6%; Iron 10%
Diet Exchanges: 1 starch, 1 medium-fat meat, 1 vegetable, 2 fat

Seafood Stew with Rosamarina

LO CAL / LO FAT / HI FIB

PREP: 25 MIN; COOK: 35 MIN

4 SERVINGS

Fresh mussels should be refrigerated and used within one or two days.

8	mussels in shells
8	medium green onions, chopped (1/2 cup)
1	clove garlic, finely chopped
1	large tomato, chopped (1 cup)
1	medium carrot, thinly sliced (1/2 cup)
1/3	cup uncooked rosamarina (orzo) pasta
1 3/4	cups chicken broth
1	bottle (8 ounces) clam juice
1/2	cup dry white wine or chicken broth
1	tablespoon chopped fresh or 1 teaspoon dried thyme leaves
2	teaspoons chopped fresh or 1/2 teaspoon dried dill weed
6	drops red pepper sauce
1/2	pound red snapper, flounder or cod fillets, skinned and cut into 1/2-inch pieces
8	uncooked medium shrimp, peeled and deveined
1	package (8 ounces) sliced mushrooms (3 cups)
	Chopped fresh parsley
	Lemon wedges

Discard any broken-shell or open (dead) mussels. Scrub mussels in cold water, removing any barnacles with a dull paring knife or oyster knife. Remove beards. (Pull beard by giving it a tug; using a paper towel may help. If you still have trouble removing it, use a pliers to grip and pull gently.) Set mussels aside.

Spray 4-quart saucepan with cooking spray; heat over medium heat. Cook onions and garlic in saucepan 5 minutes, stirring occasionally. Stir in tomato, carrot, pasta, broth, clam juice, wine, thyme, dill weed and pepper sauce. Heat to boiling; reduce heat. Cover and simmer about 20 minutes, stirring occasionally, until pasta is almost tender.

Stir in mussels, fish, shrimp and mushrooms. Cover and heat to boiling; reduce heat. Simmer 6 to 8 minutes, stirring occasionally, until fish flakes easily with fork and mussels open (remove mussels as they open; reserve). Discard any unopened mussels. Return reserved mussels to stew. Sprinkle with parsley. Serve with lemon wedges.

1 Serving: Calories 220 (Calories from Fat 30); Fat 3g (Saturated 1g); Cholesterol 60mg; Sodium 790mg; Carbohydrate 29g (Dietary Fiber 5g); Protein 24g
% Daily Value: Vitamin A 30%; Vitamin C 22%; Calcium 8%; Iron 40%
Diet Exchanges: 1 starch, 3 very lean meat, 2 vegetable

Louisiana Oyster Gumbo

LO CAL / HI FIB

PREP: 10 MIN; COOK: 24 MIN

4 SERVINGS

You'll know the flour and oil mixture is cooked to the right stage when it's the color of a penny.

   2   tablespoons all-purpose flour

   2   tablespoons olive or vegetable oil

   3   large onions, coarsely chopped (3 cups)

   1   medium red or green bell pepper, coarsely chopped (1 cup)

   3   cups chicken broth

   2   teaspoons red pepper sauce

1½   teaspoons dried thyme leaves

   ⅓   cup all-purpose flour

   1   pint shucked large oysters, undrained, or 2 cans (8 ounces each) whole oysters, undrained

       Hot cooked rice, if desired

Heat 2 tablespoons flour and the oil in Dutch oven over medium heat 5 to 10 minutes, stirring constantly, until mixture is dark brown. Stir in onions and bell pepper. Cook uncovered about 6 minutes, stirring frequently, until vegetables are tender.

Gradually stir in 2½ cups of the broth. Stir in pepper sauce and thyme. Heat to boiling; reduce heat. Cover and simmer 3 minutes.

Beat remaining ½ cup broth and ⅓ cup flour with wire whisk. Stir into broth mixture until smooth. Heat to boiling. Stir in oysters; reduce heat. Cover and simmer about 3 minutes or until oysters are heated through. Serve gumbo over rice.

1 Serving: Calories 260 (Calories from Fat 100); Fat 11g (Saturated 3g); Cholesterol 60mg; Sodium 1040mg; Carbohydrate 28g (Dietary Fiber 3g); Protein 15g
% Daily Value: Vitamin A 20%; Vitamin C 56%; Calcium 8%; Iron 52%
Diet Exchanges: 1 starch, 1 medium-fat meat, 2 vegetable, 1 fat

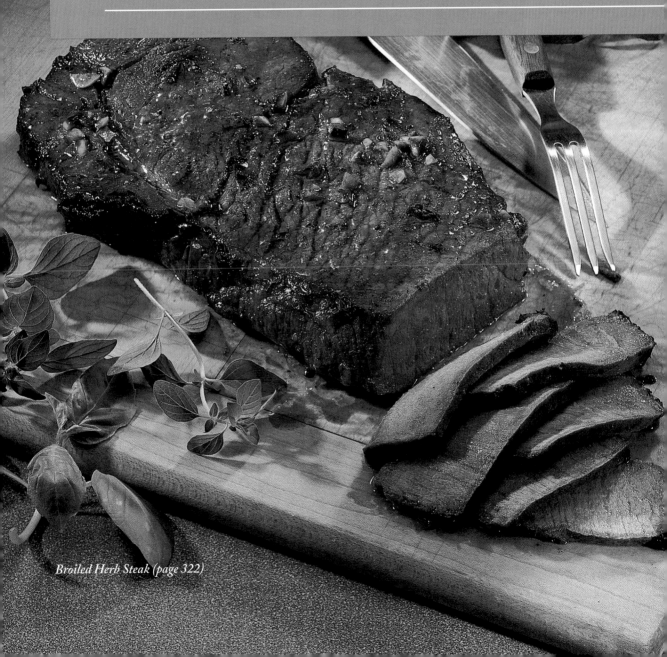

MAKE MINE MEAT

Broiled Herb Steak (page 322)

Savory Beef Tenderloin

LOW CALORIE

PREP: 15 MIN; COOK: 10 MIN

4 SERVINGS

You can still be mad about meat! By choosing the tenderloin cut, you get the protein, iron and other benefits of beef without the added fat that comes with some of the other cuts.

³⁄₄	pound beef tenderloin
2	teaspoons chopped fresh or ¹⁄₂ teaspoon dried marjoram leaves
2	teaspoons sugar
1	teaspoon coarsely ground pepper
1	tablespoon margarine
1	package (8 ounces) sliced mushrooms (3 cups)
1	small onion, thinly sliced
³⁄₄	cup beef broth
¹⁄₄	cup dry red wine or beef broth
1	tablespoon cornstarch

Remove fat from beef. Cut beef into four ³⁄₄-inch slices. (Beef is easier to cut if partially frozen, about 1¹⁄₂ hours.) Mix marjoram, sugar and pepper; rub on both sides of beef slices.

Melt margarine in 10-inch nonstick skillet over medium heat. Cook beef in margarine 3 to 5 minutes, turning once, until brown. Remove beef to platter; keep warm.

Cook mushrooms and onion in drippings in skillet over medium heat about 2 minutes, stirring occasionally, until onion is crisp-tender. Mix broth, wine and cornstarch; stir into mushroom mixture. Cook over medium heat, stirring constantly, until mixture thickens and boils. Boil and stir 1 minute. Pour over beef.

1 Serving: Calories 165 (Calories from Fat 70); Fat 8g (Saturated 3g); Cholesterol 35mg; Sodium 260mg; Carbohydrate 9g (Dietary Fiber 1g); Protein 15g
% Daily Value: Vitamin A 4%; Vitamin C 2%; Calcium 2%; Iron 12%
Diet Exchanges: ¹⁄₂ starch, 2 very lean meat

Broiled Sirloin Steak with Italian-Seasoned Vegetables

LO CAL / LO FAT

PREP: 10 MIN; BROIL: 10 MIN

4 SERVINGS

For easy cleanup, line the broiler pan with aluminum foil before putting the rack in place.

1 pound beef boneless sirloin steak, 1 inch thick

1/2 pound fresh portabella mushrooms, cut into 1/2-inch slices

1 medium yellow summer squash or zucchini, cut into 1-inch diagonal slices

1 medium onion, cut into 8 wedges

1/3 cup fat-free Italian dressing

3 tablespoons balsamic vinegar

1/2 teaspoon cracked black pepper

2 tablespoons chopped fresh flat-leaf Italian or regular parsley

Set oven control to broil. Spray broiler pan rack with cooking spray. Remove fat from beef. Place beef, mushrooms, squash and onion on rack in broiler pan. Mix dressing, vinegar and pepper; brush over beef and vegetables.

Broil with top of beef and vegetables 3 to 4 inches from heat 5 minutes. Turn beef; brush dressing mixture over beef and vegetables. Broil about 5 minutes longer or until beef is desired doneness and vegetables are crisp-tender. Discard any remaining dressing mixture. Cut beef into 4 serving pieces. Sprinkle parsley over beef and vegetables.

1 Serving: Calories 165 (Calories from Fat 35); Fat 4g (Saturated 1g); Cholesterol 60mg; Sodium 230mg; Carbohydrate 9g (Dietary Fiber 2g); Protein 25g
% Daily Value: Vitamin A 2%; Vitamin C 8%; Calcium 2%; Iron 18%
Diet Exchanges: 3 very lean meat, 2 vegetable

Mustard-Marinated Steak

LOW CALORIE

PREP: 10 MIN; MARINATE: 4 HR; BROIL: 20 MIN

8 SERVINGS

Dijon mustard has become an American favorite with a clean, sharp flavor that can range from mild to hot. Dijon is made with brown or black mustard seed, white wine, unfermented grape juice and a variety of seasonings.

- 2 pound beef bone-in chuck steak, about $3/4$ inch thick
- 2 tablespoons lemon juice
- 1 tablespoon olive or vegetable oil
- 1 tablespoon Dijon mustard
- $1/4$ teaspoon pepper
- 2 tablespoons water

Remove fat from beef. Pierce beef on both sides with fork. Mix lemon juice, oil, mustard and pepper in shallow glass or plastic dish. Add beef; turn to coat with marinade. Cover and refrigerate, turning occasionally, at least 4 hours but no longer than 24 hours.

Set oven control to broil. Remove beef from marinade; reserve marinade. Place beef on rack in broiler pan. Broil with top about 3 inches from heat about 10 minutes on each side for medium doneness (160°).

Heat marinade and water to boiling in 1-quart saucepan, stirring occasionally; pour over beef.

1 Serving: Calories 150 (Calories from Fat 90); Fat 10g (Saturated 4g); Cholesterol 45mg; Sodium 60mg; Carbohydrate 0g (Dietary Fiber 0g); Protein 15g
% Daily Value: Vitamin A 0%; Vitamin C 0%; Calcium 0%; Iron 8%
Diet Exchanges: 2 medium-fat meat

Saucy Italian Steak

LO CAL / LO FAT

PREP: 10 MIN; BAKE: $1\frac{1}{2}$ HR

6 SERVINGS

Italian green beans are flatter and wider than regular green beans, and they are usually available frozen.

- $1\frac{1}{2}$ pound beef round steak, $3/4$ to 1 inch thick
- 2 tablespoons all-purpose flour
- $1/4$ teaspoon pepper
- 1 tablespoon olive or vegetable oil
- 1 jar (14 ounces) fat-free spaghetti sauce (any variety)
- 1 package (9 ounces) frozen Italian or regular cut green beans
- $1/4$ cup sliced ripe olives

Heat oven to 375°. Remove fat from beef. Mix flour and pepper; rub over both sides of beef, shaking off excess. Cut beef into 6 serving pieces.

Heat oil in 12-inch nonstick skillet over medium heat. Cook beef in oil about 5 minutes, turning once, until brown. Place beef in ungreased rectangular baking dish, 11 × 7 × $1\frac{1}{2}$ inches. Pour spaghetti sauce over beef. Cover and bake $1\frac{1}{2}$ hours or until beef is tender. During last 30 minutes of cooking place frozen green beans in sauce around beef. Cover and continue to bake as directed. Sprinkle with olives.

1 Serving: Calories 175 (Calories from Fat 55); Fat 6g (Saturated 2g); Cholesterol 55mg; Sodium 300mg; Carbohydrate 10g (Dietary Fiber 2g); Protein 22g
% Daily Value: Vitamin A 4%; Vitamin C 4%; Calcium 2%; Iron 14%
Diet Exchanges: 3 lean meat, 2 vegetable

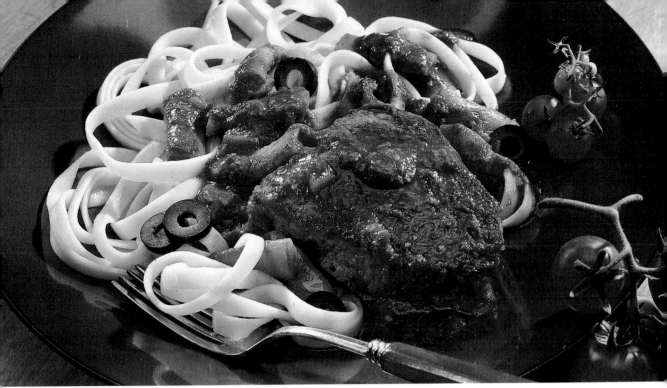

Saucy Italian Steak

Three-Pepper Beef Tenderloin

LO CAL / LO FAT

PREP: 10 MIN; MARINATE: 2 HR; ROAST: 40 MIN;

STAND: 5 MIN

6 SERVINGS

*This spicy peppered steak is not for timid taste buds!
Serve with a baked potato and a crisp green salad to
help balance the spiciness.*

1½ pound beef tenderloin

1 tablespoon freshly ground black pepper

2 teaspoons white pepper

2 teaspoons fennel seed, crushed

½ teaspoon salt

½ teaspoon ground thyme

¼ teaspoon ground red pepper (cayenne)

Remove fat from beef. Mix remaining ingredients;
rub over beef. Cover and refrigerate 2 hours but no
longer than 24 hours.

Heat oven to 350°. Spray shallow roasting pan with
cooking spray. Place beef in pan. Roast uncovered
about 40 minutes for medium doneness (160°). Let
stand 5 minutes. Cut beef across grain at slanted
angle into thin slices.

1 Serving: Calories 130 (Calories from Fat 55); Fat 6g
(Saturated 3g); Cholesterol 50mg; Sodium 240mg; Car-
bohydrate 1g (Dietary Fiber 0g); Protein 18g
% Daily Value: Vitamin A 0%; Vitamin C 0%; Calcium
0%; Iron 10%
Diet Exchanges: 2½ lean meat

Broiled Herb Steak

LO CAL / LO FAT

PREP: 15 MIN; MARINATE: 5 HR; BROIL: 20 MIN

8 SERVINGS

Reduced-sodium soy sauce has 50 percent less sodium than regular soy sauce, but still has all the great taste (photo, page 317).

2	pound beef bone-in round steak, about 1 inch thick
1	tablespoon chopped fresh or 1 teaspoon dried basil leaves
2	tablespoons reduced-sodium soy sauce
1	tablespoon vegetable oil
1	tablespoon ketchup
2	teaspoons chopped fresh or $^1/_2$ teaspoon dried oregano leaves
$^1/_2$	teaspoon salt
$^1/_2$	teaspoon coarsely ground pepper
1	clove garlic, finely chopped

Remove fat from beef. Place beef on large piece of plastic wrap. Mix remaining ingredients; brush over both sides of beef. Fold plastic wrap over beef and secure tightly. Refrigerate at least 5 hours but no longer than 24 hours.

Set oven control to broil. Place beef on rack in broiler pan. Broil with top about 3 inches from heat 8 to 10 minutes on each side for medium doneness (160°). Cut into $^1/_4$-inch slices.

1 Serving: Calories 135 (Calories from Fat 45); Fat 5g (Saturated 2g); Cholesterol 55mg; Sodium 340mg; Carbohydrate 1g (Dietary Fiber 0g); Protein 21g
% Daily Value: Vitamin A 0%; Vitamin C 0%; Calcium 0%; Iron 10%
Diet Exchanges: $2^1/_2$ lean meat

Lemon Steak Diane

LO CAL / LO FAT

PREP: 5 MIN; COOK: 15 MIN

4 SERVINGS

Worcestershire sauce gets its name from the fact it was first bottled in Worcester, England. What's in Worcestershire sauce? Garlic, soy sauce, tamarind, onions, molasses, lime, anchovies, vinegar and a variety of other seasonings. There is also a white Worcestershire sauce, which is light colored and less pungent.

1	pound beef top sirloin steak, about $^3/_4$ inch thick
$^1/_4$	teaspoon coarsely ground pepper
1	cup beef broth
1	tablespoon all-purpose flour
2	teaspoons Dijon mustard
2	teaspoons Worcestershire sauce
$^1/_2$	teaspoon grated lemon peel
2	tablespoons chopped fresh chives

Remove fat from beef. Cut beef into 4 pieces. Spray 12-inch nonstick skillet with cooking spray; heat over medium heat. Sprinkle both sides of beef with pepper. Cook beef in skillet 9 to 11 minutes for medium doneness (160°), turning once. Remove beef from skillet; keep warm.

Mix remaining ingredients except chives until smooth; add to skillet. Heat to boiling. Boil 1 minute, stirring constantly. Stir in chives. Serve over beef.

1 Serving: Calories 120 (Calories from Fat 25); Fat 3g (Saturated 1g); Cholesterol 55mg; Sodium 350mg; Carbohydrate 2g (Dietary Fiber 0g); Protein 21g
% Daily Value: Vitamin A 0%; Vitamin C 0%; Calcium 0%; Iron 12%
Diet Exchanges: 3 very lean meat, $^1/_2$ fat

Hungarian Swiss Steak

LO CAL / LO FAT

PREP: 5 MIN; COOK: 30 MIN

4 SERVINGS

Paprika is an important flavoring in Hungarian cuisine, and many believe that Hungarian paprika is superior to all others. Paprika is made from ground sweet red pepper pods and can range from mild to hot. The color can vary as well, from bright orange to deep red.

1   pound beef boneless sirloin steak, about ³/₄ inch thick

¹/₄   teaspoon peppered seasoned salt

1   can (14¹/₂ ounces) stewed tomatoes, undrained

1   tablespoon paprika

2   tablespoons ketchup

¹/₄   teaspoon caraway seed, if desired

¹/₂   cup reduced-fat sour cream

Chopped fresh chives, if desired

Remove fat from beef. Cut beef into 4 serving pieces. Sprinkle both sides of beef with seasoned salt.

Spray 12-inch nonstick skillet with cooking spray; heat over medium-high heat. Cook beef in skillet 4 to 8 minutes, turning once, until brown.

Stir in tomatoes, paprika, ketchup and caraway seed; reduce heat. Cover and simmer 15 to 20 minutes or until beef is tender. Top each serving with sour cream and chives.

1 Serving: Calories 190 (Calories from Fat 45); Fat 5g (Saturated 2g); Cholesterol 65mg; Sodium 530mg; Carbohydrate 14g (Dietary Fiber 1g); Protein 23g
% Daily Value: Vitamin A 20%; Vitamin C 12%; Calcium 6%; Iron 14%
Diet Exchanges: 1 starch, 2 lean meat

Veal and Potato Strata with Roasted Peppers

LO CAL / HI FIB

PREP: 10 MIN; COOK: 10 MIN; BAKE: 40 MIN

6 SERVINGS

If you can't find tenderized veal cutlets already packaged in the meat case, ask the butcher to tenderize slices of veal for you.

1½   pounds tenderized boneless veal cutlets

1   bag (1 pound 4 ounces) refrigerated shredded hash brown potatoes

1   jar (12 ounces) roasted red bell peppers, drained

½   teaspoon salt

3   medium onions, cut lengthwise in half, then cut crosswise into thin slices

3   cloves garlic, finely chopped

½   teaspoon dried oregano leaves

½   teaspoon cracked black pepper

4   ounces feta cheese, crumbled (⅔ cup)

Heat oven to 350°. Spray rectangular baking dish, 13 × 9 × 2 inches, with cooking spray. Remove fat from veal. Cut veal into 6 serving pieces.

Layer potatoes and bell peppers in dish. Sprinkle salt over potatoes. Cover and bake 15 minutes. While potatoes are baking, spray 12-inch nonstick skillet with cooking spray; heat over medium-high heat. Cook veal in skillet about 5 minutes, turning once, until slightly pink in center. Remove veal from skillet.

Cook onions and garlic in same skillet over medium heat about 5 minutes, stirring frequently, until onions are tender.

Place veal on potato mixture. Layer onion mixture over veal. Sprinkle with oregano and pepper. Sprinkle with feta. Cover and bake 20 to 25 minutes or until heated through.

1 Serving: Calories 295 (Calories from Fat 70); Fat 8g (Saturated 4g); Cholesterol 90mg; Sodium 640mg; Carbohydrate 36g (Dietary Fiber 4g); Protein 24g
% Daily Value: Vitamin A 18%; Vitamin C 72%; Calcium 14%; Iron 10%
Diet Exchanges: 2½ starch, 2 lean meat

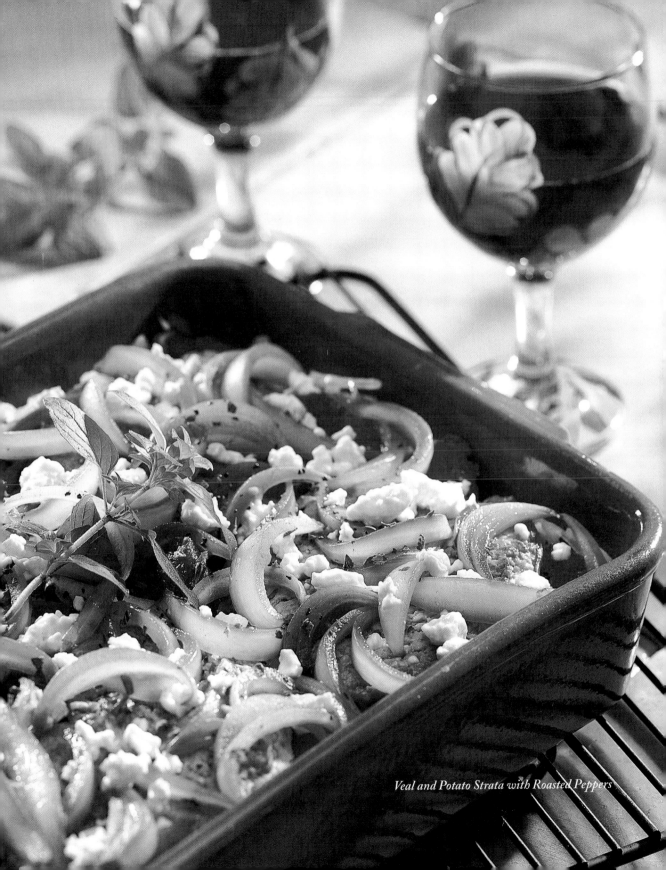

Veal and Potato Strata with Roasted Peppers

Mexican Steak Stir-Fry

LO CAL / LO FAT / HI FIB

PREP: 15 MIN; COOK: 10 MIN

4 SERVINGS

Pinto beans are two-toned, kidney-shaped beans widely used in Central and South American cooking. They turn completely pink when cooked and are best known for their use in refried beans.

- ³⁄₄ pound beef boneless sirloin
- 1 medium onion, chopped (¹⁄₂ cup)
- 1 small green bell pepper, chopped (¹⁄₂ cup)
- 1 clove garlic, finely chopped
- 1 cup frozen whole kernel corn
- ¹⁄₂ cup salsa
- 1 medium zucchini, sliced (2 cups)
- 1 can (15 to 16 ounces) pinto beans, rinsed and drained
- 1 can (14¹⁄₂ ounces) whole tomatoes, undrained

Remove fat from beef. Cut beef into ¹⁄₄ × ¹⁄₂-inch strips. (Beef is easier to cut if partially frozen, about 1¹⁄₂ hours.)

Spray 12-inch nonstick skillet or wok with cooking spray; heat over medium-high heat. Add beef, onion, bell pepper and garlic; stir-fry 4 to 5 minutes or until beef is brown.

Stir in remaining ingredients, breaking up tomatoes. Cook about 5 minutes, stirring occasionally, until zucchini is tender and mixture is hot.

1 Serving: Calories 240 (Calories from Fat 25); Fat 3g (Saturated 1g); Cholesterol 40mg; Sodium 390mg; Carbohydrate 38g (Dietary Fiber 10g); Protein 25g
% Daily Value: Vitamin A 12%; Vitamin C 46%; Calcium 10%; Iron 26%
Diet Exchanges: 2 starch, 1 lean meat, 2 vegetable

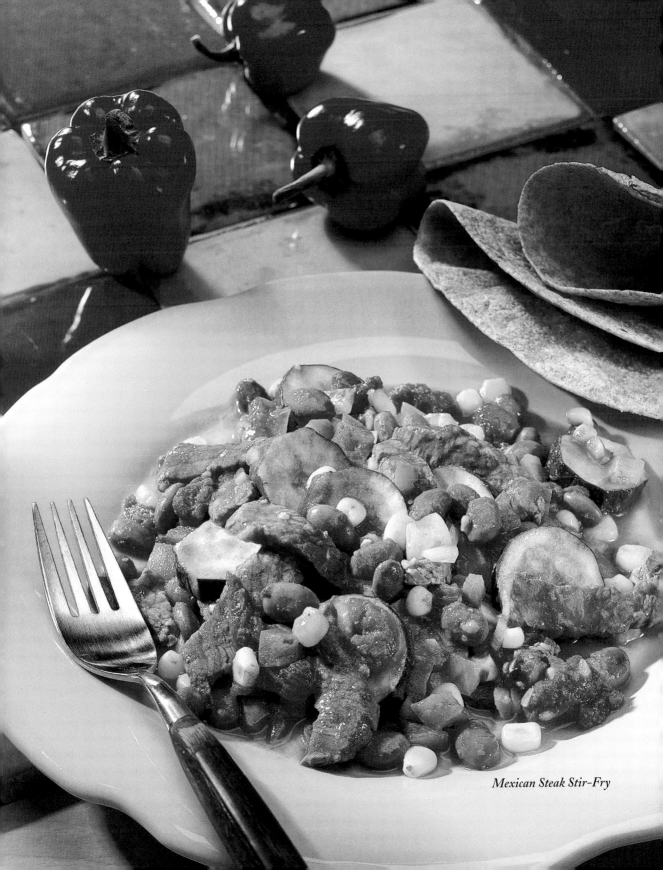

Mexican Steak Stir-Fry

Spicy Stir-Fried Beef

LO CAL / HI FIB

PREP: 25 MIN; MARINATE: 30 MIN; COOK: 10 MIN

6 SERVINGS

Bamboo shoots are the young, tender, ivory-colored shoots from the tropical bamboo plant, and they are eaten as a vegetable.

1½ pound beef flank or boneless sirloin steak

1 tablespoon cornstarch

2 tablespoons reduced-sodium soy sauce

1 teaspoon sugar

¼ teaspoon pepper

1 tablespoon reduced-sodium soy sauce

½ teaspoon crushed red pepper

1 tablespoon vegetable oil

1 teaspoon finely chopped gingerroot

2 cloves garlic, finely chopped

1 large bell pepper, cut into ¼-inch strips

1 cup shredded carrots (1½ medium)

1 can (8 ounces) sliced bamboo shoots, drained

1 can (8 ounces) sliced water chestnuts, drained

6 medium green onions, cut into 2-inch pieces

Remove fat from beef. Cut beef lengthwise into 2-inch strips; cut strips crosswise into ⅛-inch slices. Stack slices and cut into julienne strips. (Beef is easier to cut if partially frozen, about 1½ hours.)

Toss beef, cornstarch, 2 tablespoons soy sauce, the sugar and pepper in glass or plastic bowl. Cover and refrigerate 30 minutes. Mix 1 tablespoon soy sauce and the red pepper; let stand at room temperature.

Heat oil in wok or 12-inch nonstick skillet over high heat. Add beef mixture, gingerroot and garlic; stir-fry about 5 minutes or until beef is brown. Add bell pepper, carrots, bamboo shoots and water chestnuts; stir-fry 3 minutes. Add onions and red pepper mixture; cook and stir 1 minute.

1 Serving: Calories 230 (Calories from Fat 90); Fat 10g (Saturated 4g); Cholesterol 60mg; Sodium 340mg; Carbohydrate 13g (Dietary Fiber 3g); Protein 25g
% Daily Value: Vitamin A 34%; Vitamin C 26%; Calcium 4%; Iron 16%
Diet Exchanges: 3 lean meat, 2 vegetable

German-Style Meat Loaf

LOW CALORIE

PREP: 10 MIN; BAKE: 40 MIN

6 SERVINGS

Before baking, try spreading the meat loaf with a mixture of ¼ cup each packed brown sugar and spicy brown mustard. Serve the meat loaf with spaetzle, the traditional German noodle side dish. You'll find dried spaetzle in the pasta section of the supermarket.

1½	pounds diet-lean or extra-lean ground beef
1	cup lower-calorie beer, nonalcoholic beer or skim milk
¼	cup fat-free cholesterol-free egg product or 2 egg whites, slightly beaten
2	tablespoons packed brown sugar
2	tablespoons spicy brown mustard
1	teaspoon onion salt
3	slices rye or pumpernickel bread, torn into small pieces*
1	can (8 ounces) sauerkraut, very well drained and chopped

Heat oven to 350°. Mix all ingredients. Spread mixture in ungreased square pan, 9 × 9 × 2 inches. Insert meat thermometer so tip is in center of meat loaf.

Bake uncovered about 40 minutes or until no longer pink in center and juice is clear (meat thermometer should reach at least 160°). Let stand 5 minutes before serving.

*½ cup dry bread crumbs or ¾ cup quick-cooking oats can be substituted for the 3 slices bread.

1 Serving: Calories 250 (Calories from Fat 120); Fat 13g (Saturated 5g); Cholesterol 70mg; Sodium 350mg; Carbohydrate 9g (Dietary Fiber 1g); Protein 25g
% Daily Value: Vitamin A 0%; Vitamin C 0%; Calcium 2%; Iron 18%
Diet Exchanges: ½ starch, 3 lean meat, 1 fat

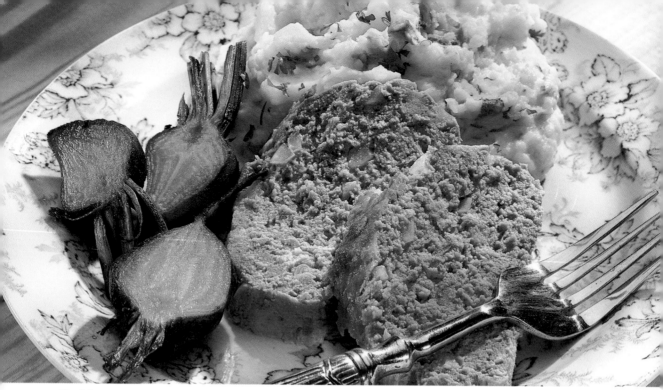

Healthy Meat Loaf

Healthy Meat Loaf

LOW CALORIE

PREP: 15 MIN; BAKE: 1 HR

6 SERVINGS

Ground turkey isn't necessarily less fatty than ground beef; be sure to check the label to see what percentage of fat it contains. Ground turkey breast is the leanest ground turkey product you can buy—it's 99 percent fat free.

$^3/_4$ pound ground turkey breast

$^3/_4$ pound extra-lean ground beef

1   large onion, finely chopped (1 cup)

$^1/_2$ cup soft bread crumbs

2   tablespoons ketchup or tomato puree

2   tablespoons Dijon mustard

$^1/_2$ teaspoon salt

$^1/_4$ cup fat-free cholesterol-free egg product or 2 egg whites

2   cloves garlic, finely chopped

Heat oven to 375°. Spray loaf pan, $8^1/_2 \times 4^1/_2 \times 2^1/_2$ inches, with cooking spray. Mix all ingredients. Spread in pan. Bake uncovered about 1 hour or until no longer pink in center and juice is clear (meat thermometer should reach at least 160°). Drain immediately.

1 Serving: Calories 225 (Calories from Fat 90); Fat 10g (Saturated 4g); Cholesterol 70mg; Sodium 390mg; Carbohydrate 9g (Dietary Fiber 1g); Protein 26g
% Daily Value: Vitamin A 0%; Vitamin C 0%; Calcium 4%; Iron 12%
Diet Exchanges: 3 lean meat, 2 vegetable

Bacon Cheeseburgers

LOW CALORIE

PREP: 10 MIN; BROIL: 10 MIN

6 SERVINGS

If you've given up bacon cheeseburgers because you think they're too high in fat and calories, bite into this mouth-watering burger. Made with extra-lean ground beef, reduced-fat cheese, fat-free cholesterol-free egg product and fat-free bacon-flavor bits, this burger lets you indulge without a twinge of guilt. Add a little fire to the burger by using hot-style ketchup.

1/4 cup fat-free cholesterol-free egg product or 2 egg whites

1 tablespoon ketchup

1 tablespoon Dijon mustard

1/4 cup dry bread crumbs

2 tablespoons imitation bacon-flavor bits or chips

1/4 teaspoon ground red pepper (cayenne)

1 pound diet-lean or extra-lean ground beef

3 slices (3/4 ounce each) reduced-fat process Cheddar- or American-flavored cheese product, cut diagonally in half

Lettuce leaves, if desired

Tomato slices, if desired

Hamburger buns, split and toasted, if desired

Set oven control to broil. Spray broiler pan rack with cooking spray.

Mix egg product, ketchup and mustard in large bowl. Stir in bread crumbs, bacon bits and red pepper. Stir in beef. Shape mixture into 6 patties, each about 1/2 inch thick.

Place patties on rack in broiler pan. Broil with tops about 5 inches from heat about 5 minutes on each side for medium, turning once, until no longer pink in center and juice is clear. Immediately top with cheese. Serve with lettuce and tomato on buns.

1 Serving: Calories 185 (Calories from Fat 90); Fat 10g (Saturated 4g); Cholesterol 45mg; Sodium 260mg; Carbohydrate 5g (Dietary Fiber 1g); Protein 20g
% Daily Value: Vitamin A 2%; Vitamin C 0%; Calcium 6%; Iron 12%
Diet Exchanges: 2 1/2 lean meat, 1 fat

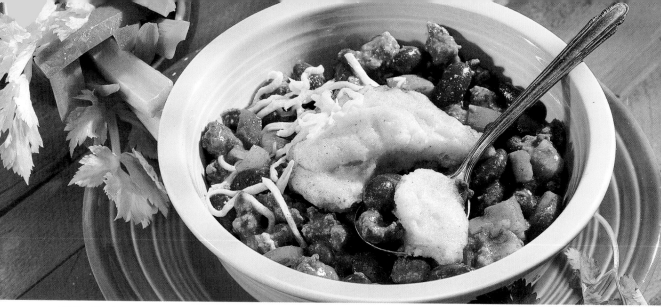

Skillet Hot Tamale Pie

Skillet Hot Tamale Pie

LO CAL / HI FIB

PREP: 10 MIN; COOK: 15 MIN

6 SERVINGS

With this cornmeal-topped pie, you can enjoy tamale-like flavor without the time-consuming work of filling and steaming authentic tamales. If you like, substitute ground turkey breast or lean ground pork for the ground beef.

1/2 cup yellow cornmeal

1/2 cup cold water

1 1/3 cups water

1 pound diet-lean or extra-lean ground beef

1 large onion, chopped (1 cup)

1 medium green or red bell pepper, chopped (1 cup)

1 can (15 to 16 ounces) reduced-sodium kidney beans, rinsed and drained

1 can (10 ounces) enchilada sauce

1/2 cup shredded reduced-fat Cheddar cheese (2 ounces)

Mix cornmeal and 1/2 cup cold water; set aside. Heat 1 1/3 cups water to boiling in 2-quart saucepan. Gradually add cornmeal mixture to boiling water, stirring constantly to make sure it does not lump. Heat to boiling, stirring constantly; reduce heat to low. Simmer uncovered about 10 minutes, stirring occasionally, until very thick.

While cornmeal mixture is cooking, cook beef, onion and bell pepper in 12-inch nonstick skillet over medium heat about 6 minutes, stirring occasionally, until beef is brown; drain. Stir in kidney beans and enchilada sauce.

Spoon hot cornmeal mixture on beef mixture in a ring around edge of skillet. Cover and simmer about 5 minutes longer or until heated through. Sprinkle with cheese.

1 Serving: Calories 290 (Calories from Fat 90); Fat 10g (Saturated 4g); Cholesterol 45mg; Sodium 390mg; Carbohydrate 31g (Dietary Fiber 7g); Protein 26g
% Daily Value: Vitamin A 14%; Vitamin C 40%; Calcium 8%; Iron 26%
Diet Exchanges: 1 1/2 starch, 1 1/2 lean meat, 1 vegetable, 1 fat

Giant Oven Burger

LOW CALORIE

PREP: 10 MIN; BAKE: 50 MIN; STAND: 5 MIN

6 SERVINGS

This easy baked burger is fun to make and to eat. Serve it with your favorite baked potato chips, and carrot and celery sticks for healthy crunch.

1   **pound diet lean or extra-lean ground beef**

1   **small bell pepper, finely chopped (¹/₂ cup)**

1   **small onion, finely chopped (¹/₄ cup)**

1   **tablespoon prepared horseradish**

1   **tablespoon mustard**

¹/₂   **teaspoon salt**

¹/₃   **cup chili sauce or ketchup**

1   **unsliced round loaf Italian or sourdough bread (8 inches in diameter)**

Heat oven to 350°. Mix all ingredients except chili sauce and bread. Press beef mixture in ungreased pie plate, 9 × 1¹/₄ inches. Spread chili sauce over top.

Bake uncovered 45 to 50 minutes or until no longer pink in center and juice is clear (meat thermometer should reach at least 160°); drain. Let stand 5 minutes. Cut bread horizontally in half. Carefully place burger between halves. Cut into wedges.

1 Serving: Calories 195 (Calories from Fat 80); Fat 9g (Saturated 3g); Cholesterol 45mg; Sodium 510mg; Carbohydrate 12g (Dietary Fiber 1g); Protein 17g
% Daily Value: Vitamin A 2%; Vitamin C 12%; Calcium 2%; Iron 12%
Diet Exchanges: 3 starch, 2¹/₂ medium-fat meat

Yummy Pork Chops

LOW CALORIE

PREP: 5 MIN; BAKE: 50 MIN

4 SERVINGS

For a bit of a kick, substitute chili sauce or chili puree with garlic for the ketchup.

- 4 pork loin chops, $1/2$ inch thick (about $1^1/4$ pounds)
- 3 tablespoons reduced-sodium soy sauce
- 3 tablespoons ketchup
- 2 teaspoons honey

Heat oven to 350°. Remove fat from pork. Place pork in ungreased square baking dish, $8 \times 8 \times 2$ inches. Mix remaining ingredients; pour over pork.

Cover and bake about 45 minutes or until pork is slightly pink when cut near bone. Uncover and bake 5 minutes longer.

1 Serving: Calories 190 (Calories from Fat 70); Fat 8g (Saturated 3g); Cholesterol 65mg; Sodium 570mg; Carbohydrate 7g (Dietary Fiber 0g); Protein 23g
% Daily Value: Vitamin A 0%; Vitamin C 0%; Calcium 0%; Iron 6%
Diet Exchanges: 3 lean meat, $1/2$ fruit

Pork Chop Dinner

LOW CAL / HI FIB

PREP: 10 MIN; COOK: 40 MIN

4 SERVINGS

Carrots offer good nutrition, as they are an excellent source of vitamin A and contain beta-carotene.

- 4 pork loin or rib chops, 1 inch thick (about $1^1/2$ pounds)
- $1/4$ cup beef or chicken broth
- 4 medium potatoes, peeled and cut into fourths
- 4 small carrots, cut into 1-inch pieces
- 4 medium onions, cut into fourths
- $3/4$ teaspoon salt
- $1/4$ teaspoon pepper

Remove fat from pork. Spray 12-inch nonstick skillet with cooking spray; heat over medium-high heat. Cook pork in skillet about 5 minutes, turning once, until brown.

Add broth, potatoes, carrots and onions to skillet. Sprinkle with salt and pepper. Heat to boiling; reduce heat. Cover and simmer about 30 minutes or until vegetables are tender and pork is slightly pink when cut near bone.

1 Serving: Calories 335 (Calories from Fat 90); Fat 10g (Saturated 4g); Cholesterol 75mg; Sodium 510mg; Carbohydrate 36g (Dietary Fiber 5g); Protein 30g
% Daily Value: Vitamin A 76%; Vitamin C 20%; Calcium 4%; Iron 10%
Diet Exchanges: 2 starch, 3 lean meat, 1 vegetable

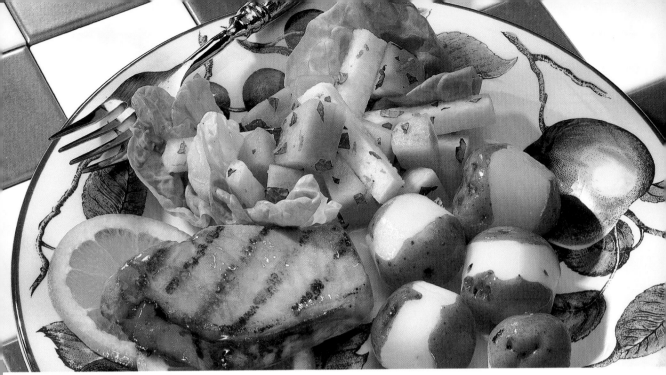

Grilled Honey-Mustard Pork Chops

Grilled Honey-Mustard Pork Chops

LOW CALORIE

PREP: 5 MIN; GRILL: 15 MIN

4 SERVINGS

Serve these chops with boiled new potatoes and the Crunchy Jicama and Melon Salad on page 361.

4	pork boneless butterfly loin chops, 1 inch thick (about 1 pound)
1/4	cup honey
2	tablespoons Dijon mustard
1	tablespoon orange juice
1	teaspoon cider vinegar
1/2	teaspoon Worcestershire sauce
	Dash of onion powder

Heat coals or gas grill. Remove fat from pork. Mix remaining ingredients.

Cover and grill pork 4 to 6 inches from medium heat 14 to 16 minutes, brushing occasionally with honey mixture and turning once, until pork is slightly pink in center. Discard any remaining honey mixture.

1 Serving: Calories 235 (Calories from Fat 70); Fat 8g (Saturated 3g); Cholesterol 65mg; Sodium 145mg; Carbohydrate 19g (Dietary Fiber 0g); Protein 22g
% Daily Value: Vitamin A 0%; Vitamin C 0%; Calcium 0%; Iron 6%
Diet Exchanges: 3 lean meat, 1 vegetable, 1 fruit

Ginger-Sherry Pork Chops

LOW CALORIE

PREP: 10 MIN; MARINATE: 1 HR; BROIL: 15 MIN

4 SERVINGS

Butterfly in cooking terms means to split a food down the center, cutting almost but not completely through. The two halves are then opened flat to resemble a butterfly shape.

4 pork boneless butterfly loin chops, about 1 inch thick (about 1 pound)

1/3 cup sherry or apple juice

1 tablespoon finely chopped gingerroot

2 tablespoons reduced-sodium soy sauce

1 teaspoon honey

1 clove garlic, finely chopped

Remove fat from pork. Mix remaining ingredients in shallow glass or plastic dish. Add pork; turn to coat with marinade. Cover and refrigerate at least 1 hour but no longer than 24 hours.

Set oven control to broil. Remove pork from marinade; reserve marinade. Place pork on rack in broiler pan. Brush with marinade. Broil with tops about 4 inches from heat about 7 minutes or until brown. Turn pork; brush with marinade. Broil 5 to 7 minutes longer or until pork is slightly pink in center. Discard any remaining marinade.

1 Serving: Calories 180 (Calories from Fat 70); Fat 8g (Saturated 3g); Cholesterol 65mg; Sodium 310mg; Carbohydrate 5g (Dietary Fiber 0g); Protein 22g **% Daily Value:** Vitamin A 0%; Vitamin C 0%; Calcium 0%; Iron 6% **Diet Exchanges:** 3 lean meat, 1/2 fruit

Tangy Barbecued Pork

LO CAL / LO FAT / HI FIB

PREP: 10 MIN; COOK: 20 MIN

6 SERVINGS

All you need to complete this meal is coleslaw for a salad and your favorite bread or dinner rolls.

3 pork boneless butterfly loin chops, 1/2 inch thick (about 3/4 pound)

2 medium onions, cut lengthwise in half, then cut crosswise into thin slices

1/2 cup apricot spreadable fruit

1/2 cup fat-free sweet-spicy French dressing

3 tablespoons reduced-sodium onion soup mix (from 1 1/2 ounce packet)

1 teaspoon red pepper sauce

Hot cooked brown rice, if desired

Remove fat from pork. Spray 12-inch nonstick skillet with cooking spray; heat over medium heat. Cook pork in skillet about 5 minutes, turning once, until brown. Remove pork from skillet.

Cook onions in same skillet over medium heat about 5 minutes, stirring frequently, until tender. Stir in spreadable fruit, dressing, soup mix (dry) and pepper sauce. Heat to boiling; reduce heat. Simmer uncovered 5 minutes, stirring occasionally.

Place pork on sauce. Spoon sauce over pork to cover. Cover and simmer about 5 minutes or until pork is slightly pink in center. Serve over rice.

1 Serving: Calories 185 (Calories from Fat 35); Fat 4g (Saturated 1g); Cholesterol 30mg; Sodium 530mg; Carbohydrate 28g (Dietary Fiber 2g); Protein 11g **% Daily Value:** Vitamin A 0%; Vitamin C 4%; Calcium 4%; Iron 4% **Diet Exchanges:** 2 starch, 1/2 lean meat

Pork Chops Smothered with Cabbage

LOW CAL / LO FAT / HI FIB

PREP: 15 MIN; COOK: 1 HR 20 MIN

6 SERVINGS

Serve with slices of Oat-Potato Sandwich Bread (page 389) or your favorite store-bought or bakery bread.

- 6 pork rib or loin chops, about ¾ inch thick (about 1½ pounds)
- ½ teaspoon salt
- ¼ teaspoon pepper
- 1 bag (16 ounces) coleslaw mix (6 cups)
- 3 medium baking apples, chopped (3 cups)
- 1 large red onion, sliced
- 1 cup chicken broth
- ¼ cup cider vinegar or red wine vinegar
- ¼ cup packed brown sugar

Remove fat from pork. Sprinkle both sides of pork with salt and pepper. Spray 12-inch nonstick skillet with cooking spray; heat over medium-high heat. Cook pork in skillet, turning once, until brown. Remove pork from skillet.

Mix remaining ingredients in skillet. Heat to boiling, stirring occasionally. Place pork on top; reduce heat. Cover and simmer about 45 minutes or until pork is slightly pink when cut near bone.

1 Serving: Calories 220 (Calories from Fat 55); Fat 6g (Saturated 2g); Cholesterol 45mg; Sodium 400mg; Carbohydrate 28g (Dietary Fiber 5g); Protein 18g
% Daily Value: Vitamin A 2%; Vitamin C 46%; Calcium 6%; Iron 10%
Diet Exchanges: 2 lean meat, 2 vegetable, 1 fruit

Parmesan Breaded Pork Chops

LOW CALORIE

PREP: 10 MIN; COOK: 20 MIN

4 SERVINGS

Italian-style bread crumbs are seasoned with a variety of herbs and spices. If you can't find the Italian-style, you can substitute seasoned bread crumbs (also available at grocery stores).

- 4 pork boneless butterfly loin chops, about ½ inch thick (about 1 pound)
- ⅓ cup Italian-style dry bread crumbs
- 2 tablespoons grated Parmesan cheese
- ¼ cup fat-free cholesterol-free egg product or 2 egg whites
- 1 can (14½ ounces) chunky tomatoes with olive oil, garlic and spices, undrained
- 1 can (8 ounces) tomato sauce
- 1 small green bell pepper, chopped (½ cup)

Remove fat from pork. Mix bread crumbs and cheese. Dip pork into egg product, then coat with crumb mixture. Spray 12-inch nonstick skillet with cooking spray; heat over medium heat. Cook pork in skillet about 5 minutes, turning once, until brown.

Stir in remaining ingredients. Heat to boiling; reduce heat. Cover and simmer 10 to 12 minutes, stirring occasionally, until pork is slightly pink in center.

1 Serving: Calories 300 (Calories from Fat 125); Fat 14g (Saturated 5g); Cholesterol 65mg; Sodium 810mg; Carbohydrate 19g (Dietary Fiber 2g); Protein 27g
% Daily Value: Vitamin A 12%; Vitamin C 30%; Calcium 10%; Iron 14%
Diet Exchanges: 1 starch, 2½ medium-fat meat, 1 vegetable

Pork with Apple and Parsnips

LO CAL / HI FIB

PREP: 10 MIN; COOK: 40 MIN

4 SERVINGS

Parsnips are a root vegetable. Although they are available all year, their peak seasons are fall and winter. Parsnips are shaped like jumbo carrots and are creamy white in color.

4   pork loin or rib chops, about $\frac{1}{2}$ inch thick (about 1 pound)

3   medium parsnips, cut crosswise into $\frac{1}{2}$-inch slices

1   medium onion, sliced

$\frac{1}{2}$ cup chicken broth

1   teaspoon ground mustard (dry)

$\frac{1}{4}$ teaspoon salt

$\frac{1}{4}$ teaspoon ground allspice or cinnamon

$\frac{1}{8}$ teaspoon pepper

1   medium apple, cut into $\frac{1}{4}$-inch wedges

2   tablespoons chopped fresh parsley

Remove fat from pork. Cook pork in 10-inch nonstick skillet over medium heat, turning once, until brown; drain.

Place parsnips and onion on pork. Mix broth, mustard, salt, allspice and pepper; pour over vegetables and pork. Heat to boiling; reduce heat. Cover and simmer about 30 minutes or until pork is tender.

Place apple wedges on vegetables. Cover and simmer about 3 minutes or just until apple is tender. Sprinkle with parsley.

1 Serving: Calories 220 (Calories from Fat 65); Fat 7g (Saturated 3g); Cholesterol 50mg; Sodium 320mg; Carbohydrate 23g (Dietary Fiber 4g); Protein 20g
% Daily Value: Vitamin A 0%; Vitamin C 12%; Calcium 4%; Iron 8%
Diet Exchanges: 1 starch, 2 lean meat, $\frac{1}{2}$ fruit

Pork with Stuffed Yams

LOW CALORIE

PREP: 10 MIN; BAKE: 1 HR

4 SERVINGS

All you need to complete this hearty meal is a simple side dish of your favorite cooked green vegetable.

2	medium yams or sweet potatoes
4	pork loin or rib chops, about $3/4$ inch thick (about $1^1/2$ pounds)
$^1/_2$	teaspoon salt
$^1/_4$	teaspoon paprika
$^1/_8$	teaspoon garlic powder
$^1/_8$	teaspoon pepper
$^1/_2$	cup orange juice
2	tablespoons orange juice
$^1/_2$	cup chopped apple
2	tablespoons finely chopped onion
2	tablespoons finely chopped celery

Heat oven to 350°. Pierce yams with fork to allow steam to escape. Bake 55 to 60 minutes or until tender. Remove fat from pork chops. About 30 minutes before yams are done, place pork in ungreased rectangular pan, 13 × 9 × 2 inches. Mix salt, paprika, garlic powder and pepper; sprinkle half of the salt mixture over pork. Turn pork; sprinkle with remaining salt mixture. Pour $^1/_2$ cup orange juice into pan. Cover and bake 30 minutes.

Cut each yam lengthwise in half. Scoop out pulp, leaving $^1/_4$-inch shell. Mash pulp until no lumps remain. Beat in 2 tablespoons orange juice until light and fluffy. Stir in apple, onion and celery. Fill shells with pulp mixture.

Move pork to one end of pan; place yams in other end of pan. Bake uncovered about 30 minutes or until yams are hot and pork is slightly pink when cut near bone.

1 Serving: Calories 280 (Calories from Fat 90); Fat 10g (Saturated 4g); Cholesterol 75mg; Sodium 350mg; Carbohydrate 21g (Dietary Fiber 2g); Protein 28g
% Daily Value: Vitamin A 100%; Vitamin C 24%; Calcium 2%; Iron 8%
Diet Exchanges: 1 starch, 3 lean meat, 1 vegetable

Caribbean Pork Roast

LOW CALORIE

PREP: 20 MIN; MARINATE: 4 HR; ROAST: 2¼ HR;

STAND: 15 MIN

8 SERVINGS

Allspice isn't a blend of numerous spices, as its name implies, but is a single spice. Popular in Caribbean cuisine, allspice tastes like a combination of cinnamon, nutmeg and clove.

2- to 2½- pound pork boneless center loin roast

1	cup orange juice
½	cup lime juice
1½	teaspoons ground cumin
1½	teaspoons red pepper sauce
¾	teaspoon ground allspice
1	medium green bell pepper, cut into eighths
1	medium onion, cut into fourths
4	cloves garlic, finely chopped
	Salt and pepper to taste
1½	teaspoons sugar
½	teaspoon salt

Remove fat from pork. Pierce pork deeply all over with meat fork or skewer. Place pork in heavy resealable plastic food-storage bag. Place remaining ingredients except salt and pepper, sugar and ½ teaspoon salt in blender or food processor. Cover and blend on medium speed until smooth. Pour blended mixture over pork. Seal bag; place in dish. Refrigerate, turning bag occasionally, at least 4 hours but no longer than 24 hours.

Heat oven to 325°. Remove pork from marinade; refrigerate marinade. Sprinkle pork with salt and pepper to taste. Place pork on rack in shallow roasting pan. Insert meat thermometer so tip is in center of thickest part of pork and does not rest in fat. Roast uncovered 1 to 1½ hours for medium doneness (160°). Remove pork from pan. Cover and let stand about 15 minutes before slicing.

Pour marinade into 1½-quart saucepan. Stir in sugar and ½ teaspoon salt. Heat to boiling; reduce heat. Simmer uncovered about 5 minutes, stirring occasionally, until mixture thickens slightly. Serve sauce with pork.

1 Serving: Calories 165 (Calories from Fat 65); Fat 7g (Saturated 3g); Cholesterol 50mg; Sodium 480mg; Carbohydrate 8g (Dietary Fiber 1g); Protein 19g
% Daily Value: Vitamin A 2%; Vitamin C 24%; Calcium 2%; Iron 6%
Diet Exchanges: 2½ lean meat, ½ fruit

Stacked Pork Enchiladas with Salsa Verde

LO CAL / HI FIB

PREP: 20 MIN; BAKE: 10 MIN

5 SERVINGS

Green salsa is often made with tomatillos, which sometimes are called green tomatoes. In truth, they're not tomatoes at all but a completely different fruit, the tomatillo.

- 3/4 pound pork tenderloin
- 1 jar (16 ounces) green salsa (salsa verde)
- 1 container (8 ounces) reduced-fat sour cream
- 1 large onion, chopped (1 cup)
- 1 medium yellow or green bell pepper, chopped (1 cup)
- 3 cloves garlic, finely chopped
- 3/4 cup shredded reduced-fat mozzarella cheese (3 ounces)
- 4 fat-free flour tortillas (6 to 8 inches in diameter)

Heat oven to 400°. Spray square baking dish, 9 × 9 × 2 inches, with cooking spray. Remove fat from pork. Cut pork into 3/4-inch cubes.

Mix salsa and sour cream; set aside. Spray 10-inch nonstick skillet with cooking spray; heat over medium-high heat. Cook pork, onion, bell pepper and garlic in skillet about 6 minutes, stirring occasionally, until pork is no longer pink.

Stir 2 cups of the salsa mixture into pork mixture. Cook uncovered over medium heat 1 minute, stirring frequently; remove from heat. Stir in 1/2 cup of the cheese.

Place 1 tortilla in baking dish. Top with one-third of the pork mixture. Repeat layers twice more. Top with remaining tortilla. Spoon remaining salsa mixture on top; sprinkle with remaining 1/4 cup cheese. Cover loosely with aluminum foil and bake about 10 minutes or until heated through.

1 Serving: Calories 335 (Calories from Fat 80); Fat 9g (Saturated 5g); Cholesterol 65mg; Sodium 440mg; Carbohydrate 41g (Dietary Fiber 4g); Protein 27g
% Daily Value: Vitamin A 18%; Vitamin C 56%; Calcium 24%; Iron 10%
Diet Exchanges: 2 starch, 2 lean meat, 2 vegetable

Italian Roasted Pork Tenderloin

LO CAL / LO FAT

PREP: 10 MIN; ROAST: 30 MIN

6 SERVINGS

Pork has slimmed down! Once thought of as a fatty meat, pork today is leaner than it's ever been. For the leanest pork cut, choose the tenderloin.

2   pork tenderloins, about $3/4$ pound each

1   teaspoon olive or vegetable oil

$1/2$ teaspoon salt

$1/2$ teaspoon fennel seed, crushed

$1/4$ teaspoon pepper

1   clove garlic, finely chopped

Heat oven to 375°. Spray roasting pan rack with cooking spray. Remove fat from pork. Mash remaining ingredients into a paste. Rub paste on pork.

Place pork on rack in shallow roasting pan. Insert meat thermometer so tip is in thickest part of pork. Roast uncovered about 35 minutes for medium doneness (160°).

1 Serving: Calories 140 (Calories from Fat 45); Fat 5g (Saturated 2g); Cholesterol 65mg; Sodium 240mg; Carbohydrate 0g (Dietary Fiber 0g); Protein 24g
% Daily Value: Vitamin A 0%; Vitamin C 0%; Calcium 0%; Iron 6%
Diet Exchanges: 3 lean meat

Caramelized Pork Slices

LO CAL / LO FAT

PREP: 10 MIN; COOK: 10 MIN

4 SERVINGS

Serve this slightly sweet roast pork with corn and baked or mashed sweet potatoes.

1   pound pork tenderloin

2   cloves garlic, finely chopped

2   tablespoons packed brown sugar

1   tablespoon orange juice

1   tablespoon molasses

$1/2$ teaspoon salt

$1/4$ teaspoon pepper

Remove fat from pork. Cut pork into $1/2$-inch slices. Spray 10-inch nonstick skillet with cooking spray; heat over medium-high heat.

Cook pork and garlic in skillet 6 to 8 minutes, turning occasionally, until pork is slightly pink in center. Drain if necessary. Stir in remaining ingredients. Cook until mixture thickens and coats pork.

1 Serving: Calories 175 (Calories from Fat 35); Fat 4g (Saturated 2g); Cholesterol 65mg; Sodium 350mg; Carbohydrate 11g (Dietary Fiber 0g); Protein 24g
% Daily Value: Vitamin A 0%; Vitamin C 2%; Calcium 2%; Iron 10%
Diet Exchanges: 3 lean meat, $1/2$ fruit

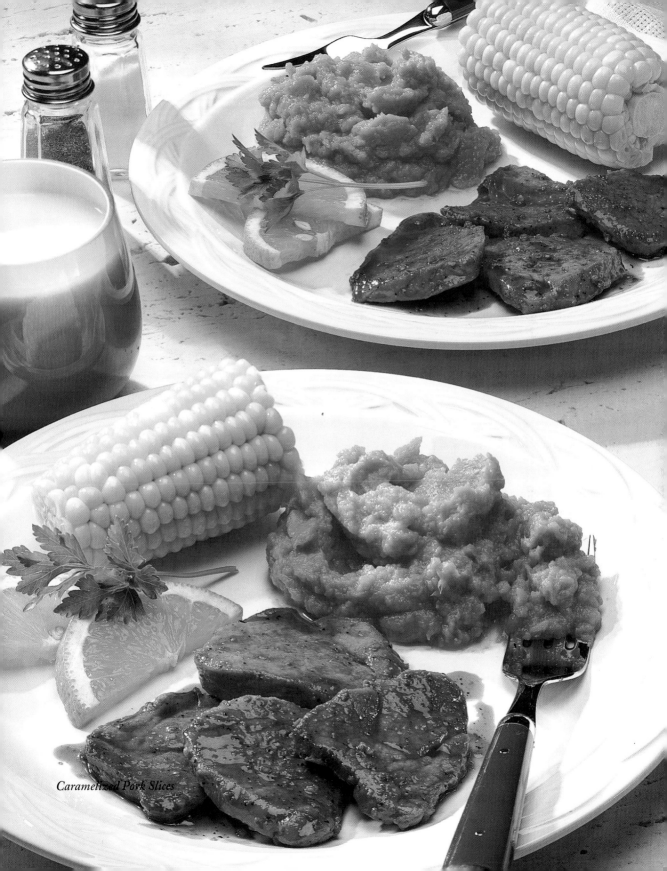

Caramelized Pork Slices

Stir-Fried Pork

LO CAL / LO FAT

PREP: 15 MIN; COOK: 15 MIN

4 SERVINGS

Mirin, also called rice wine, is a low-alcohol, sweet rice wine used in Japanese cooking.

- 1 **pound pork tenderloin**
- 2 **cans (8 ounces each) pineapple chunks in juice, drained and juice reserved**
- 3 **tablespoons white vinegar**
- 3 **tablespoons mirin (rice wine) or sweet white wine or water**
- 3 **tablespoons reduced-sodium soy sauce**
- 2 **teaspoons cornstarch**
- 1 **teaspoon sesame or vegetable oil**
- 1 **small onion, chopped (¹/₄ cup)**
- 1 **medium green bell pepper, cut into 1-inch pieces**

Remove fat from pork. Cut pork into 1-inch cubes. Mix reserved pineapple juice, the vinegar, mirin, soy sauce and cornstarch.

Spray 12-inch nonstick skillet with cooking spray; heat over medium-high heat. Add oil and pork; stir-fry 6 to 8 minutes or until pork is no longer pink. Remove pork from skillet.

Spray skillet with cooking spray. Add onion and bell pepper; stir-fry about 5 minutes or until onion is tender. Stir in pork, pineapple and juice mixture. Heat to boiling. Boil about 45 seconds, stirring constantly, until thickened.

1 Serving: Calories 220 (Calories from Fat 45); Fat 5g (Saturated 2g); Cholesterol 65mg; Sodium 450mg; Carbohydrate 20g (Dietary Fiber 1g); Protein 25g
% Daily Value: Vitamin A 2%; Vitamin C 30%; Calcium 2%; Iron 10%
Diet Exchanges: 2¹/₂ lean meat, 1 vegetable, 1 fruit

Mustard Lamb Chops

LOW CALORIE

PREP: 10 MIN; BROIL: 10 MIN

6 SERVINGS

Chopped fresh chives can be used in place of the thyme leaves.

- 6 **lamb sirloin or shoulder chops, about ³/₄ inch thick (about 2 pounds)**
- 1 **tablespoon chopped fresh or 1 teaspoon dried thyme leaves**
- 2 **tablespoons Dijon mustard**
- ¹/₄ **teaspoon salt**

Set oven control to broil. Remove fat from lamb. Place lamb on rack in broiler pan. Mix remaining ingredients. Brush half of the mustard mixture evenly over lamb.

Broil lamb with tops 3 to 4 inches from heat about 4 minutes or until brown. Turn lamb; brush with remaining mustard mixture. Broil 5 to 7 minutes longer for medium doneness (160°).

1 Serving: Calories 145 (Calories from Fat 65); Fat 7g (Saturated 3g); Cholesterol 65mg; Sodium 210mg; Carbohydrate 0g (Dietary Fiber 0g); Protein 20g
% Daily Value: Vitamin A 0%; Vitamin C 0%; Calcium 0%; Iron 8%
Diet Exchanges: 2¹/₂ lean meat

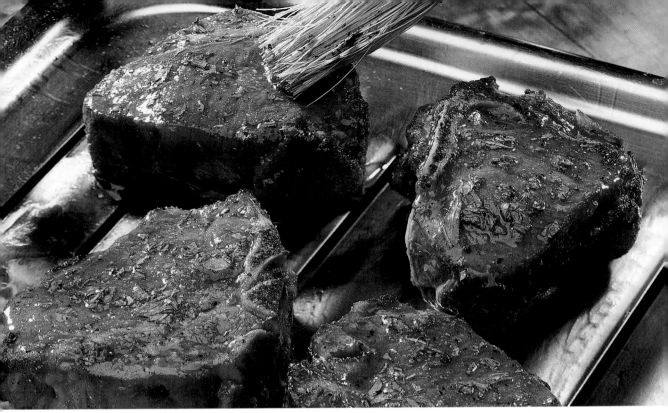

Mint-Wine Lamb Chops

Mint-Wine Lamb Chops

LO CAL / LO FAT / LO SODIUM

PREP: 10 MIN; BROIL: 10 MIN

8 SERVINGS

Lamb is a great source of protein. Protein is important because it helps build new cells and hormones that keep our bodies running smoothly.

8   lamb rib or loin chops, about 1 inch thick (about 2 pounds)

2   tablespoons dry white wine or apple juice

2   tablespoons honey

1   teaspoon chopped fresh or $\frac{1}{4}$ teaspoon dried mint leaves

$\frac{1}{4}$ teaspoon salt

$\frac{1}{8}$ teaspoon pepper

Set oven control to broil. Remove fat from lamb. Mix remaining ingredients. Place lamb on rack in broiler pan; brush with wine mixture.

Broil lamb with tops 3 to 4 inches from heat about 4 minutes or until brown. Brush with wine mixture. Turn lamb; brush with wine mixture. Broil 5 to 7 minutes longer for medium doneness (160°). Discard any remaining wine mixture.

1 Serving: Calories 100 (Calories from Fat 45); Fat 5g (Saturated 2g); Cholesterol 35mg; Sodium 105mg; Carbohydrate 4g (Dietary Fiber 0g); Protein 10g
% Daily Value: Vitamin A 0%; Vitamin C 0%; Calcium 0%; Iron 4%
Diet Exchanges: 2 lean meat

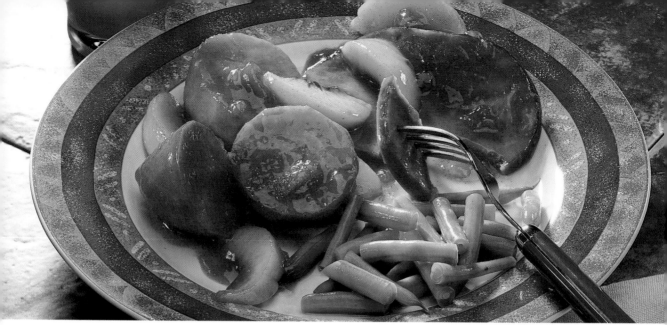

Ham with Spiced Sweet Potatoes and Peaches

Ham with Spiced Sweet Potatoes and Peaches

LO FAT / HI FIB

PREP: 10 MIN; BAKE: 25 MIN

6 SERVINGS

Using canned sweet potatoes saves you the work of peeling and cooking the fresh potatoes.

6 slices fully cooked lower-fat, lower-sodium ham slices, ¼ inch thick (about 1 pound)

6 medium sweet potatoes or yams (2 pounds), peeled and cut into 1½-inch slices*

½ cup water

1 jar (10 ounces) apricot or orange marmalade spreadable fruit

¼ cup brown sugar

½ teaspoon ground cinnamon

⅛ teaspoon ground red pepper (cayenne)

1 bag (16 ounces) frozen sliced peaches, partially thawed and drained

Heat oven to 375°. Arrange ham in ungreased rectangular baking dish, 13 × 9 × 2 inches.

Heat sweet potatoes and water to boiling in 3-quart saucepan; reduce heat. Cover and simmer about 10 minutes or until potatoes are almost tender; drain.

While sweet potatoes are cooking, heat spreadable fruit, brown sugar, cinnamon and red pepper in 1-quart saucepan over medium heat about 5 minutes, stirring constantly, until hot and bubbly. Arrange sweet potatoes and peaches on ham. Pour sauce over top. Cover and bake 15 minutes. Bake uncovered about 5 to 10 minutes longer until heated through.

*1 can (23 ounces) sweet potatoes in light syrup, drained, can be substituted for the fresh sweet potatoes; do not cook.

1 Serving: Calories 370 (Calories from Fat 25); Fat 3g (Saturated 1g); Cholesterol 35mg; Sodium 580mg; Carbohydrate 85g (Dietary Fiber 8g); Protein 15g
% Daily Value: Vitamin A 100%; Vitamin C 22%; Calcium 8%; Iron 12%
Diet Exchanges: 2½ starch, 1½ very lean meat, 2 fruit

Ham with Cabbage and Apples

LO CAL / HI FIB

PREP: 10 MIN; COOK: 15 MIN

4 SERVINGS

Serve this quick dish with instant mashed potatoes.

4 cups coleslaw mix or shredded cabbage

1 tablespoon packed brown sugar

1 tablespoon cider vinegar

$1/8$ teaspoon pepper

1 large onion, chopped (1 cup)

1 large green cooking apple, sliced

1 pound fully cooked ham slice, about $1/2$ inch thick

Spray 10-inch nonstick skillet with cooking spray; heat over medium heat. Cook all ingredients except ham in skillet about 5 minutes, stirring frequently, until apple is crisp-tender.

Place ham on cabbage mixture; reduce heat. Cover and cook about 10 minutes or until ham is hot.

1 Serving: Calories 215 (Calories from Fat 70); Fat 8g (Saturated 3g); Cholesterol 50mg; Sodium 1240mg; Carbohydrate 19g (Dietary Fiber 3g); Protein 20g
% Daily Value: Vitamin A 0%; Vitamin C 22%; Calcium 4%; Iron 10%
Diet Exchanges: $2^1/2$ lean meat, 1 vegetable, 1 fruit

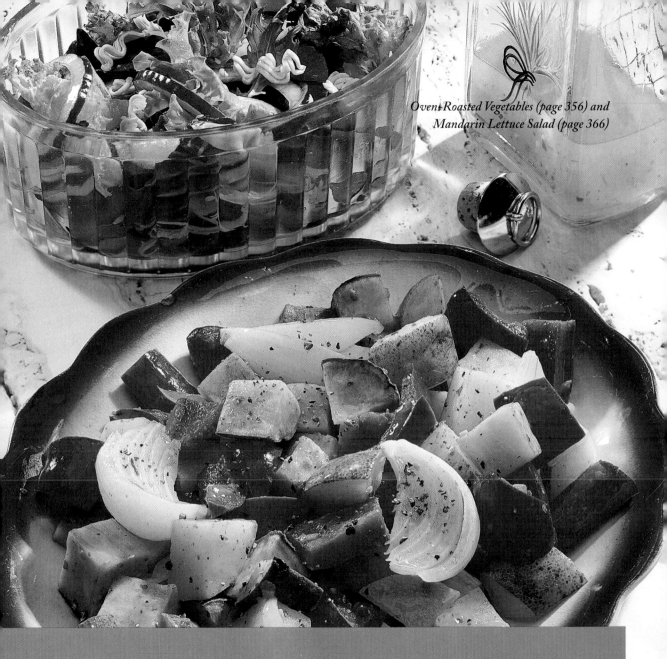

Oven-Roasted Vegetables (page 356) and
Mandarin Lettuce Salad (page 366)

VEGETABLES
AND SIDE DISHES

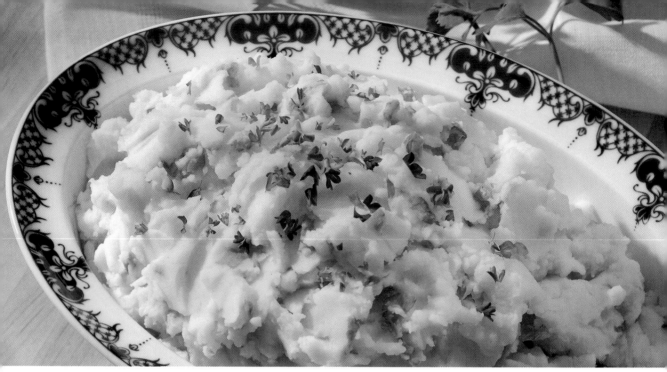

Horseradish Mashed Potatoes

Horseradish Mashed Potatoes

LO CAL / LO FAT / LO CHOL / HI FIB

PREP: 10 MIN; COOK: 20 MIN

4 SERVINGS

If you prefer a milder flavor, use horseradish sauce in place of the prepared horseradish and decrease the yogurt to ¹/₄ cup. Horseradish sauce looks like mayonnaise and is higher in calories and fat than prepared horseradish. You can find it next to the bottled tartar sauce and mayonnaise in your supermarket.

　4　**medium unpeeled boiling potatoes (about 1¹/₂ pounds), cut into ¹/₂-inch slices**

¹/₃　**cup plain low-fat or fat-free yogurt**

　1　**tablespoon prepared horseradish**

¹/₂　**teaspoon salt**

2 to 4　**tablespoons skim milk**

　Chopped fresh parsley, if desired

Heat 1 inch water to boiling in 3-quart saucepan. Add potatoes. Heat to boiling. Reduce heat to low and cook about 15 minutes or until tender; drain. Return potatoes to saucepan. Shake pan with potatoes over low heat to dry; remove from heat.

Mash potatoes until no lumps remain. Beat in yogurt, horseradish and salt. Add milk in small amounts, beating after each addition (amount of milk needed to make potatoes smooth and fluffy depends on the kind of potatoes used). Beat vigorously until potatoes are light and fluffy. Sprinkle with parsley.

1 Serving: Calories 130 (Calories from Fat 0); Fat 0g (Saturated 0g); Cholesterol 1mg; Sodium 180mg; Carbohydrate 31g (Dietary Fiber 3g); Protein 4g
% Daily Value: Vitamin A 0%; Vitamin C 12%; Calcium 6%; Iron 8%
Diet Exchanges: 2 starch

Sweet Potato Surprise

LO CAL / LO FAT / LO CHOL / LO SODIUM

PREP: 15 MIN; BAKE: 10 MIN

6 SERVINGS

The surprise in this side dish is the marshmallow hidden inside a ball of mashed sweet potato! To top it off, the balls are brushed with melted margarine and rolled in cornflake crumbs for a buttery-crisp coating.

1   can (18 ounces) vacuum-pack sweet potatoes

1   tablespoon packed brown sugar

6   large marshmallows

1   tablespoon margarine, melted

$1/3$ cup cornflake crumbs

Heat oven to 450°. Grease square pan, 8 × 8 × 2 inches. Mash sweet potatoes and brown sugar. Shape $1/3$ cup potato mixture around each marsh-mallow into a ball.

Brush 1 sweet potato ball at a time with margarine; roll in cornflake crumbs to coat. Place in pan. Bake uncovered 8 to 10 minutes or until coating is light brown.

1 Serving: Calories 135 (Calories from Fat 20); Fat 2g (Saturated 0g); Cholesterol 0mg; Sodium 95mg; Carbo-hydrate 28g (Dietary Fiber 1g); Protein 2g
% Daily Value: Vitamin A 72%; Vitamin C 18%; Cal-cium 2%; Iron 8%
Diet Exchanges: 1 starch, 2 vegetable

Italian Potatoes

LO CAL / LO FAT / LO CHOL / LO SODIUM

PREP: 15 MIN; COOK: 30 MIN

6 SERVINGS

You may think all spaghetti sauces are low in calories and nearly fat free, but check the label on several of your favorite brands and note the differences. Added sugar and oils can drive up calories and fat.

3   medium unpeeled potatoes (1 pound), cut into 1-inch cubes (2 cups)

$1 1/2$ medium onions, finely chopped ($3/4$ cup)

1   medium carrot, finely chopped ($1/2$ cup)

$1/2$ cup chicken broth

2   tablespoons fat-free spaghetti sauce or tomato sauce

$1/4$ teaspoon pepper

2   cloves garlic, finely chopped

2   tablespoons chopped fresh parsley

Cook all ingredients except parsley in 2-quart saucepan over medium-low heat 20 to 30 minutes, stirring occasionally, until potatoes are tender. Stir in parsley.

1 Serving: Calories 80 (Calories from Fat 0); Fat 0g (Saturated 0g); Cholesterol 0mg; Sodium 90mg; Carbo-hydrate 20g (Dietary Fiber 2g); Protein 2g
% Daily Value: Vitamin A 16%; Vitamin C 10%; Cal-cium 2%; Iron 6%
Diet Exchanges: 1 starch, 1 vegetable

Zesty Salsa Corn

LO CAL / LO FAT / LO CHOL / LO SODIUM / HI FIB

PREP: 5 MIN; COOK: 5 MIN

5 SERVINGS

Salsa is a great boon to those trying to watch their waistlines; it not only tastes great, it is low in calories, and also fat free.

> 1   bag (16 ounces) frozen whole kernel corn
>
> 1/2 cup salsa
>
> 1/4 cup sliced ripe olives

Cook corn as directed on package. Stir in salsa and olives; cook until hot.

1 Serving: Calories 85 (Calories from Fat 10); Fat 1g (Saturated 0g); Cholesterol 0mg; Sodium 130mg; Carbohydrate 19g (Dietary Fiber 3g); Protein 3g
% Daily Value: Vitamin A 4%; Vitamin C 6%; Calcium 2%; Iron 4%
Diet Exchanges: 1 starch

Baked Corn on the Cob with Herbs

LO CAL / LO FAT / LO CHOL / HI FIB

PREP: 5 MIN; BAKE: 25 MIN

4 SERVINGS

For a tantalizing blend of flavors, team two herbs together with the corn—basil and rosemary or thyme and dill weed are especially good combinations.

> 4   ears corn
>
>   Butter-flavored cooking spray
>
> 1/4 teaspoon salt
>
> 1/8 teaspoon pepper
>
> 20 to 24 sprigs fresh basil, rosemary, thyme, dill weed, marjoram or sage

Heat oven to 450°. Husk corn and remove silk. Place each ear on 12-inch square of aluminum foil. Spray on all sides with cooking spray. Sprinkle with salt and pepper. Place 5 or 6 sprigs of fresh herb around each ear. Seal foil.

Place sealed ears of corn directly on oven rack. Bake about 20 minutes or until corn is tender.

1 Serving: Calories 110 (Calories from Fat 10); Fat 1g (Saturated 0g); Cholesterol 0mg; Sodium 160mg; Carbohydrate 25g (Dietary Fiber 3g); Protein 3g
% Daily Value: Vitamin A 2%; Vitamin C 5%; Calcium 0%; Iron 4%
Diet Exchanges: 1 1/2 starch

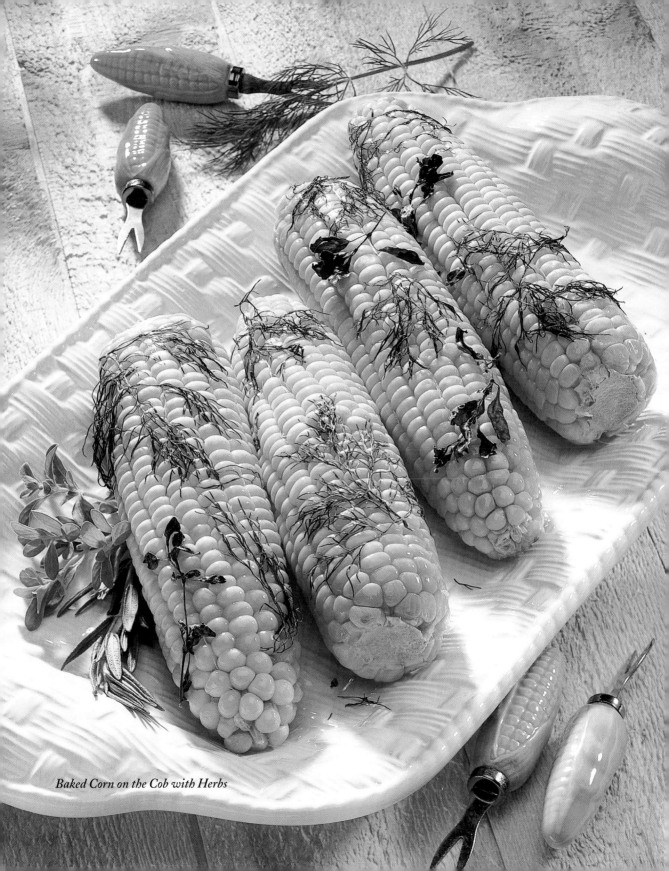

Baked Corn on the Cob with Herbs

Sesame Pea Pods

LO CAL / LO FAT / LO SODIUM / LO CHOL

PREP: 10 MIN; COOK: 5 MIN

6 SERVINGS

Bell peppers are a good C source. Vitamin C, or ascorbic acid, is key for healthy gums and teeth. Don't cook peppers too long, though, because heat easily destroys vitamin C.

1 tablespoon sesame or vegetable oil

1/2 pound snow (Chinese) pea pods, strings removed (2 cups)

1 tablespoon sesame seed

1 medium red or yellow bell pepper, cut into thin strips

Heat oil in 10-inch nonstick skillet over medium-high heat. Cook pea pods and sesame seed in oil about 2 minutes, stirring occasionally, until pea pods are crisp-tender.

Stir in bell pepper. Cook about 2 minutes, stirring occasionally, until bell pepper is crisp-tender.

1 Serving: Calories 40 (Calories from Fat 25); Fat 3g (Saturated 1g); Cholesterol 0mg; Sodium 2mg; Carbohydrate 3g (Dietary Fiber 1g); Protein 1g
% Daily Value: Vitamin A 12%; Vitamin C 38%; Calcium 0%; Iron 2%
Diet Exchanges: 1 vegetable

Orange-Glazed Snap Peas with Carrot

LO CAL / LO FAT / LO CHOL /

LO SODIUM / HI FIB

PREP: 5 MIN; COOK: 12 MIN

4 SERVINGS

Although closely related to snow peas, snap pea pods are sweeter and have more rounded and fully developed peas inside. You'll find them in your supermarket during the spring and fall.

1 bag (16 ounces) frozen snap pea pods

1 medium carrot, shredded (2/3 cup)

1/2 cup orange juice

1 1/2 teaspoons cornstarch

1/2 teaspoon grated orange peel

1/4 teaspoon ground ginger

1/8 teaspoon salt

Cook pea pods as directed on package—except add carrot to the pea pods.

While pea pods and carrot are cooking, heat remaining ingredients to boiling in 1-quart saucepan, stirring constantly. Boil and stir 1 minute.

Drain vegetables. Pour sauce over vegetables; toss until evenly coated.

1 Serving: Calories 55 (Calories from Fat 0); Fat 0g (Saturated 0g); Cholesterol 0mg; Sodium 85mg; Carbohydrate 13g (Dietary Fiber 3g); Protein 4g
% Daily Value: Vitamin A 24%; Vitamin C 50%; Calcium 4%; Iron 12%
Diet Exchanges: 1/2 starch, 1 vegetable

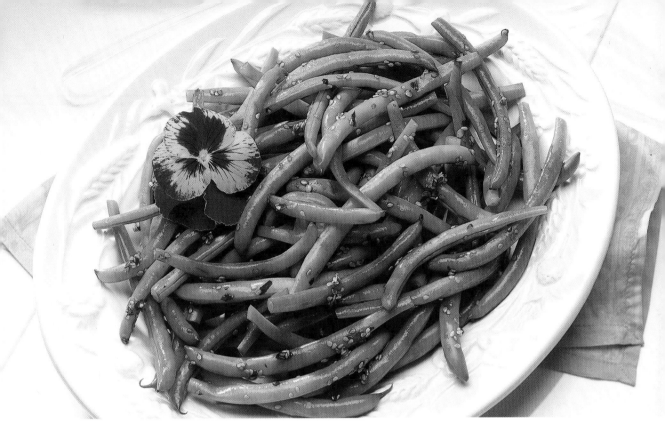

Sesame Green Beans

Sesame Green Beans

LO CAL / LO FAT / LO CHOL / LO SODIUM / HI FIB

PREP: 10 MIN; COOK: 15 MIN

4 SERVINGS

Nothing beats fresh green beans, especially when they're tossed with a tongue-tingling sesame seed-and-soy sauce dressing. If you like your vegetables with lots of zing, be sure to use the ¹/₂ teaspoon crushed red pepper.

1	pound green beans
2	teaspoons sesame seed
1	tablespoon rice vinegar
1	tablespoon reduced-sodium soy sauce
1	teaspoon sugar
¹/₂	teaspoon crushed red pepper

Heat 1 inch water to boiling in 2-quart saucepan. Add beans. Boil uncovered 5 minutes. Cover and boil about 5 minutes longer or until crisp-tender.

While beans are cooking, heat sesame seed in 6-inch skillet over medium heat about 2 minutes, stirring frequently until browning begins, then stirring constantly until golden brown. Stir in remaining ingredients; heat through.

Drain beans. Pour sauce over beans; toss until evenly coated.

1 Serving: Calories 40 (Calories from Fat 10); Fat 1g (Saturated 0g); Cholesterol 0mg; Sodium 140mg; Carbohydrate 8g (Dietary Fiber 3g); Protein 2g
% Daily Value: Vitamin A 4%; Vitamin C 2%; Calcium 4%; Iron 6%
Diet Exchanges: 1¹/₂ vegetable

Honey-Glazed Carrots

LO CAL / LO FAT / LO CHOL / LO SODIUM

PREP: 5 MIN; COOK: 15 MIN

6 SERVINGS

Carrots are A-OK! They are an excellent source of vitamin A, which we need for proper vision and healthy hair and skin.

- 1   bag (16 ounces) baby-cut carrots
- 2   tablespoons honey
- 1   tablespoon margarine
      Ground nutmeg

Place carrots in 1 inch water in 2-quart saucepan. Heat to boiling; reduce heat. Cover and simmer 10 to 15 minutes or until tender. Drain well.

Add honey and margarine to carrots in saucepan; heat to boiling. Cook carrots, stirring frequently, until margarine is melted and carrots are glazed. Sprinkle with nutmeg.

1 Serving: Calories 70 (Calories from Fat 20); Fat 2g (Saturated 0g); Cholesterol 0mg; Sodium 50mg; Carbohydrate 14g (Dietary Fiber 2g); Protein 1g
% Daily Value: Vitamin A 100%; Vitamin C 6%; Calcium 2%; Iron 2%
Diet Exchanges: 3 vegetable

Oven-Roasted Vegetables

LO CAL / LO FAT / LO CHOL / LO SODIUM / HI FIB

PREP: 10 MIN; BAKE: 25 MIN

6 SERVINGS

Roasting the baking potatoes and sweet potato with their skins on not only saves time but also provides more fiber, iron, calcium and B vitamins than unpeeled potatoes (photo, page 349).

- 2   medium unpeeled baking potatoes, cut into 1-inch chunks (1 1/3 cups)
- 1   medium unpeeled sweet potato, cut into 1-inch chunks (1 cup)
- 2   medium onions, cut crosswise in half, then cut into wedges
- 1/3 cup fat-free Italian dressing
- 1/4 teaspoon ground red pepper (cayenne)
- 1   medium bell pepper, cut into 1-inch squares

Move oven rack to position slightly above middle of oven. Heat oven to 500°.

Generously spray rectangular pan, 13 × 9 × 2 inches, with cooking spray. Place baking potatoes, sweet potato and onions in pan. Mix dressing and red pepper; pour over vegetables. Cover and bake 10 minutes.

Stir bell pepper into vegetables. Cover and bake 5 minutes; stir vegetables. Bake uncovered 10 minutes longer.

1 Serving: Calories 80 (Calories from Fat 0); Fat 0g (Saturated 0g); Cholesterol 0mg; Sodium 125mg; Carbohydrate 21g (Dietary Fiber 3g); Protein 2g
% Daily Value: Vitamin A 42%; Vitamin C 24%; Calcium 2%; Iron 4%
Diet Exchanges: 1 starch, 1 vegetable

Leeks au Gratin

LO CAL / LO CHOL

PREP: 10 MIN; COOK: 5 MIN; BAKE: 25 MIN

4 SERVINGS

Leeks look like giant green onions and have a very mild onion flavor. Before using, slit the leeks lengthwise from top to bottom and rinse thoroughly to remove all of the dirt trapped between the leaf layers.

4	medium leeks with tops (2 pounds), cut into $1/2$-inch pieces
1	tablespoon margarine
1	tablespoon plus 1 teaspoon all-purpose flour
$1/4$	teaspoon salt
	Dash of pepper
$2/3$	cup skim milk
$1/4$	cup finely shredded Gruyère or Swiss cheese
2	tablespoons dry bread crumbs
	Cooking spray

Heat 1 inch water to boiling in 3-quart saucepan. Add leeks. Cover and cook over medium heat about 5 minutes or until crisp-tender; drain.

Heat oven to 325°. Spray shallow 1-quart casserole with cooking spray. Melt margarine in 2-quart saucepan over low heat. Stir in flour, salt and pepper. Cook, stirring constantly, until margarine is absorbed; remove from heat. Gradually stir in milk. Heat to boiling, stirring constantly. Boil and stir 1 minute. Stir in cheese until melted.

Stir leeks into sauce. Pour into casserole. Sprinkle with bread crumbs; spray lightly with cooking spray. Bake uncovered about 25 minutes or until heated through.

1 Serving: Calories 145 (Calories from Fat 70); Fat 8g (Saturated 3g); Cholesterol 15mg; Sodium 280mg; Carbohydrate 13g (Dietary Fiber 2g); Protein 7g
% Daily Value: Vitamin A 12%; Vitamin C 14%; Calcium 24%; Iron 8%
Diet Exchanges: 1 vegetable, $1/2$ skim milk, 2 fat

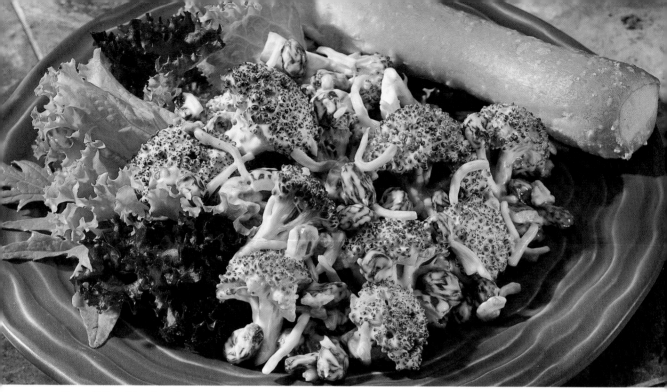

Broccoli Sunshine Salad

Broccoli Sunshine Salad

LO CAL / LO CHOL / HI FIB

PREP: 15 MIN

4 SERVINGS

This healthy adaptation of a community cookbook favorite will bring a sunshiny smile to the face of everyone who tries it. Stir the salad just before serving. If the dressing is too thick, thin it with a little vinegar.

- 1/2 cup reduced-fat mayonnaise or salad dressing
- 1 tablespoon sugar
- 2 tablespoons cider vinegar
- 3 cups broccoli flowerets (1/2 pound)
- 1/3 cup raisins
- 1/4 cup shredded reduced-fat Cheddar cheese
- 2 tablespoons imitation bacon-flavor bits or chips
- 2 tablespoons chopped red onion

Mix mayonnaise, sugar and vinegar in large bowl. Add remaining ingredients; toss until evenly coated.

1 Serving: Calories 185 (Calories from Fat 100); Fat 11g (Saturated 2g); Cholesterol 10mg; Sodium 350mg; Carbohydrate 25g (Dietary Fiber 3g); Protein 5g
% Daily Value: Vitamin A 8%; Vitamin C 42%; Calcium 6%; Iron 6%
Diet Exchanges: 4 vegetable, 2 fat

Marinated Harvest Salad

LO CAL / LO FAT / LO CHOL / HI FIB

PREP: 20 MIN; COOK: 10 MIN; CHILL: 2 HR

8 SERVINGS

You've got to love them! Sweet potatoes are naturally rich tasting and sweet, and they are a good source of vitamins A and C.

2	tablespoons vegetable oil
2	cloves garlic, finely chopped
1	cup julienne strips yams or sweet potatoes
1	cup julienne strips jicama
1	cup julienne strips zucchini
1	cup julienne strips unpeeled red apple
1	small fennel bulb, thinly sliced
2	medium green onions, sliced (2 tablespoons)
1/4	cup cider vinegar
1/4	cup water
1	teaspoon Dijon mustard
3/4	teaspoon salt
	Freshly ground pepper

Heat oil in 10-inch nonstick skillet over medium heat. Cover and cook garlic and yams in oil about 5 minutes, stirring occasionally, until yams are crisp-tender. Stir in jicama, zucchini, apple, fennel and onions.

Mix vinegar, water, mustard and salt; stir into vegetables. Cook 1 minute. Place vegetables in bowl. Cover and refrigerate about 2 hours or until chilled. Serve with pepper.

1 Serving: Calories 75 (Calories from Fat 35); Fat 4g (Saturated 1g); Cholesterol 0mg; Sodium 250mg; Carbohydrate 12g (Dietary Fiber 3g); Protein 1g
% Daily Value: Vitamin A 48%; Vitamin C 24%; Calcium 2%; Iron 2%
Diet Exchanges: 2 vegetable, 1/2 fat

Creamy Country Potato Salad

LO CAL / LO FAT / LO CHOL

PREP: 5 MIN; COOK: 25 MIN; CHILL: 2 HR

6 SERVINGS

Red potatoes rule when making potato salad. Their waxy texture allows them to stay firmer after cooking, so they don't turn into mashed potatoes when you mix up the salad.

1	pound medium red potatoes, cubed (2$\frac{1}{2}$ cups)
$\frac{1}{2}$	cup reduced-fat buttermilk
$\frac{1}{4}$	cup lemon juice
2	tablespoons reduced-fat mayonnaise or salad dressing
1	tablespoon Dijon mustard
1	tablespoon chopped fresh or 1 teaspoon dried thyme leaves
$\frac{1}{2}$	teaspoon salt
1	medium stalk celery, chopped ($\frac{1}{2}$ cup)
1	small bell pepper, chopped ($\frac{1}{2}$ cup)

Heat 1$\frac{1}{2}$ quarts water to boiling in 2-quart saucepan. Add potatoes. Cover and heat to boiling; reduce heat. Simmer 10 to 15 minutes or until tender; drain.

Mix buttermilk, lemon juice, mayonnaise, mustard, thyme and salt in large glass or plastic bowl. Add potatoes, celery and bell pepper; toss. Cover and refrigerate about 2 hours or until chilled.

1 Serving: Calories 80 (Calories from Fat 20); Fat 2g (Saturated 1g); Cholesterol 5mg; Sodium 290mg; Carbohydrate 16g (Dietary Fiber 2g); Protein 2g
% Daily Value: Vitamin A 2%; Vitamin C 18%; Calcium 4%; Iron 4%
Diet Exchanges: 1 starch

Crunchy Jicama and Melon Salad

LO CAL / LO FAT / LO CHOL / LO SODIUM

PREP: 15 MIN; CHILL: 2 HR

6 SERVINGS

Get to know jicama! It may look ugly on the outside, but it's terrific on the inside. Jicama stays crisp and crunchy and tastes somewhat like water chestnuts, only moister and sweeter.

1½ cups julienne strips jicama (½ medium)

1½ cups ½-inch cubes cantaloupe (½ medium)

1 teaspoon grated lime peel

3 tablespoons lime juice

2 tablespoons chopped fresh or 1 tablespoon dried mint leaves

1 teaspoon honey

¼ teaspoon salt

Mix all ingredients in glass or plastic bowl. Cover and refrigerate about 2 hours or until chilled.

1 Serving: Calories 30 (Calories from Fat 0); Fat 0g (Saturated 0g); Cholesterol 0mg; Sodium 105mg; Carbohydrate 8g (Dietary Fiber 2g); Protein 1g
% Daily Value: Vitamin A 10%; Vitamin C 42%; Calcium 0%; Iron 2%
Diet Exchanges: ½ fruit

Oriental Coleslaw

LO CAL / LO FAT / LO CHOL / LO SODIUM

PREP: 15 MIN

4 SERVINGS

Rice vinegar is light colored and quite a bit milder in flavor than either cider or distilled white vinegar. Look for it with the vinegars or Asian foods in your supermarket.

Sesame Dressing (below)

2 cups finely shredded Chinese (napa) cabbage (8 ounces)

¼ cup chopped jicama

¼ cup chopped green bell pepper

¼ cup coarsely shredded carrot

Prepare sesame dressing. Toss dressing and remaining ingredients.

Sesame Dressing

3 tablespoons rice vinegar or white wine vinegar

2 teaspoons sugar

2 teaspoons sesame seed, toasted (page 124)

2 teaspoons reduced-sodium soy sauce

1 teaspoon sesame or vegetable oil

⅛ teaspoon crushed red pepper

Mix all ingredients.

1 Serving: Calories 40 (Calories from Fat 20); Fat 2g (Saturated 0g); Cholesterol 0mg; Sodium 130mg; Carbohydrate 6g (Dietary Fiber 1g); Protein 1g
% Daily Value: Vitamin A 22%; Vitamin C 38%; Calcium 4%; Iron 2%
Diet Exchanges: 1 vegetable

Corn, Pea and Sun-Dried Tomato Salad

LO CAL / LO FAT / LO CHOL / HI FIB

PREP: 15 MIN; CHILL: 2 HR

6 SERVINGS

Corn and peas are higher in calories than are most other veggies, such as broccoli, beans or carrots. As do potatoes, corn and peas contain more starch than their more watery relatives, and that increases the calorie count.

1	cup frozen whole kernel corn, thawed
1	cup frozen green peas, thawed
1/2	cup thinly sliced red onion
1	small tomato, chopped (1/2 cup)
5	medium green onions, chopped (1/3 cup)
2	tablespoons chopped fresh parsley
1	tablespoon finely chopped sun-dried tomato (not oil-packed)
3	tablespoons lime juice
2	tablespoons white vinegar
1/2	teaspoon salt
1/4	teaspoon pepper
3	cups bite-size pieces lettuce

Mix all ingredients except lettuce in glass or plastic bowl. Cover and refrigerate about 2 hours or until chilled. Serve on lettuce.

1 Serving: Calories 60 (Calories from Fat 10); Fat 1g (Saturated 0g); Cholesterol 0mg; Sodium 300mg; Carbohydrate 13g (Dietary Fiber 3g); Protein 3g
% Daily Value: Vitamin A 4%; Vitamin C 24%; Calcium 2%; Iron 6%
Diet Exchanges: 3 vegetable

Bean and Hominy Medley

LO CAL / LO FAT / LO CHOL / HI FIB

PREP: 5 MIN; COOK: 10 MIN

6 SERVINGS

Ideal for impromptu picnics or barbecues, this tangy basil-accented side dish is the perfect partner for grilled burgers or kabobs.

1	package (9 ounces) frozen Italian or regular cut green beans
1	can (15 to 16 ounces) reduced-sodium kidney beans, rinsed and drained
1	can (14 to 15 ounces) hominy or 1 can (15 to 16 ounces) garbanzo beans, rinsed and drained
1/2	cup fat-free red wine vinegar dressing
3/4	teaspoon dried basil leaves
4	medium green onions, sliced (1/4 cup)

Cook and drain green beans as directed on package. Place cooked beans in colander. Rinse with cold water to chill; drain well.

Toss green beans and remaining ingredients in large bowl until evenly coated.

1 Serving: Calories 140 (Calories from Fat 10); Fat 1g (Saturated 0g); Cholesterol 0mg; Sodium 360mg; Carbohydrate 32g (Dietary Fiber 8g); Protein 8g
% Daily Value: Vitamin A 2%; Vitamin C 2%; Calcium 6%; Iron 16%
Diet Exchanges: 1 starch, 3 vegetable

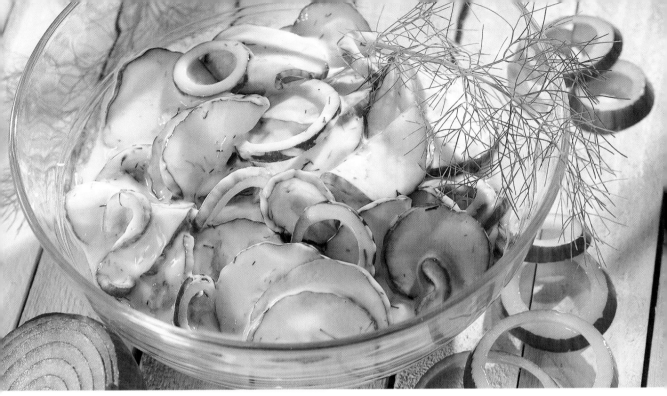

Creamy Dilled Cucumbers

Creamy Dilled Cucumbers

LO CAL / LO FAT / LO CHOL

PREP: 10 MIN; CHILL: 4 HR

6 SERVINGS

Fresh or dried basil can be substituted for the dill weed.

- $^1/_2$ **cup plain fat-free yogurt**
- 1 **teaspoon chopped fresh or $^1/_4$ teaspoon dried dill weed**
- $^1/_2$ **teaspoon salt**
- $^1/_8$ **teaspoon pepper**
- 2 **small cucumbers, sliced (2 cups)**
- 1 **small red onion, thinly sliced and separated into rings**

Mix all ingredients. Cover and refrigerate at least 4 hours to blend flavors.

1 Serving: Calories 25 (Calories from Fat 0); Fat 0g (Saturated 0g); Cholesterol 0mg; Sodium 210mg; Carbohydrate 4g (Dietary Fiber 0g); Protein 2g
% Daily Value: Vitamin A 0%; Vitamin C 6%; Calcium 4%; Iron 0%
Diet Exchanges: 1 vegetable

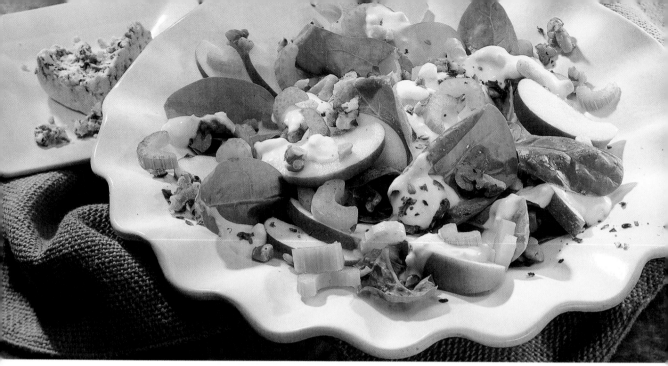

Blue Cheese Waldorf Salad

Blue Cheese Waldorf Salad

LO CAL / LO FAT / LO CHOL / LO SODIUM

PREP: 5 MIN; CHILL: 1 HR

4 SERVINGS

Although high in calories and fat, nuts provide lots of vitamin E. We need vitamin E as a protective agent against cell damage. The key is just not to go nuts!

Blue Cheese Dressing (right)

4 **medium unpeeled red eating apples, cut into ¼-inch slices**

Lemon juice

2 **cups tightly packed spinach leaves**

2 **medium stalks celery, thinly sliced (1 cup)**

2 **tablespoons chopped walnuts, toasted (page 242)**

Prepare Blue Cheese Dressing. Sprinkle apple slices with lemon juice. Toss apples and spinach in large bowl. Spoon dressing over salad. Sprinkle with celery and walnuts.

Blue Cheese Dressing

⅓ **cup plain fat-free yogurt**

1 **tablespoon reduced-fat mayonnaise or salad dressing**

1 **tablespoon finely crumbled blue cheese**

Mix all ingredients. Cover and refrigerate at least 1 hour to blend flavors.

1 Serving: Calories 85 (Calories from Fat 25); Fat 3g (Saturated 1g); Cholesterol 2mg; Sodium 110mg; Carbohydrate 14g (Dietary Fiber 2g); Protein 2g
% Daily Value: Vitamin A 8%; Vitamin C 12%; Calcium 6%; Iron 2%
Diet Exchanges: 1 fruit, ½ fat

Greek Salad

LO CAL / LO FAT / LO CHOL

PREP: 10 MIN

4 SERVINGS

If cucumbers have a habit of chasing after you all day, look for burpless cukes in your produce department.

1	medium unpeeled cucumber
2	cups bite-size pieces spinach
2	cups bite-size pieces lettuce
1/3	cup fat-free Caesar dressing
1/4	cup crumbled feta cheese
1	tablespoon sliced ripe olives
1	medium tomato, cut into thin wedges
1	medium green onion, sliced (1 tablespoon)

Score cucumber by running tines of fork lengthwise down sides; cut into slices. Toss cucumber and remaining ingredients.

1 Serving: Calories 65 (Calories from Fat 25); Fat 3g (Saturated 3g); Cholesterol 10mg; Sodium 430mg; Carbohydrate 8g (Dietary Fiber 2g); Protein 3g
% Daily Value: Vitamin A 28%; Vitamin C 30%; Calcium 10%; Iron 8%
Diet Exchanges: 2 vegetable

Mandarin Lettuce Salad

LO CAL / LO FAT / LO CHOL

PREP: 15 MIN

6 SERVINGS

Transform this savory salad into a main dish by grilling or broiling four chicken breast halves, slicing them and tossing them with the greens (photo, page 349).

- 1 bag (10 ounces) salad mix
- 1 small red onion, cut lengthwise in half, then cut crosswise into thin slices
- 1 can (11 ounces) mandarin orange segments, chilled and drained
- 1 package (3 ounces) Oriental-flavor reduced-fat baked ramen noodle soup mix
- 1/3 cup fat-free Italian dressing
- 1/4 cup water
- 1 teaspoon sugar
- 1 teaspoon sesame seed

Mix salad greens, onion and orange segments in large bowl. Shake seasoning packet from soup mix, dressing, water, sugar and sesame seed in tightly covered container.

Coarsely crumble noodles; sprinkle over salad greens mixture. Shake dressing. Pour dressing over salad; toss until evenly coated.

1 Serving: Calories 95 (Calories from Fat 10); Fat 1g (Saturated 0g); Cholesterol 0mg; Sodium 390mg; Carbohydrate 21g (Dietary Fiber 2g); Protein 3g
% Daily Value: Vitamin A 2%; Vitamin C 10%; Calcium 2%; Iron 6%
Diet Exchanges: 1/2 starch, 1 vegetable, 1/2 fruit

Three-Fruit Salad with Papaya Dressing

LO CAL / LO FAT / LO CHOL / LO SODIUM / HI FIB

PREP: 15 MIN

4 SERVINGS

This versatile fresh-fruit dressing makes a delightful topper for slices of angel food or sponge cake, too.

- 1 medium papaya, peeled, seeded and chopped (1 1/2 cups)
- 1/2 cup plain low-fat or fat-free yogurt
- 1/4 cup packed brown sugar
- 8 strawberries, cut in half
- 2 medium oranges, peeled and sliced
- 4 kiwifruits, peeled and sliced

Place papaya, yogurt and brown sugar in blender or food processor. Cover and blend on high speed about 30 seconds or until smooth.

Arrange strawberries, oranges and kiwifruits on 4 salad plates. Pour dressing over fruits.

1 Serving: Calories 175 (Calories from Fat 10); Fat 1g (Saturated 0g); Cholesterol 2mg; Sodium 35mg; Carbohydrate 44g (Dietary Fiber 6g); Protein 4g
% Daily Value: Vitamin A 4%; Vitamin C 100%; Calcium 14%; Iron 4%
Diet Exchanges: 3 fruit

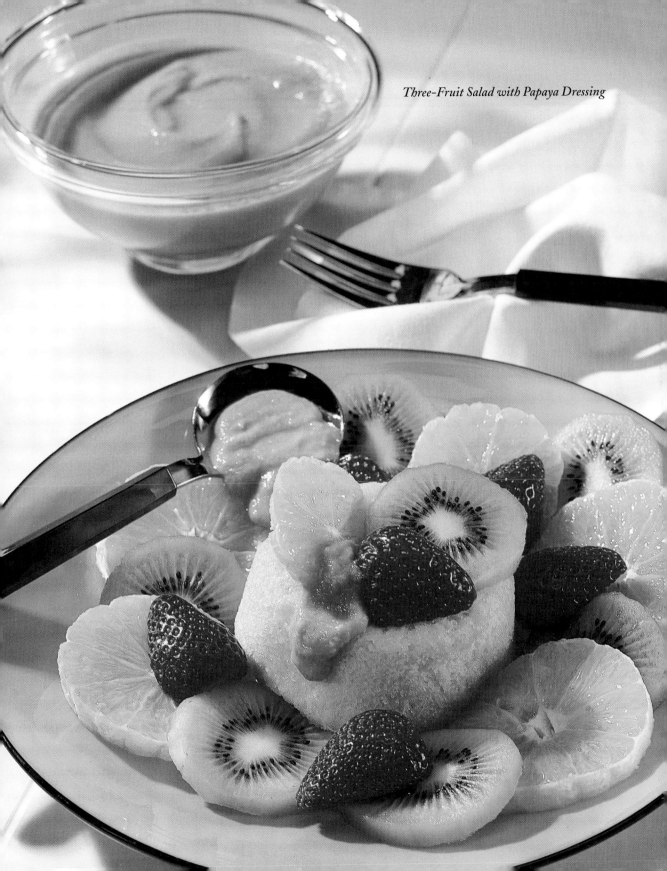

Three-Fruit Salad with Papaya Dressing

Bacon-Spinach Salad

LO CAL / LO FAT / LO CHOL

PREP: 5 MIN; COOK: 10 MIN

4 SERVINGS

Spinach has to plead guilty. What's the charge? Being a nutrition powerhouse. Spinach is a good source of vitamins A and C and the mineral iron. It's a good source of calcium, too.

- 4 slices bacon, diced
- 1/4 cup white vinegar
- 4 teaspoons sugar
- 1/4 teaspoon salt
- 1/8 teaspoon pepper
- 1 bag (10 ounces) washed fresh spinach
- 5 medium green onions, chopped (1/3 cup)

Cook bacon in 12-inch nonstick skillet over low heat, stirring occasionally, until crisp. Stir in vinegar, sugar, salt and pepper. Heat through, stirring constantly, until sugar is dissolved; remove from heat.

Add spinach and onions to bacon mixture. Toss 1 to 2 minutes or until spinach is wilted.

1 Serving: Calories 70 (Calories from Fat 10); Fat 3g (Saturated 1g); Cholesterol 5mg; Sodium 300mg; Carbohydrate 8g (Dietary Fiber 2g); Protein 4g
% Daily Value: Vitamin A 48%; Vitamin C 18%; Calcium 6%; Iron 10%
Diet Exchanges: 2 vegetable, 1/2 fat

Pineapple Fruit and Rice Salad

LO CAL / LO FAT / LO CHOL / LO SODIUM

PREP: 20 MIN

6 SERVINGS

Come summertime, try this potluck and buffet classic with coarsely chopped nectarines and sliced strawberries in place of the apple and pear.

- 1 cup uncooked instant rice
- 1/2 cup pineapple or piña colada low-fat yogurt
- 1/4 teaspoon ground cinnamon
- 1 cup frozen (thawed) whipped topping
- 1 medium unpeeled eating apple, coarsely chopped
- 1 medium unpeeled pear, coarsely chopped
- 1 cup seedless grape halves

Cook rice as directed on package. Place cooked rice in wire mesh strainer or colander with small holes. Rinse with cold water to chill; drain well.

Mix yogurt and cinnamon in medium bowl. Fold in whipped topping. Gently stir in rice and remaining ingredients.

1 Serving: Calories 155 (Calories from Fat 20); Fat 2g (Saturated 2g); Cholesterol 1mg; Sodium 20mg; Carbohydrate 33g (Dietary Fiber 2g); Protein 3g
% Daily Value: Vitamin A 0%; Vitamin C 4%; Calcium 4%; Iron 4%
Diet Exchanges: 1/2 starch, 2 fruit

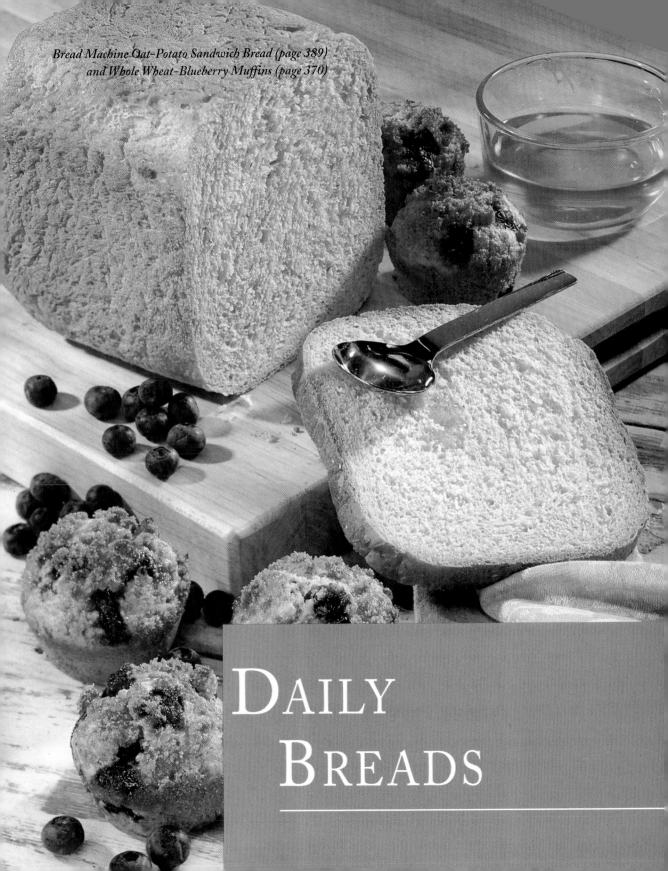

Bread Machine Oat–Potato Sandwich Bread (page 389)
and Whole Wheat–Blueberry Muffins (page 370)

DAILY
BREADS

Whole Wheat-Blueberry Muffins

LO CAL / LO CHOL

PREP: 15 MIN; BAKE: 20 MIN

12 MUFFINS

Don't get tough with your muffins! Our muffin batter directions say to stir "just until flours are moistened (batter will be lumpy)" because overmixing the batter results in tough muffins (photo, page 369).

¼	cup packed brown sugar
½	teaspoon ground cinnamon
¾	cup skim milk
¼	cup vegetable oil
¼	cup honey
½	cup fat-free cholesterol-free egg product or 2 egg whites
1	cup all-purpose flour
1	cup whole wheat flour
3	teaspoons baking powder
½	teaspoon salt
1	cup fresh or frozen (thawed and well drained) blueberries

Heat oven to 400°. Spray 12 medium muffin cups, 2½ × 1¼ inches, with cooking spray, or line with paper baking cups. Mix brown sugar and cinnamon; set aside.

Beat milk, oil, honey and egg product in large bowl with spoon. Stir in flours, baking powder and salt just until flours are moistened (batter will be lumpy). Fold in blueberries.

Divide batter evenly among muffin cups (cups will be full). Sprinkle with brown sugar mixture. Bake about 20 minutes or until golden brown. Immediately remove from pan.

1 Muffin: Calories 160 (Calories from Fat 45); Fat 5g (Saturated 1g); Cholesterol 0mg; Sodium 240mg; Carbohydrate 28g (Dietary Fiber 2g); Protein 3g
% Daily Value: Vitamin A 0%; Vitamin C 0%; Calcium 10%; Iron 6%
Diet Exchanges: 2 starch

Honey-Bran Muffins

LO CAL / LO CHOL

PREP: 15 MIN; BAKE: 25 MIN

6 MUFFINS

Oat bran or wheat germ can be used instead of the wheat bran. No matter which you choose, they all add a bit of a coarse texture and extra fiber.

- ¼   cup wheat bran
- 3   tablespoons boiling water
- ¼   cup skim milk
- 2   tablespoons packed brown sugar
- 2   tablespoons vegetable oil
- 2   tablespoons honey
- ¼   cup fat-free cholesterol-free egg product or 2 egg whites
- ⅔   cup all-purpose flour
- 1½   teaspoons baking powder
- ¼   teaspoon salt
   Sugar, if desired

Heat oven to 400°. Spray 6 medium muffin cups, 2½ × 1¼ inches, with cooking spray, or line with paper baking cups. Mix wheat bran and boiling water; set aside.

Beat milk, brown sugar, oil, honey and egg product in medium bowl with spoon. Stir in bran mixture, flour, baking powder and salt just until flour is moistened (batter will be lumpy).

Divide batter evenly among muffin cups (cups will be about ¾ full). Sprinkle with sugar. Bake 20 to 25 minutes or until golden brown. Immediately remove from pan.

1 Muffin: Calories 145 (Calories from Fat 45); Fat 5g (Saturated 1g); Cholesterol 0mg; Sodium 200mg; Carbohydrate 23g (Dietary Fiber 1g); Protein 3g
% Daily Value: Vitamin A 0%; Vitamin C 0%; Calcium 8%; Iron 6%
Diet Exchanges: 1½ starch, ½ fat

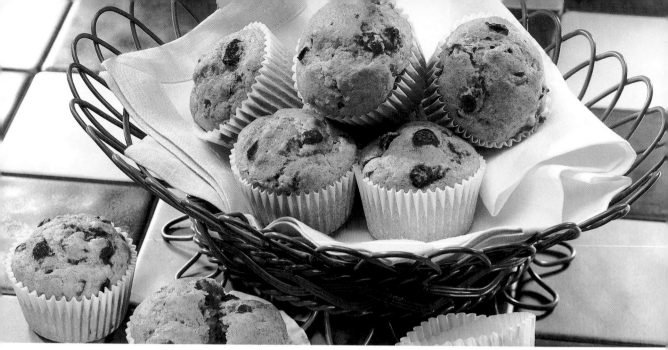

Cranberry-Orange Muffins

Cranberry-Orange Muffins

LO CAL / LO CHOL

PREP: 15 MIN; BAKE: 25 MIN

12 MUFFINS

For extra orange flavor, substitute ¹/₂ cup of orange juice for half of the milk. For the orange peel, grate only the orange part of the peel; the white part, or pith, is bitter.

1   cup skim milk

¹/₄   cup vegetable oil

1   tablespoon grated orange peel

¹/₄   cup fat-free cholesterol-free egg product
     or 2 egg whites

1   cup all-purpose flour

1   cup whole wheat flour

¹/₃   cup sugar

3   teaspoons baking powder

¹/₂   teaspoon salt

³/₄   cup fresh or frozen cranberries, chopped

    Sugar, if desired

Heat oven to 400°. Spray 12 medium muffin cups, 2¹/₂ × 1¹/₄ inches, with cooking spray, or line with paper baking cups.

Beat milk, oil, orange peel and egg product in large bowl with spoon. Stir in flours, ¹/₃ cup sugar, the baking powder and salt just until flour is moistened (batter will be lumpy). Fold in cranberries.

Divide batter evenly among muffin cups (cups will be full). Sprinkle with sugar. Bake 20 to 25 minutes or until golden brown. Immediately remove from pan.

1 Muffin: Calories 145 (Calories from Fat 45); Fat 5g (Saturated 1g); Cholesterol 0mg; Sodium 240mg; Carbohydrate 23g (Dietary Fiber 2g); Protein 4g
% Daily Value: Vitamin A 0%; Vitamin C 0%; Calcium 10%; Iron 6%
Diet Exchanges: 1¹/₂ starch, ¹/₂ fat

Banana-Gingerbread Muffins

LO CAL / LO FAT / LO CHOL

PREP: 5 MIN; BAKE: 20 MIN

16 MUFFINS

The best bananas to use for baking have skins turning brown with black spots, and they are soft to the touch. Why? They will provide more moistness and full banana flavor.

1   package (14.5 ounces) gingerbread cake and cookie mix

1   cup mashed very ripe bananas (2 medium)

³⁄₄   cup quick-cooking or old-fashioned oats

³⁄₄   cup water

¹⁄₄   cup fat-free cholesterol-free egg product or 2 egg whites

Heat oven to 375°. Grease bottoms only of 16 medium muffin cups, 2¹⁄₂ × 1¹⁄₄ inches, or line with paper baking cups. Mix gingerbread mix (dry) and remaining ingredients until well blended.

Divide batter evenly among muffin cups. Bake 15 to 20 minutes or until toothpick inserted in center comes out clean. Immediately remove from pan.

1 Muffin: Calories 135 (Calories from Fat 25); Fat 3g (Saturated 1g); Cholesterol 0mg; Sodium 180mg; Carbohydrate 26g (Dietary Fiber 1g); Protein 2g
% Daily Value: Vitamin A 0%; Vitamin C 0%; Calcium 0%; Iron 4%
Diet Exchanges: 1 starch, 1 fruit

Morning Glory Muffins

LO CAL / LO FAT / LO CHOL / HI FIB

PREP: 15 MIN; BAKE: 25 MIN

12 MUFFINS

Both crushing the cereal and allowing it to stand in milk for five minutes are necessary to keep these muffins moist. The fresh apple and carrot also help with their moistness.

1	cup Fiber One® cereal
²⁄₃	cup skim milk
1³⁄₄	cups all-purpose flour
³⁄₄	cup chopped unpeeled apple
¹⁄₂	cup packed brown sugar
¹⁄₂	cup finely shredded carrot
¹⁄₄	cup granulated sugar
¹⁄₄	cup flaked coconut
¹⁄₂	cup fat-free cholesterol-free egg product or 3 egg whites
1	tablespoon vegetable oil
3	teaspoons baking powder
2	teaspoons ground cinnamon
1	teaspoon vanilla
¹⁄₂	teaspoon salt

Heat oven to 375°. Grease bottoms only of 12 medium muffin cups, 2¹⁄₂ × 1¹⁄₄ inches, or line with paper baking cups.

Crush cereal.* Mix cereal and milk in large bowl; let stand about 5 minutes or until cereal is softened. Stir in remaining ingredients.

Divide batter evenly among muffin cups (cups will be almost full). Bake 22 to 25 minutes or until golden brown. Immediately remove from pan.

*Place cereal between sheets of waxed paper or plastic wrap or in plastic bag; crush with rolling pin. Or crush in blender or food processor.

1 Muffin: Calories 160 (Calories from Fat 20); Fat 2g (Saturated 1g); Cholesterol 0mg; Sodium 280mg; Carbohydrate 35g (Dietary Fiber 3g); Protein 4g
% Daily Value: Vitamin A 14%; Vitamin C 0%; Calcium 10%; Iron 12%
Diet Exchanges: 2 starch

Double-Oat Scones

LO CAL / LO CHOL / HI FIB

PREP: 15 MIN; BAKE: 18 MIN

8 SCONES

Oats are a good source of soluble fiber. Research shows that oats can be helpful in lowering blood cholesterol, which is good news for your heart.

1	cup all-purpose flour
¼	cup packed brown sugar
1½	teaspoons baking powder
¼	teaspoon baking soda
¼	teaspoon salt
3	tablespoons firm margarine
½	cup quick-cooking or old-fashioned oats
½	cup oat bran
½	cup dried cranberries or raisins
¼	cup fat-free cholesterol-free egg product or 2 egg whites

About ½ cup reduced-fat buttermilk

Heat oven to 400°. Mix flour, brown sugar, baking powder, baking soda and salt in large bowl. Cut in margarine, using pastry blender or crisscrossing 2 knives, until mixture resembles fine crumbs. Stir in oats, oat bran and cranberries. Stir in egg product and just enough buttermilk so dough leaves side of bowl and forms a ball.

Turn dough onto lightly floured surface; gently roll in flour to coat. Knead lightly 10 times. Pat into 8-inch circle on ungreased cookie sheet. Cut into 8 wedges with floured knife, but do not separate.

Bake 16 to 18 minutes or until golden brown. Remove from cookie sheet; separate wedges. Serve warm.

1 Scone: Calories 190 (Calories from Fat 45); Fat 5g (Saturated 1g); Cholesterol 0mg; Sodium 290mg; Carbohydrate 35g (Dietary Fiber 4g); Protein 5g
% Daily Value: Vitamin A 6%; Vitamin C 6%; Calcium 8%; Iron 8%
Diet Exchanges: 2 starch, ½ fruit

Tropical Banana Tea Wedges

LO CAL / LO FAT / LO CHOL

PREP: 25 MIN; BAKE: 30 MIN

16 WEDGES

Wow, these tea wedges, or scones, are jam-packed with all sorts of good stuff! Dried apricots not only add a tart and tangy flavor, they also provide vitamin A and iron.

- 1 cup all-purpose flour
- 1 cup whole wheat flour
- 1 cup chopped dried apricots
- 1/2 cup oat bran
- 1/4 cup packed brown sugar
- 2 teaspoons baking powder
- 1 teaspoon ground cinnamon
- 1/2 teaspoon ground cloves
- 1/2 teaspoon baking soda
- 1/4 teaspoon salt
- 3 tablespoons firm margarine
- 3/4 cup mashed very ripe bananas (1 1/2 medium)
- 1/4 cup vanilla fat-free yogurt
- 1/4 cup fat-free cholesterol-free egg product or 2 egg whites

Heat oven to 375°. Spray cookie sheet with cooking spray. Mix flours, apricots, oat bran, brown sugar, baking powder, cinnamon, cloves, baking soda and salt in large bowl. Cut in margarine, using pastry blender or crisscrossing 2 knives, until mixture resembles fine crumbs. Mix remaining ingredients until smooth; stir into flour mixture until dough leaves side of bowl.

Turn dough onto lightly floured surface; gently roll in flour to coat. Knead lightly 10 times. Pat into 12-inch circle on cookie sheet. Cut into 16 wedges with floured knife, but do not separate.

Bake about 30 minutes or until light brown. Remove from cookie sheet; separate wedges. Serve warm.

1 Wedge: Calories 130 (Calories from Fat 25); Fat 3g (Saturated 1g); Cholesterol 0mg; Sodium 170mg; Carbohydrate 25g (Dietary Fiber 2g); Protein 3g
% Daily Value: Vitamin A 8%; Vitamin C 0%; Calcium 4%; Iron 8%
Diet Exchanges: 1 starch, 1/2 fruit, 1/2 fat

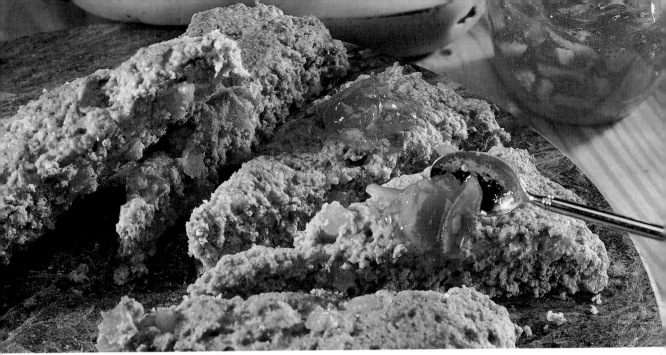

Tropical Banana Tea Wedges

Whole Wheat Popovers

LO CAL / LO FAT / LO SODIUM / HI FIB

PREP: 5 MIN; BAKE: 40 MIN

6 POPOVERS

It's not the popovers that are fattening, it's the butter you put on them that makes them less healthy! If you can't pass up the delectable flavor of butter, make small changes toward choices with less fat. In this case, try light butter instead of regular and use less of it than you normally would.

¾ cup all-purpose flour

¼ cup whole wheat flour

1 cup skim milk

¼ teaspoon salt

2 eggs

Heat oven to 450°. Spray six 6-ounce custard cups or 6-cup popover pan with cooking spray. Mix all ingredients with hand beater just until smooth (do not overbeat).

Fill cups about half full. Bake 20 minutes. Reduce oven temperature to 350°. Bake 20 minutes longer. Immediately remove from cups. Serve hot.

1 Popover: Calories 115 (Calories from Fat 20); Fat 2g (Saturated 1g); Cholesterol 70mg; Sodium 140mg; Carbohydrate 18g (Dietary Fiber 1g); Protein 6g
% Daily Value: Vitamin A 4%; Vitamin C 0%; Calcium 6%; Iron 6%
Diet Exchanges: 1 starch, ½ lean meat

Crunchy Oven French Toast

LO CAL / LO FAT / LO CHOL

PREP: 15 MIN; BAKE: 18 MIN

12 SLICES

If you love the flavor of 100 percent pure maple syrup, use it in place of the honey.

2	tablespoons margarine
5	tablespoons wheat germ
1/4	cup orange juice
2	tablespoons honey
3/4	cup fat-free cholesterol-free egg product or 6 egg whites
12	slices French bread, each 1 inch thick

Heat oven to 450°. Melt margarine in jelly roll pan, 15½ × 10½ × 1 inch, in oven; spread evenly in pan. Sprinkle 3 tablespoons of the wheat germ evenly over margarine.

Beat orange juice, honey and egg product with hand beater until foamy, using a bowl large enough for all the bread. Soak each side of bread in egg mixture for 5 minutes. Drizzle any remaining egg mixture over bread. Sprinkle remaining 2 tablespoons wheat germ evenly over bread.

Place bread in prepared jelly roll pan. Bake about 10 minutes or until bottoms are golden brown; turn. Bake 6 to 8 minutes longer or until bottoms are golden brown.

1 Slice: Calories 115 (Calories from Fat 25); Fat 3g (Saturated 1g); Cholesterol 0mg; Sodium 200mg; Carbohydrate 18g (Dietary Fiber 1g); Protein 5g
% Daily Value: Vitamin A 2%; Vitamin C 2%; Calcium 2%; Iron 6%
Diet Exchanges: 1 starch, ½ fat

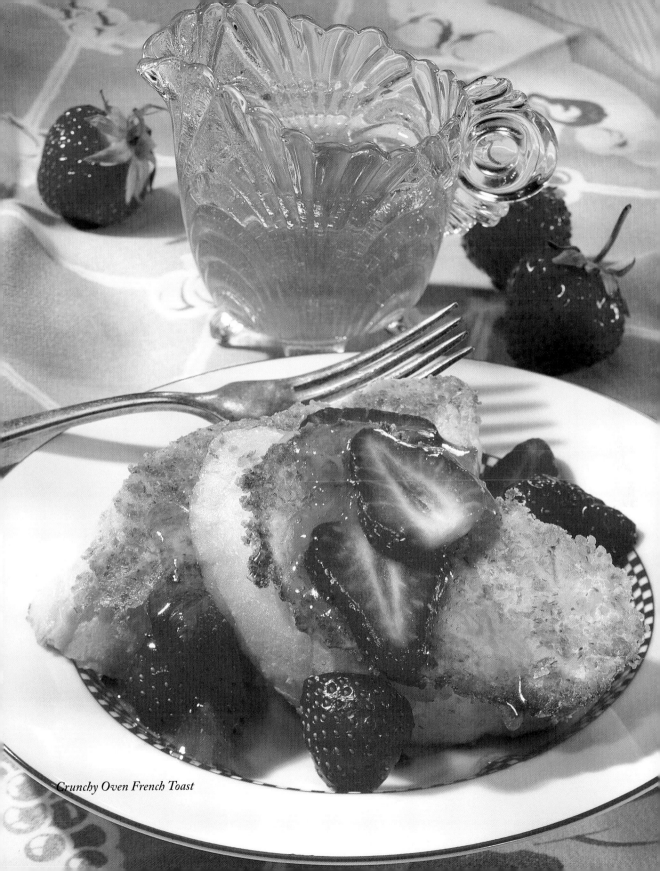

Crunchy Oven French Toast

Apple-Oat Coffee Cake

LO CHOL / HI FIB

PREP: 20 MIN; BAKE: 45 MIN

12 SERVINGS

Choose your favorite baking apple for this yummy coffee cake. Don't have a favorite? Try Granny Smith, Brae-burn, Cortland, Haralson or Rome Beauty.

Oat Streusel (right)

1 cup all-purpose flour

1 cup whole wheat flour

¾ cup sugar

¼ cup margarine, softened

1 cup skim milk

3 teaspoons baking powder

1 teaspoon ground cinnamon

½ teaspoon salt

¼ teaspoon ground nutmeg

¼ teaspoon ground allspice

¼ cup fat-free cholesterol-free egg product or 2 egg whites

2 medium apples, chopped (2 cups)

Apple slices, if desired

Heat oven to 350°. Grease square pan, 9 × 9 × 2 inches. Prepare Oat Streusel; set aside.

Beat remaining ingredients except apples in large bowl with electric mixer on low speed 30 seconds, scraping bowl frequently. Beat on medium speed 2 minutes, scraping bowl occasionally. Stir in chopped apples.

Spread half of the batter in pan; sprinkle with half of the streusel. Top with remaining batter; sprinkle with remaining streusel. Bake 40 to 45 minutes or until toothpick inserted in center comes out clean. Serve warm. Garnish with apple slices.

Oat Streusel

3 tablespoons firm margarine

1 cup quick-cooking or old-fashioned oats

¼ cup all-purpose flour

¼ cup packed brown sugar

¼ cup chopped nuts

Cut margarine into oats, flour and brown sugar, using pastry blender or fork, until crumbly. Stir in nuts.

1 Serving: Calories 270 (Calories from Fat 80); Fat 9g (Saturated 1g); Cholesterol 0mg; Sodium 330mg; Carbohydrate 44g (Dietary Fiber 3g); Protein 6g
% Daily Value: Vitamin A 10%; Vitamin C 0%; Calcium 10%; Iron 8%
Diet Exchanges: 3 starch, 1 fat

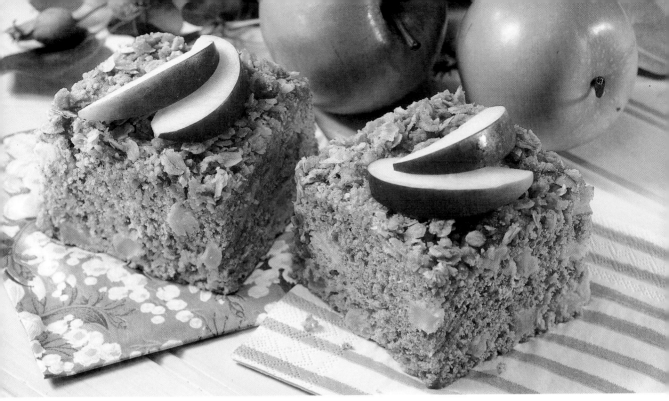

Apple-Oat Coffee Cake

Whole Wheat Waffles

LO CAL / LO CHOL / HI FIB

PREP: 10 MIN; BAKE: 15 MIN

TWELVE 4-INCH WAFFLE SQUARES

Instead of the usual butter and syrup, try serving these waffles with fresh sliced strawberries and fat-free whipped topping.

2 cups whole wheat flour

1/4 cup margarine, melted, or vegetable oil

1 3/4 cups skim milk

1/2 cup fat-free cholesterol-free egg product or 4 egg whites

1 tablespoon sugar

3 teaspoons baking powder

1/2 teaspoon salt

6 tablespoons wheat germ

Heat nonstick waffle iron; spray with cooking spray. Beat all ingredients except wheat germ with hand beater or wire whisk just until smooth.

For each waffle, pour about one-third of batter onto center of hot waffle iron; sprinkle with 2 table-spoons of the wheat germ. Bake about 5 minutes or until steaming slows. Carefully remove waffle.

One 4-inch Waffle Square: Calories 135 (Calories from Fat 45); Fat 5g (Saturated 1g); Cholesterol 0mg; Sodium 300mg; Carbohydrate 19g (Dietary Fiber 3g); Protein 6g **% Daily Value:** Vitamin A 6%; Vitamin C 0%; Calcium 12%; Iron 6%
Diet Exchanges: 1 starch, 1/2 lean meat, 1/2 fat

Raisin-Spice Coffee Cake

LO CAL / LO CHOL / HI FIB

PREP: 15 MIN; BAKE: 45 MIN

9 SERVINGS

Raisins, the most common form of dried fruit, are a good source of fiber and the mineral magnesium.

Streusel (right)

1 cup all-purpose flour

1 cup whole wheat flour

1 cup sugar

$^1/_4$ cup margarine, softened

1 cup skim milk

$^1/_4$ cup fat-free cholesterol-free egg product or 2 egg whites

3 teaspoons baking powder

1 teaspoon ground cinnamon

$^1/_2$ teaspoon salt

$^1/_4$ teaspoon ground allspice or cloves

$^1/_4$ teaspoon ground nutmeg

$^1/_2$ cup raisins

Heat oven to 350°. Spray square pan, 9 × 9 × 2 inches, with cooking spray. Prepare Streusel; set aside.

Beat remaining ingredients except raisins with electric mixer on low speed 30 seconds. Beat on medium speed 2 minutes, scraping bowl occasionally. Stir in raisins.

Spread batter in pan. Sprinkle with Streusel. Bake 40 to 45 minutes or until toothpick inserted in center comes out clean. Serve warm.

Streusel

2 tablespoons firm margarine

$^1/_4$ cup all-purpose flour

2 tablespoons packed brown sugar or granulated sugar

$^1/_2$ teaspoon ground cinnamon

$^1/_4$ cup chopped nuts

Cut margarine into flour, brown sugar and cinnamon, using pastry blender or fork, until crumbly. Stir in nuts.

1 Serving: Calories 335 (Calories from Fat 90); Fat 10g (Saturated 2g); Cholesterol 0mg; Sodium 410mg; Carbohydrate 58g (Dietary Fiber 3g); Protein 6g
% Daily Value: Vitamin A 12%; Vitamin C 0%; Calcium 14%; Iron 10%
Diet Exchanges: not recommended

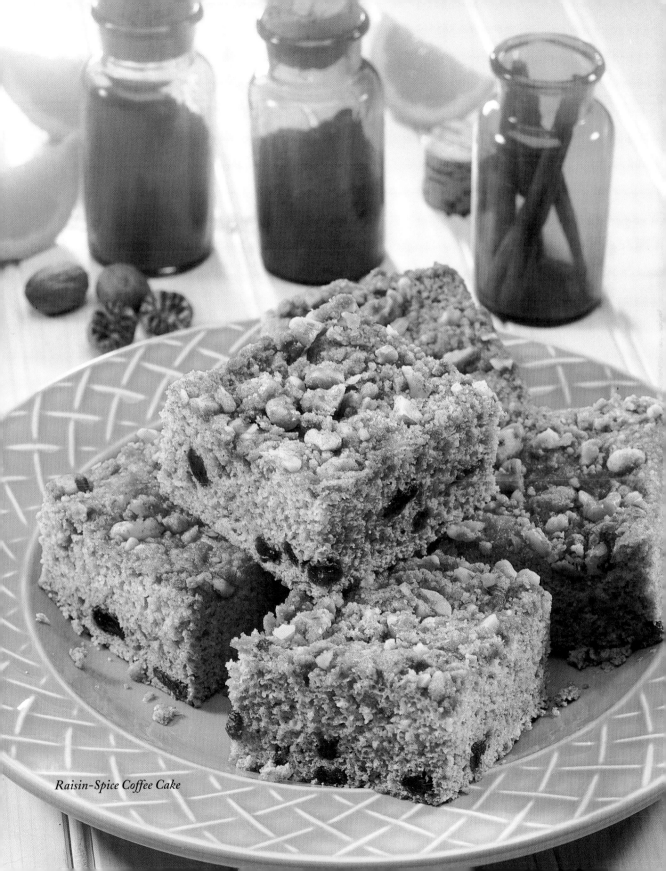

Raisin-Spice Coffee Cake

Buttermilk-Raisin Breakfast Buns

LO CAL / LO FAT / LO CHOL / HI FIB

PREP: 25 MIN; BAKE: 25 MIN

8 BUNS

Any flavor of spreadable fruit can be used in this recipe—be adventurous!

2	teaspoons margarine
3 to 3½	cups all-purpose flour
1	tablespoon baking powder
½	teaspoon salt
1	cup reduced-fat buttermilk
½	cup fat-free cholesterol-free egg product or 4 egg whites
1½	cups golden or regular raisins
1	container (6 ounces) unsweetened applesauce (¾ cup)
2	teaspoons ground cinnamon
2	tablespoons strawberry spreadable fruit, melted

Heat oven to 400°. Spray rectangular pan, 13 × 9 × 2 inches, with cooking spray. Cut margarine into flour, baking powder and salt in large bowl, using pastry blender or crisscrossing 2 knives, until mixture resembles fine crumbs. Mix in buttermilk and egg product.

Turn dough onto lightly floured surface. Gently knead in enough flour to make dough easy to handle (dough will be soft). Roll dough into 8-inch square. Mix raisins, applesauce and cinnamon; spread over dough. Roll up dough; pinch edge of dough into roll to seal. Cut roll into 8 slices. Place 1 inch apart in pan.

Bake 20 to 25 minutes or until light brown. Brush with spreadable fruit. Remove from pan. Cool on wire rack.

1 Bun: Calories 305 (Calories from Fat 20); Fat 2g (Saturated 1g); Cholesterol 0mg; Sodium 400mg; Carbohydrate 67g (Dietary Fiber 3g); Protein 8g
% Daily Value: Vitamin A 2%; Vitamin C 0%; Calcium 16%; Iron 18%
Diet Exchanges: 2½ starch, 2 fruit

High-Fiber Honey-Whole Wheat Loaf

LO CAL / LO FAT / LO CHOL / LO SODIUM / HI FIB

PREP: 25 MIN; PROOF: 2 HR; BAKE: 35 MIN

1 LOAF (16 SLICES)

When making yeast bread, it's important to stick to the temperature given for the liquid in the recipe. If the liquid is too cold, it won't activate the yeast and your bread won't rise. If it's too hot, it kills the yeast, also resulting in bread that won't rise. Use an instant-read thermometer or candy thermometer to take the temperature of the liquid.

$2^1/_2$ to $2^3/_4$	cups all-purpose flour
$^1/_2$	teaspoon salt
1	package regular or quick* active dry yeast
$1^1/_2$	cups very warm water (120° to 130°)
$^1/_4$	cup honey
1	tablespoon olive or vegetable oil
1	cup whole wheat flour
1	cup Fiber One® cereal

Mix $1^3/_4$ cups of the all-purpose flour, the salt and yeast in large bowl. Add warm water, honey and oil. Beat with electric mixer on low speed 1 minute, scraping bowl frequently. Beat on medium speed 1 minute, scraping bowl frequently. Stir in whole wheat flour and cereal. Stir in enough remaining all-purpose flour, $^1/_4$ cup at a time, to make dough easy to handle.

Turn dough onto lightly floured surface; gently roll in flour to coat. Knead about 10 minutes or until smooth and elastic. Spray large bowl with cooking spray. Place dough in bowl, and turn greased side up. Cover and let rise in warm place about $1^1/_4$ hours or until double. (Dough is ready if indentation remains when touched.)

Spray cookie sheet with cooking spray. Punch down dough. Shape into about 9-inch round loaf. Place on cookie sheet. Cover and let rise in warm place about 40 minutes or until double.

Heat oven to 350°. Bake 30 to 35 minutes or until loaf is golden brown and sounds hollow when tapped. Remove from cookie sheet to wire rack; cool.

*If using quick active yeast, let dough rest 10 minutes after kneading, and omit first rising time.

1 Slice: Calories 120 (Calories from Fat 10); Fat 1g (Saturated 0g); Cholesterol 0mg; Sodium 95mg; Carbohydrate 28g (Dietary Fiber 3g); Protein 3g
% Daily Value: Vitamin A 0%; Vitamin C 0%; Calcium 0%; Iron 10%
Diet Exchanges: $1^1/_2$ starch

Rosemary Focaccia

LO CAL / LO FAT / LO CHOL / LO SODIUM

PREP: 30 MIN; PROOF: 2 HR; BAKE: 35 MIN

16 SERVINGS

The saying "a little goes a long way" certainly applies to this recipe. Although many focaccia recipes call for more olive oil, we call for just 1 tablespoon. To get the most flavor, use extra-virgin olive oil.

$4^1/_2$ to 5 cups all-purpose flour

1 large onion, chopped (1 cup)

1 tablespoon olive or vegetable oil

1 teaspoon dried rosemary leaves, crumbled

$^1/_2$ teaspoon salt

1 package regular or quick* active dry yeast

2 cups very warm water (120° to 130°)

Cornmeal

Olive or vegetable oil

2 teaspoons dried rosemary leaves, crumbled

Mix 2 cups of the flour, the onion, 1 tablespoon oil, 1 teaspoon rosemary, the salt and yeast in large bowl. Add warm water. Beat with electric mixer on low speed 1 minute, scraping bowl frequently. Beat on medium speed 1 minute, scraping bowl frequently. Stir in enough remaining flour, 1 cup at a time, to make dough easy to handle.

Turn dough onto lightly floured surface; gently roll in flour to coat. Knead about 10 minutes or until smooth and elastic. Spray large bowl with cooking spray. Place dough in bowl, and turn greased side up. Cover and let rise in warm place about $1^1/_2$ hours or until double. (Dough is ready if indentation remains when touched.)

Spray jelly roll pan, $15^1/_2 \times 10^1/_2 \times 1$ inch, with cooking spray; sprinkle lightly with cornmeal. Punch down dough. Press in pan. Cover and let rise in warm place about 30 minutes or until almost double.

Heat oven to 400°. Press dough to edges of pan. Brush lightly with oil; sprinkle with 2 teaspoons rosemary. Bake 30 to 35 minutes or until golden brown. Remove from pan to wire rack; cool.

*If using quick active yeast, let dough rest 10 minutes after kneading, and omit first rising time.

1 Serving: Calories 140 (Calories from Fat 20); Fat 2g (Saturated 0g); Cholesterol 0mg; Sodium 75mg; Carbohydrate 28g (Dietary Fiber 1g); Protein 4g
% Daily Value: Vitamin A 0%; Vitamin C 0%; Calcium 0%; Iron 10%
Diet Exchanges: $1^1/_2$ starch, $^1/_2$ fat

Oatmeal Pancakes

LO CAL / LO FAT / LO CHOL

PREP: 10 MIN; COOK: 5 MIN

9 PANCAKES

The richness of buttermilk paired with the gentle sweetness of oats makes these pancakes delicious, and the whole wheat flour adds subtle, yet hearty texture.

- 1/2 cup quick-cooking or old-fashioned oats
- 1/4 cup all-purpose flour
- 1/4 cup whole wheat flour
- 3/4 cup reduced-fat buttermilk
- 1/4 cup skim milk
- 1/4 cup fat-free cholesterol-free egg product or 2 egg whites
- 1 tablespoon sugar
- 2 tablespoons vegetable oil
- 1 teaspoon baking powder
- 1/2 teaspoon baking soda
- 1/2 teaspoon salt

Beat all ingredients with hand beater or whisk just until smooth. (For thinner pancakes, stir in additional 2 to 4 tablespoons milk.)

Spray griddle or 10-inch nonstick skillet with cooking spray. Heat griddle over medium heat or to 375°. (To test griddle, sprinkle with a few drops of water. If bubbles skitter around, heat is just right.)

For each pancake, pour about 1/4 cup batter onto hot griddle. Cook pancakes until puffed and dry around edges. Turn and cook other sides until golden brown.

1 Pancake: Calories 65 (Calories from Fat 25); Fat 3g (Saturated 1g); Cholesterol 0mg; Sodium 220mg; Carbohydrate 8g (Dietary Fiber 1g); Protein 2g
% Daily Value: Vitamin A 0%; Vitamin C 0%; Calcium 4%; Iron 2%
Diet Exchanges: 1/2 starch, 1/2 fat

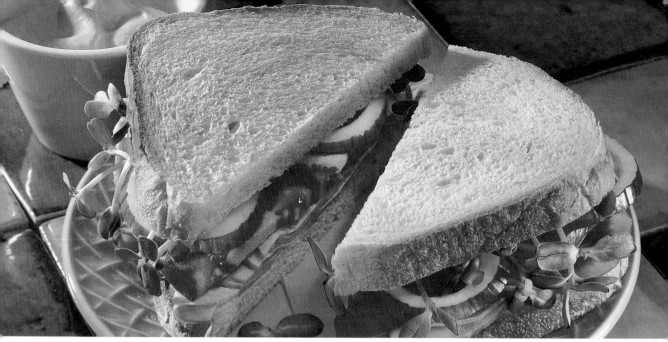

Bread Machine Honey-Mustard Bread

Bread Machine Honey-Mustard Bread

LO CAL / LO FAT / LO CHOL

Ingredient	1½-LB Recipe (12 slices)	2-LB Recipe (16 slices)
Water	¾ cup plus 1 tablespoon	1 cup
Honey	2 tablespoons	3 tablespoons
Mustard	2 tablespoons	3 tablespoons
Margarine, softened	2 tablespoons	3 tablespoons
Bread flour	3 cups	4 cups
Salt	½ teaspoon	¾ teaspoon
Paprika	½ teaspoon	1 teaspoon
Bread machine yeast	1½ teaspoons	1¾ teaspoons

Make 1½-Pound Recipe with bread machines that use 3 cups flour, or make 2-Pound Recipe with bread machines that use 4 cups flour.

Measure carefully, placing all ingredients in bread machine pan in the order recommended by the manufacturer.

Select Basic/White cycle. Use Medium or Light crust color. Do not use delay cycles. Remove baked bread from pan, and cool on wire rack.

1 Slice: Calories 145 (Calories from Fat 20); Fat 2g (Saturated 0g); Cholesterol 0mg; Sodium 150mg; Carbohydrate 29g (Dietary Fiber 1g); Protein 4g
% Daily Value: Vitamin A 2%; Vitamin C 0%; Calcium 0%; Iron 10%
Diet Exchanges: 2 starch

Bread Machine Oat-Potato Sandwich Bread

LO CAL / LO FAT / LO CHOL

This bread is great for making sandwiches. Try using fat-free smoked turkey or ham and slices of fat-free or reduced-fat cheese along with crisp lettuce, onions and tomatoes (photo, page 369).

INGREDIENT	1½-LB RECIPE (12 SLICES)	2-LB RECIPE (16 SLICES)
Water	1¼ cups	1½ cups plus 1 tablespoon
Vegetable or olive oil	1 tablespoon	1 tablespoon
Honey	2 tablespoons	3 tablespoons
Bread flour	3 cups	4 cups
Potato Buds® mashed potatoes (dry)	½ cup	⅔ cup
Old-fashioned or quick-cooking oats	¾ cup	1 cup
Grated lemon peel	½ teaspoon	1 teaspoon
Dried thyme leaves	½ teaspoon	1 teaspoon
Salt	1½ teaspoons	2 teaspoons
Bread machine yeast	1½ teaspoons	2 teaspoons

Make 1½-Pound Recipe with bread machines that use 3 cups flour, or make 2-Pound Recipe with bread machines that use 4 cups flour.

Measure carefully, placing all ingredients in bread machine pan in the order recommended by the manufacturer.

Select Basic/White cycle. Use Medium or Light crust color. Do not use delay cycles. Remove baked bread from pan, and cool on wire rack.

1 Slice: Calories 165 (Calories from Fat 20); Fat 2g (Saturated 0g); Cholesterol 0mg; Sodium 300mg; Carbohydrate 34g (Dietary Fiber 2g); Protein 5g
% Daily Value: Vitamin A 0%; Vitamin C 0%; Calcium 0%; Iron 10%
Diet Exchanges: 2 starch, 1 vegetable

Bread Machine French Baguettes

LO CAL / LO FAT / LO CHOL / LO SODIUM

2 LOAVES (12 SLICES EACH)

To make these loaves ahead of time, prepare dough as directed—except after making slashes across loaves, cover with plastic wrap. Refrigerate at least 4 hours but no longer than 48 hours. Before baking, remove from refrigerator and let rise covered in warm place about 2 hours or until double. Continue as directed.

1	cup water
2¾	cups bread flour
1	tablespoon sugar
1	teaspoon salt
1½	teaspoons bread machine yeast
1	egg yolk
1	tablespoon water

Measure carefully, placing all ingredients except egg yolk and 1 tablespoon water in bread machine pan in the order recommended by the manufacturer.

Select Dough/Manual cycle. Spray large bowl with cooking spray. When done, remove dough from pan, using lightly floured hands. Place dough in bowl, and turn to coat with cooking spray. Cover and let rise in warm place about 30 minutes or until double. (Dough is ready if indentation remains when touched.)

Spray cookie sheet with cooking spray. Punch down dough. Roll dough into rectangle, 16 × 12 inches, on lightly floured surface. Cut dough crosswise in half. Roll up each half tightly, beginning at 12-inch side. Gently roll back and forth to taper ends.

Place loaves 3 inches apart on cookie sheet. Make ¼-inch-deep diagonal slashes across loaves every 2 inches, or make 1 lengthwise slash on each loaf. Cover and let rise in warm place 30 to 40 minutes or until double.

Heat oven to 375°. Mix egg yolk and 1 tablespoon water; brush over tops of loaves. Bake 20 to 25 minutes or until golden brown. Serve warm, or cool on wire rack.

1 Slice: Calories 60 (Calories from Fat 0); Fat 0g (Saturated 0g); Cholesterol 10mg; Sodium 100mg; Carbohydrate 13g (Dietary Fiber 0g); Protein 2g
% Daily Value: Vitamin A 0%; Vitamin C 0%; Calcium 0%; Iron 4%
Diet Exchanges: 1 starch

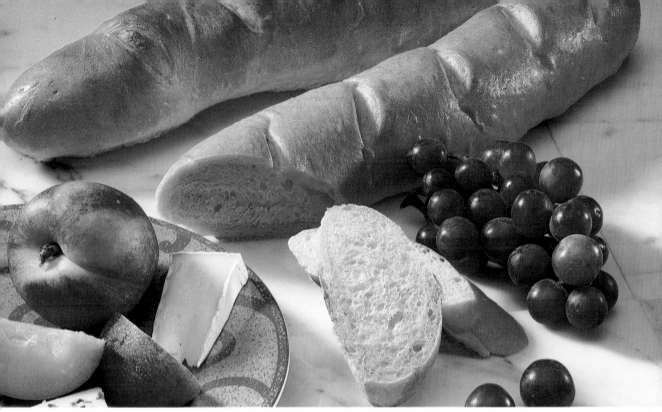

Bread Machine French Baguettes

Cutting Bread Machine Loaves

For best results when cutting warm bread loaves, we recommend using an electric knife. Also, a sharp serrated or sawtooth bread knife works well.

There are several ways to cut bread machine loaves:

➤ For square slices, place the loaf on its side and cut down through the loaf. We find this to be the easiest way to cut loaves.

➤ For rectangular slices, place the loaf upright and cut from the top down. Slices may be cut in half, either lengthwise or crosswise.

➤ For wedges, place the loaf upright and cut down from the center into wedges. Or cut loaf in half from the top down, then place each half cut side down and cut lengthwise into wedges.

➤ For other shapes, use your imagination! Bread slices can be cut into triangles, fingerlike strips and chunks. Or slices can be cut into other interesting shapes with cookie cutters.

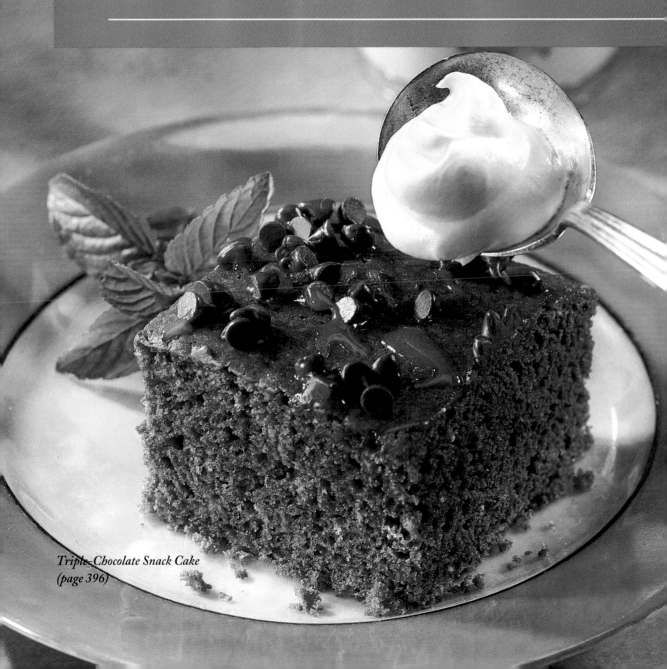

GO FOR DESSERT!

Triple-Chocolate Snack Cake
(page 396)

Chocolate Chip Cookies

LO CAL / LO FAT / LO CHOL / LO SODIUM

PREP: 15 MIN; BAKE: 10 MIN

ABOUT 2½ DOZEN COOKIES

Don't try to substitute vegetable-oil spreads or whipped margarine for the stick variety. These products have a high water content and will greatly affect the success of your recipe.

½ cup granulated sugar

¼ cup packed brown sugar

¼ cup margarine, softened

1 teaspoon vanilla

2 tablespoons fat-free cholesterol-free egg product or 1 egg white

½ cup all-purpose flour

½ cup whole wheat flour

½ teaspoon baking soda

¼ teaspoon salt

½ cup miniature semisweet chocolate chips

Heat oven to 375°. Mix sugars, margarine, vanilla and egg product in medium bowl. Stir in flours, baking soda and salt. Stir in chocolate chips.

Drop dough by rounded teaspoonfuls about 2 inches apart onto ungreased cookie sheet. Bake 8 to 10 minutes or until golden brown. Cool slightly; remove from cookie sheet to wire rack.

1 Cookie: Calories 70 (Calories from Fat 20); Fat 2g (Saturated 1g); Cholesterol 0mg; Sodium 65mg; Carbohydrate 12g (Dietary Fiber 0g); Protein 1g
% Daily Value: Vitamin A 2%; Vitamin C 0%; Calcium 0%; Iron 2%
Diet Exchanges: ½ starch, ½ fat

Oaties

LO CAL / LO FAT / LO CHOL / LO SODIUM

PREP: 20 MIN; BAKE: 15 MIN

ABOUT 3 DOZEN COOKIES

1¼ cups all-purpose flour

1 cup quick-cooking oats

1 teaspoon ground cinnamon

½ teaspoon baking soda

⅛ teaspoon salt

½ cup fat-free cholesterol-free egg product or 3 egg whites

½ cup packed brown sugar

¼ cup granulated sugar

⅓ cup unsweetened applesauce

¼ cup margarine, softened

1 teaspoon vanilla

1 cup raisins or chopped dried fruit

Heat oven to 325°. Spray cookie sheet with cooking spray. Mix flour, oats, cinnamon, baking soda and salt; set aside. Beat egg product in large bowl with electric mixer on medium speed until foamy. Add sugars, applesauce, margarine and vanilla. Beat on medium speed until smooth. Add flour mixture; beat on low speed just until mixed. Stir in raisins.

Drop dough by tablespoonfuls 2 inches apart onto cookie sheet; flatten slightly. Bake 12 to 15 minutes or until light brown. Cool slightly; remove from cookie sheet to wire rack.

1 Cookie: Calories 60 (Calories from Fat 10); Fat 1g (Saturated 0g); Cholesterol 0mg; Sodium 50mg; Carbohydrate 12g (Dietary Fiber 1g); Protein 1g
% Daily Value: Vitamin A 2%; Vitamin C 0%; Calcium 0%; Iron 2%
Diet Exchanges: 1 starch

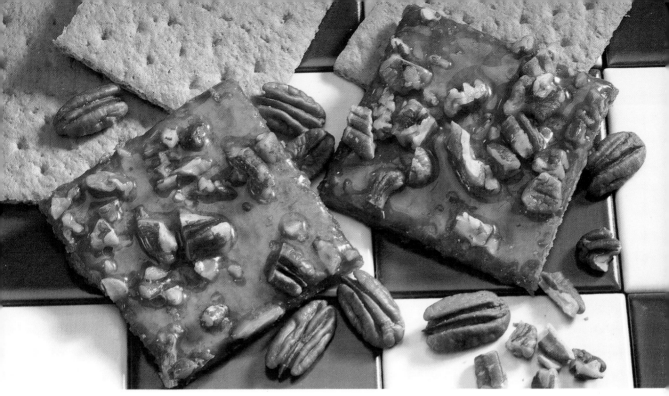

Quick Praline Bars

Quick Praline Bars

LO CAL / LO CHOL / LO SODIUM

PREP: 10 MIN; BAKE: 10 MIN

ABOUT 2 DOZEN BARS

Go nuts! Chopped almonds or cashews can be substituted for the pecans, if you wish.

24   graham cracker squares

$^1/_2$ cup packed brown sugar

$^1/_2$ cup margarine

$^1/_2$ teaspoon vanilla

$^1/_2$ cup chopped pecans

Heat oven to 350°. Arrange graham crackers in single layer in ungreased jelly roll pan, $15^1/_2 \times 10^1/_2 \times 1$ inch.

Heat brown sugar and margarine to boiling in 2-quart saucepan. Boil 1 minute, stirring constantly; remove from heat. Stir in vanilla.

Pour sugar mixture over crackers; spread evenly. Sprinkle with pecans. Bake 8 to 10 minutes or until bubbly; cool slightly.

1 Bar: Calories 95 (Calories from Fat 5); Fat 6g (Saturated 1g); Cholesterol 0mg; Sodium 90mg; Carbohydrate 10g (Dietary Fiber 0g); Protein 0g
% Daily Value: Vitamin A 4%; Vitamin C 0%; Calcium 0%; Iron 2%
Diet Exchanges: $^1/_2$ starch, 1 fat

Tiramisu Coffee Dessert

LO CAL / LO CHOL

PREP: 15 MIN; CHILL: 1 HR

15 SERVINGS

The classic recipe for tiramisu calls for mascarpone cheese, egg yolks and heavy whipping cream. We've cut the fat and calories in our version without sacrificing the flavor.

- 1 loaf (9 × 5 inches) angel food cake, cut into 8 slices
- 1 cup strong coffee (room temperature)
- 1 package (8 ounces) reduced-fat cream cheese (Neufchâtel), softened
- 1/2 cup sugar
- 1/2 cup chocolate-flavored syrup
- 1 container (8 ounces) frozen fat-free whipped topping, thawed (3 1/4 cups)

  Baking cocoa

Arrange cake slices to cover bottom of rectangular baking dish, 13 × 9 × 2 inches. Drizzle coffee over cake.

Beat cream cheese, sugar and chocolate syrup in large bowl with electric mixer on medium speed until smooth. Gently stir in whipped topping until well blended. Spread over cake.

Cover and refrigerate about 1 hour or until set. Sprinkle with cocoa before serving. Cover and refrigerate any remaining dessert.

1 Serving: Calories 185 (Calories from Fat 55); Fat 7g (Saturated 5g); Cholesterol 10mg; Sodium 230mg; Carbohydrate 28g (Dietary Fiber 0g); Protein 3g
% Daily Value: Vitamin A 4%; Vitamin C 0%; Calcium 2%; Iron 2%
Diet Exchanges: 2 starch, 1 fat

Triple-Chocolate Snack Cake

LO CAL / LO CHOL

PREP: 10 MIN; BAKE: 40 MIN; COOK: 5 MIN

9 SERVINGS

In the mood for cake? You don't have to wait long! This rich, low-calorie chocolate delight comes together quickly and is best eaten warm (photo, page 393).

- 1 3/4 cups Bisquick® Reduced Fat baking mix
- 1 cup sugar
- 1/4 cup baking cocoa
- 1/4 cup fat-free cholesterol-free egg product or 2 egg whites
- 1 cup chocolate skim milk
- 1 tablespoon vegetable oil
- 1 teaspoon vanilla
- 1/4 cup miniature semisweet chocolate chips
- 2 tablespoons caramel fat-free topping

  Frozen (thawed) fat-free whipped topping or vanilla fat-free frozen yogurt, if desired

Heat oven to 375°. Spray square pan, 8 × 8 × 2 inches, with cooking spray. Mix baking mix, sugar and cocoa in large bowl. Mix egg product, milk, oil and vanilla until blended; stir into baking mix mixture. Spread in pan.

Bake 35 to 40 minutes or until toothpick inserted in center comes out clean. Cool in pan on wire rack 5 minutes. Sprinkle chocolate chips over cake. Drizzle with caramel topping. Serve warm with whipped topping.

1 Serving: Calories 245 (Calories from Fat 45); Fat 5g (Saturated 2g); Cholesterol 0mg; Sodium 310mg; Carbohydrate 48g (Dietary Fiber 2g); Protein 4g
% Daily Value: Vitamin A 2%; Vitamin C 0%; Calcium 6%; Iron 8%
Diet Exchanges: 3 starch

Chocolate-Glazed Brownies

LO CAL / LO CHOL / LO SODIUM

PREP: 10 MIN; BAKE: 25 MIN; COOK: 15 MIN

16 BROWNIES

For an easy holiday treat, substitute peppermint extract for the vanilla in the Chocolate Glaze and sprinkle crushed hard peppermint candies over the top.

1 cup sugar

1/3 cup margarine, softened

1 teaspoon vanilla

1/2 cup fat-free cholesterol-free egg product or 4 egg whites

2/3 cup all-purpose flour

1/2 cup baking cocoa

1/2 teaspoon baking powder

1/4 teaspoon salt

Chocolate Glaze (right)

Heat oven to 350°. Spray square pan, 8 × 8 × 2 inches, with cooking spray. Mix sugar, margarine, vanilla and egg product in medium bowl. Stir in remaining ingredients except Chocolate Glaze. Spread in pan.

Bake 20 to 25 minutes or until toothpick inserted in center comes out clean; cool. Spread Chocolate Glaze evenly over brownies. Cut into about 2-inch squares.

Chocolate Glaze

2/3 cup powdered sugar

2 tablespoons baking cocoa

1/4 teaspoon vanilla

3 to 4 teaspoons hot water

Mix all ingredients until smooth and spreadable.

1 Brownie: Calories 130 (Calories from Fat 35); Fat 4g (Saturated 1g); Cholesterol 0mg; Sodium 115mg; Carbohydrate 23g (Dietary Fiber 1g); Protein 2g
% Daily Value: Vitamin A 4%; Vitamin C 0%; Calcium 2%; Iron 4%
Diet Exchanges: 1 1/2 starch, 1/2 fat

Brownie Trifle

LO CAL / LO CHOL

PREP: 15 MIN; BAKE: 30 MIN; CHILL: 4 HR

20 SERVINGS

Decrease the fat and calories even more in this decadent dessert by leaving out the English toffee bits. If you want an extra dose of chocolate, garnish with chocolate curls or sprinkle ¼ cup of miniature semisweet chocolate chips over the crowning layer of whipped topping.

- 1 package (1 pound 3.8 ounces) fudge brownie mix
- ¼ cup water
- ½ cup vegetable oil
- ½ cup fat-free cholesterol-free egg product
- 1 tablespoon freeze-dried instant coffee (dry)
- 1 package (4-serving size) chocolate fat-free sugar-free chocolate instant pudding and pie filling mix
- 2 cups skim milk
- 1 package (6-ounce) English toffee bits (reserving 2 tablespoons for garnish)
- 1 container (8 ounces) frozen fat-free whipped topping, thawed (3¼ cups)

Heat oven to 350°. Prepare brownie mix as directed on package for 13 × 9-inch rectangular pan, using water, oil and egg product and stirring coffee into batter. Bake and cool as directed.

Cut brownies into 1-inch squares. Place half of the brownie squares in bottom of 3-quart glass bowl. Prepare pudding mix as directed on package for pudding, using skim milk. Pour half of the pudding over brownies in bowl. Top with half each of the toffee bits and whipped topping. Repeat with remaining brownies, pudding, toffee bits and whipped topping. Sprinkle with reserved toffee bits.

Cover and refrigerate at least 4 hours before serving. Cover and refrigerate any remaining trifle.

1 Serving: Calories 240 (Calories from Fat 90); Fat 10g (Saturated 3g); Cholesterol 5mg; Sodium 220mg; Carbohydrate 34g (Dietary Fiber 0g); Protein 3g
% Daily Value: Vitamin A 2%; Vitamin C 0%; Calcium 6%; Iron 4%
Diet Exchanges: 2 starch, 2 fat

Saucy Raspberry Rhubarb

LO CAL / LO FAT / LO CHOL / LO SODIUM / HI FIB

PREP: 10 MIN; COOK: 15 MIN

6 SERVINGS

To enjoy this dessert year-round, chop fresh rhubarb into ½-inch pieces, place in an airtight plastic bag and freeze until ready to use.

- 3 cups chopped fresh rhubarb or 1 bag (16 ounces) frozen cut rhubarb, thawed
- ½ cup apple juice
- 3 tablespoons packed brown sugar
- 1 pint (2 cups) raspberries
- 2 tablespoons reduced-fat sour cream

Heat rhubarb, apple juice, brown sugar and 1 cup of the raspberries to boiling in 1-quart saucepan; reduce heat. Simmer uncovered about 10 minutes, stirring occasionally, until rhubarb is soft; cool.

Stir in remaining 1 cup raspberries. Spoon into dessert dishes. Top with sour cream.

1 Serving: Calories 72 (Calories from Fat 0); Fat 0g (Saturated 0g); Cholesterol 0mg; Sodium 10mg; Carbohydrate 17g (Dietary Fiber 4g); Protein 1g
% Daily Value: Vitamin A 2%; Vitamin C 12%; Calcium 14%; Iron 4%
Diet Exchanges: 1 fruit

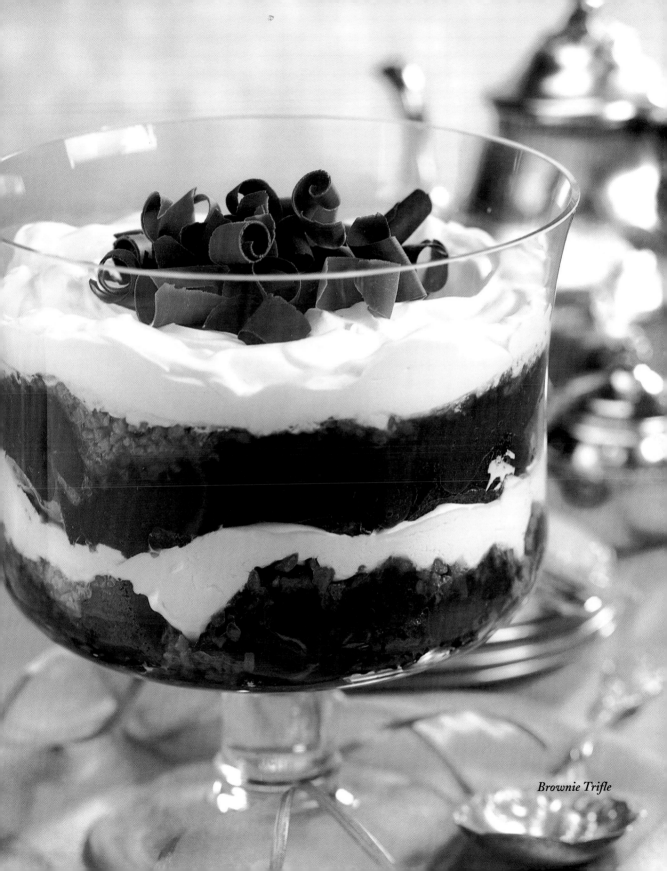

Brownie Trifle

Lemon-Topped Gingerbread

LO CAL / LO FAT / LO CHOL / LO SODIUM

PREP: 10 MIN; BAKE: 35 MIN; COOL: 10 MIN

8 SERVINGS

Want to give the gingerbread a strong, spicy flavor? Use dark molasses. Or, for a sweeter, more delicate-flavored cake, try the light variety.

½	cup all-purpose flour
½	cup whole wheat flour
¼	cup molasses
¼	cup hot water
2	tablespoons packed brown sugar
2	tablespoons shortening
2	tablespoons fat-free cholesterol-free egg product or 1 egg white
½	teaspoon baking soda
½	teaspoon ground ginger
½	teaspoon ground cinnamon
⅛	teaspoon salt
	Lemon Sauce (right)

Heat oven to 325°. Spray loaf pan, 8½ × 4½ × 2½ inches, with cooking spray. Beat all ingredients except Lemon Sauce in medium bowl with electric mixer on low speed 30 seconds, scraping bowl constantly. Beat on medium speed 3 minutes, scraping bowl occasionally. Pour into pan.

Bake 30 to 35 minutes or until toothpick inserted in center comes out clean. Cool 10 minutes; remove from pan. Serve warm or cool with Lemon Sauce.

Lemon Sauce

3	tablespoons sugar
1	tablespoon cornstarch
1	cup water
1	tablespoon grated lemon peel
1	tablespoon lemon juice

Mix sugar and cornstarch in 1-quart saucepan. Gradually stir in water. Cook over medium heat, stirring constantly, until mixture thickens and boils. Boil and stir 1 minute; remove from heat. Stir in remaining ingredients. Serve warm or cool.

1 Serving: Calories 145 (Calories from Fat 30); Fat 3g (Saturated 1g); Cholesterol 0mg; Sodium 130mg; Carbohydrate 28g (Dietary Fiber 1g); Protein 2g
% Daily Value: Vitamin A 0%; Vitamin C 0%; Calcium 2%; Iron 6%
Diet Exchanges: 2 starch

Lemon Meringue Cake with Strawberries

LOW CHOLESTEROL

PREP: 15 MIN; BAKE: 40 MIN

9 SERVINGS

When preparing the meringue for this cake, it is important to beat the egg whites until shiny and stiff but not dry. The meringue will get watery if the egg whites are underbeaten and will clump together and bake flat if overbeaten.

1	pint (2 cups) strawberries, sliced
1/4	cup sugar
1 1/4	cups all-purpose flour
1	cup sugar
1/4	cup margarine, softened
1/2	cup skim milk
1 1/2	teaspoons baking powder
1 1/2	teaspoons grated lemon peel
1	teaspoon vanilla
1/4	teaspoon salt
2	egg whites or 1/4 cup fat-free cholesterol-free egg product
2	egg whites
1/2	cup sugar

Mix strawberries and 1/4 cup sugar. Cover and refrigerate until serving.

Heat oven to 350°. Spray square pan, 9 × 9 × 2 inches, with cooking spray. Beat flour, 1 cup sugar, the margarine, milk, baking powder, lemon peel, vanilla, salt and 2 egg whites in large bowl with electric mixer on low speed 30 seconds, scraping bowl constantly. Beat on high speed 2 minutes, scraping bowl occasionally. Pour into pan. Bake 25 to 30 minutes or until toothpick inserted in center comes out clean. Cool slightly.

Increase oven temperature to 400°F. Beat 2 egg whites in medium bowl on high speed until foamy. Beat in 1/2 cup sugar, 1 tablespoon at a time; continue beating until stiff and glossy. Spread over cake. Bake 8 to 10 minutes or until meringue is light brown. Cool completely. Top each serving with strawberries.

1 Serving: Calories 280 (Calories from Fat 45); Fat 5g (Saturated 1g); Cholesterol 0mg; Sodium 240mg; Carbohydrate 56g (Dietary Fiber 1g); Protein 4g
% Daily Value: Vitamin A 8%; Vitamin C 16%; Calcium 6%; Iron 6%
Diet Exchanges: 1 starch, 2 1/2 fruit, 1 fat

Creamy Raspberry-Filled Angel Cake

LO CAL / LO FAT / LO CHOL

PREP: 1 1/2 HR

12 SERVINGS

For a fun and low-fat cake with kid appeal, use confetti angel food cake and decorate with candy sprinkles or colored sugar.

1   cup boiling water

1   package (4-serving size) sugar-free raspberry-flavored gelatin

1/2 cup cold water

1   pint (2 cups) raspberries

1   container (8 ounces) frozen fat-free whipped topping, thawed

1   round (10 inches in diameter) angel food cake

     Additional raspberries, if desired

Pour boiling water over gelatin in large bowl; stir until gelatin is dissolved. Stir in cold water. Refrigerate about 1 hour or until thickened but not set.

Fold 1 pint raspberries and half of the whipped topping into gelatin mixture. Refrigerate about 15 minutes or until thickened but not set.

Split cake horizontally to make 3 layers. (To split, mark side of cake with toothpicks and cut with long, thin serrated knife.) Fill layers with gelatin mixture. Spoon or pipe remaining whipped topping onto top of cake. Garnish with raspberries. Cover and refrigerate any remaining cake.

1 Serving: Calories 160 (Calories from Fat 0); Fat 0g (Saturated 0g); Cholesterol 0mg; Sodium 390mg; Carbohydrate 36g (Dietary Fiber 1g); Protein 4g
% Daily Value: Vitamin A 0%; Vitamin C 8%; Calcium 0%; Iron 4%
Diet Exchanges: 1 starch, 1 1/2 fruit

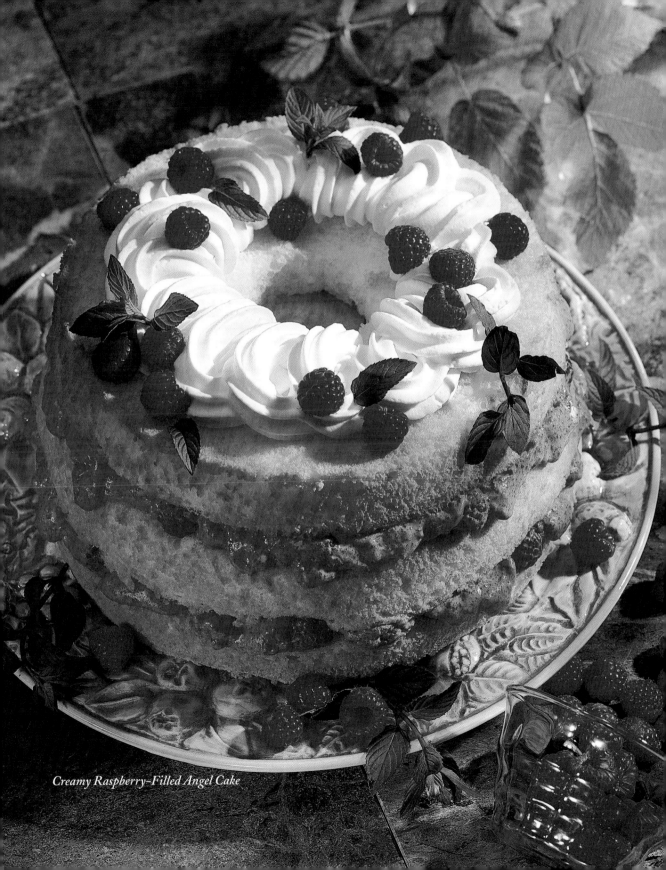

Creamy Raspberry-Filled Angel Cake

Crunch-Topped Apple Spice Cake

LO CAL / LO CHOL

PREP: 20 MIN; BAKE: 45 MIN

15 SERVINGS

Many traditional recipes for Apple Cake call for the nuts to be stirred into the batter. By replacing stirred-in nuts with the Nut Topping in this recipe, you'll get maximum flavor and a lot less fat.

- ⅓ cup boiling water
- 2 medium unpeeled cooking apples, chopped (2 cups)
- 1¼ cups packed brown sugar
- 1 cup all-purpose flour
- 1 cup whole wheat flour
- ¾ cup fat-free cholesterol-free egg product or 5 egg whites
- ⅓ cup vegetable oil
- 1¼ teaspoons baking soda
- 1 teaspoon ground cinnamon
- 1 teaspoon vanilla
- ½ teaspoon ground cloves
- ¼ teaspoon salt
  Nut Topping (right)

Heat oven to 350°. Spray rectangular pan, 13 × 9 × 2 inches, with cooking spray; dust with flour. Pour boiling water over apples in large bowl. Add remaining ingredients except Nut Topping. Beat with electric mixer on low speed 1 minute, scraping bowl constantly. Beat on medium speed 2 minutes, scraping bowl occasionally. Pour into pan.

Sprinkle Nut Topping over batter. Bake 40 to 45 minutes or until toothpick inserted in center comes out clean.

Nut Topping

- ⅓ cup finely chopped nuts
- 2 tablespoons packed brown sugar

Mix ingredients.

1 Serving: Calories 205 (Calories from Fat 60); Fat 7g (Saturated 1g); Cholesterol 0mg; Sodium 170mg; Carbohydrate 35g (Dietary Fiber 2g); Protein 3g
% Daily Value: Vitamin A 0%; Vitamin C 0%; Calcium 2%; Iron 8%
Diet Exchanges: 2 starch, 1 fat

Streusel Pumpkin Pie

LO CAL / LO FAT / LO CHOL

PREP: 15 MIN; BAKE: 55 MIN;

COOL: 15 MIN; CHILL: 4 HR

8 SERVINGS

Getting your vitamin A has never been so easy. One slice of this pie packs in 100 percent of your daily requirement for vitamin A.

Brown Sugar Topping (right)

1   can (15 ounces) pumpkin

1   can (12 ounces) evaporated skimmed milk

$1/2$ cup fat-free cholesterol-free egg product or 4 egg whites

$1/2$ cup sugar

$1/2$ cup all-purpose flour

$1^1/2$ teaspoons pumpkin pie spice

$3/4$ teaspoon baking powder

$1/8$ teaspoon salt

2   teaspoons grated orange peel

Heat oven to 350°. Spray pie plate, 10 × 1$1/2$-inches, with cooking spray. Prepare Brown Sugar Topping; set aside.

Place remaining ingredients in blender or food processor in order listed. Cover and blend on medium speed until smooth. Pour into pie plate. Sprinkle with topping.

Bake 50 to 55 minutes or until knife inserted in center comes out clean. Cool 15 minutes. Refrigerate about 4 hours or until chilled.

Brown Sugar Topping

$1/4$ cup packed brown sugar

$1/4$ cup quick-cooking oats

1   tablespoon margarine, softened

Mix all ingredients.

1 Serving: Calories 200 (Calories from Fat 20); Fat 2g (Saturated 0g); Cholesterol 2mg; Sodium 230mg; Carbohydrate 38g (Dietary Fiber 2g); Protein 7g
% Daily Value: Vitamin A 100%; Vitamin C 2%; Calcium 22%; Iron 10%
Diet Exchanges: 2 starch, 1 vegetable

Caramel-Apple Bread Pudding

LO CAL / LO FAT / LO CHOL

PREP: 15 MIN; BAKE: 45 MIN

8 SERVINGS

For a special breakfast treat, serve this dessert with warmed maple-flavored syrup in place of the caramel topping.

1	cup unsweetened applesauce
1/2	cup packed brown sugar
1	cup skim milk
1/2	cup fat-free cholesterol-free egg product
1	teaspoon vanilla
1/2	teaspoon ground cinnamon
5	cups 1-inch cubes French bread
1/2	cup caramel fat-free topping, warmed

Heat oven to 350°. Spray quiche dish, 9 × 1 1/2 inches, or pie plate, 9 × 1 1/4 inches, with cooking spray. Mix all ingredients except bread and caramel topping in large bowl with wire whisk until smooth. Fold in bread. Pour into quiche dish.

Bake 40 to 45 minutes or until golden brown and set. Cut into wedges. Drizzle caramel topping over each serving.

1 Serving: Calories 200 (Calories from Fat 10); Fat 1g (Saturated 0g); Cholesterol 0mg; Sodium 240mg; Carbohydrate 43g (Dietary Fiber 1g); Protein 5g
% Daily Value: Vitamin A 2%; Vitamin C 0%; Calcium 8%; Iron 6%
Diet Exchanges: 2 starch, 1 fruit

Rice Pudding

LO CAL / LO FAT / LO CHOL / LO SODIUM

PREP: 5 MIN; COOK: 25 MIN; STAND: 5 MIN

6 SERVINGS

To add a new twist on this traditional recipe, try substituting dried cranberries or cherries for the raisins.

1	cup uncooked regular long grain rice
3	cups skim milk
2	tablespoons packed brown sugar
2	tablespoons chopped raisins
1	teaspoon vanilla
1/2	teaspoon ground cinnamon
1/2	teaspoon ground cardamom
1/2	cup skim milk

Heat all ingredients except 1/2 cup milk to boiling in 2-quart saucepan, stirring occasionally; reduce heat to medium.

Cook 18 to 20 minutes, stirring occasionally, until rice is tender and all milk is absorbed; remove from heat. Cover and let stand 5 minutes. Stir in 1/2 cup milk. Serve warm or chilled.

1 Serving: Calories 200 (Calories from Fat 10); Fat 1g (Saturated 0g); Cholesterol 5mg; Sodium 75mg; Carbohydrate 41g (Dietary Fiber 1g); Protein 8g
% Daily Value: Vitamin A 8%; Vitamin C 0%; Calcium 18%; Iron 8%
Diet Exchanges: 2 starch, 1 skim milk

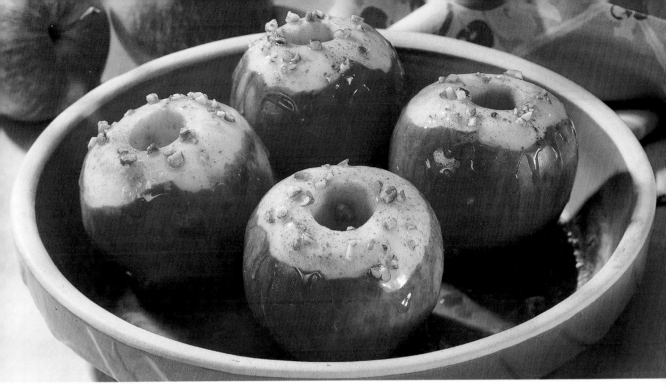

Baked Maple Apples

Baked Maple Apples

LO CAL / LO FAT / LO CHOL / LO SODIUM / HI FIB

PREP: 10 MIN; BAKE: 40 MIN

4 SERVINGS

Heading to the apple orchard? Choose apple varieties such as Rome Beauty, Imperial, Greening and Winesap, which will hold their shape during baking.

4	medium cooking apples
2	teaspoons margarine
1/4	cup reduced-calorie maple-flavored syrup
1/4	teaspoon ground cinnamon
1	tablespoon chopped nuts, if desired

Heat oven to 375°. Core apples. Peel 1-inch strip of skin from around middle of each apple, or peel upper half of each apple to prevent splitting.

Place apples upright in ungreased square baking dish, 8 × 8 × 2 inches. Place 1/2 teaspoon of the margarine and 1 tablespoon of the syrup in center of each apple. Pour water into baking dish until 1/4 inch deep.

Bake uncovered 30 to 40 minutes, spooning syrup in dish over apples several times, until apples are tender when pierced with fork. Sprinkle with cinnamon and nuts.

1 Serving: Calories 120 (Calories from Fat 20); Fat 2g (Saturated 0g); Cholesterol 0mg; Sodium 60mg; Carbohydrate 29g (Dietary Fiber 4g); Protein 0g
% Daily Value: Vitamin A 2%; Vitamin C 12%; Calcium 0%; Iron 0%
Diet Exchanges: 2 fruit

Poached Raspberry Pears

LO CAL / LO FAT / LO CHOL / LO SODIUM / HI FIB

PREP: 10 MIN; COOK: 35 MIN

6 SERVINGS

Bosc pears have a distinct tapered neck and golden rust-brown skin. Not only are they good for eating, but they are also delicious when cooked.

- 1/2 cup seedless raspberry spreadable fruit
- 1 cup apple juice
- 2 teaspoons grated lemon peel
- 2 tablespoons lemon juice
- 3 firm Bosc pears, peeled and cut into fourths

Mix all ingredients except pears in 10-inch nonstick skillet. Add pears. Heat to boiling; reduce heat. Simmer uncovered about 30 minutes, spooning juice mixture over pears and turning every 10 minutes, until pears are tender. Serve warm or chilled.

1 Serving: Calories 135 (Calories from Fat 10); Fat 1g (Saturated 0g); Cholesterol 0mg; Sodium 5mg; Carbohydrate 35g (Dietary Fiber 4g); Protein 1g
% Daily Value: Vitamin A 0%; Vitamin C 12%; Calcium 2%; Iron 2%
Diet Exchanges: 2 fruit

Cherry-Chocolate Fruit Decadence

LO CAL / LO FAT / LO CHOL / LO SODIUM

PREP: 15 MIN

8 SERVINGS

Cherry yogurt gives this velvety pudding an irresistible tang. Serve it with fruit in parfait, spoon it over reduced-fat pound cake or simply enjoy it with your favorite store-bought cookie on the side.

- 1 cup cherry low-fat yogurt
- 1/2 cup fat-free chocolate-flavored syrup
- 2 tablespoons shredded coconut
- 1 container (8 ounces) frozen fat-free whipped topping, thawed (3 1/4 cups)
- 1 pint (2 cups) strawberries, sliced, or 3 medium bananas, sliced

Mix yogurt, chocolate syrup and coconut in large bowl. Fold in whipped topping.* Arrange layer of strawberries in each of 8 dessert or parfait dishes. Top with half of the yogurt mixture. Repeat layers. Serve immediately.

*The yogurt mixture may be prepared in advance and stored in a covered container in the refrigerator up to 24 hours.

1 Serving: Calories 120 (Calories from Fat 20); Fat 2g (Saturated 1g); Cholesterol 0mg; Sodium 45mg; Carbohydrate 25g (Dietary Fiber 1g); Protein 2g
% Daily Value: Vitamin A 0%; Vitamin C 20%; Calcium 0%; Iron 4%
Diet Exchanges: 1/2 starch, 1 fruit

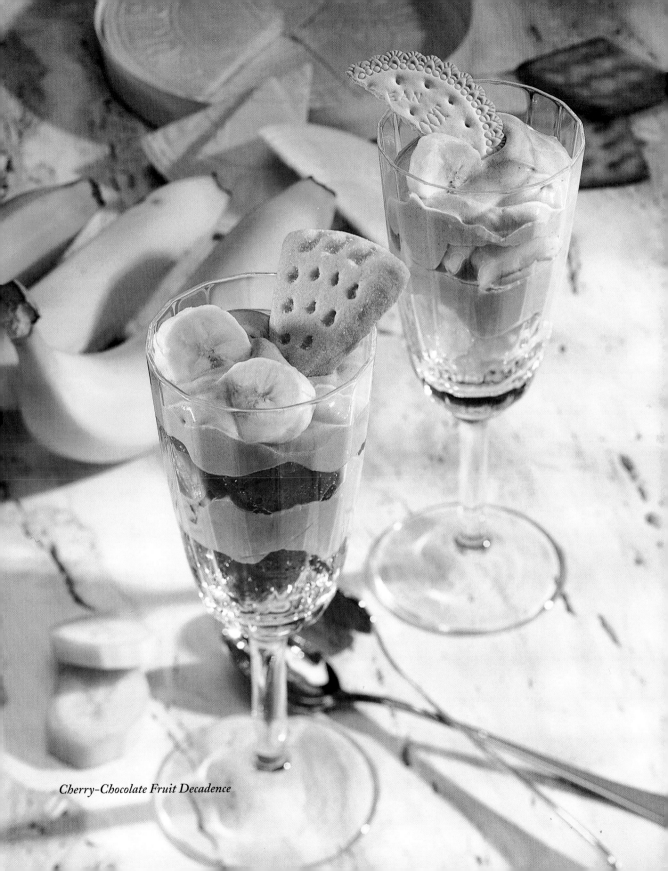

Cherry-Chocolate Fruit Decadence

Strawberry-Honey Sorbet

LO CAL / LO FAT / LO CHOL / LO SODIUM

PREP: 15 MIN; CHILL: 4 HR;

FREEZE: 2 HR; STAND: 10 MIN

8 SERVINGS

For an impressive dessert finale, use lemons as serving bowls. Simply slice lemons crosswise in half, using a serrated knife, and cut a thin slice from each end so they stand upright. Scoop out the seeds and pulp, and spoon the sorbet into each of the lemon halves.

1   pint (2 cups) strawberries, chopped

2   cups cranberry juice

1/4 cup chopped fresh or 1 tablespoon dried mint leaves

3   tablespoons honey

1   teaspoon grated lemon peel

Heat strawberries, juice, mint and honey in 1 1/2-quart saucepan over medium heat 5 minutes, stirring occasionally; remove from heat. Cover and refrigerate at least 4 hours.

Place strawberry mixture in blender or food processor. Cover and blend on high speed until smooth; strain. Cover and blend until smooth. Pour into square pan, 9 × 9 × 2 inches. Stir in lemon peel. Cover and freeze about 2 hours or until firm. (Or pour into 1-quart ice-cream freezer; freeze according to manufacturer's directions.)

Let stand 10 minutes at room temperature before spooning into dessert dishes.

1 Serving: Calories 55 (Calories from Fat 0); Fat 0g (Saturated 0g); Cholesterol 0mg; Sodium 5mg; Carbohydrate 15g (Dietary Fiber 1g); Protein 0g
% Daily Value: Vitamin A 0%; Vitamin C 44%; Calcium 0%; Iron 2%
Diet Exchanges: 1 fruit

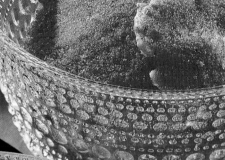

*Cantaloupe Sorbet (page 413)
and Strawberry-Honey Sorbet*

Caribbean Bananas

LO CAL / LO CHOL / LO SODIUM / HI FIB

PREP: 10 MIN; BAKE: 15 MIN

4 SERVINGS

For an indulgent treat without all the fat, serve with a scoop of vanilla fat-free ice cream or frozen yogurt.

4 medium bananas

2 tablespoons margarine, melted

1 tablespoon lemon juice

1/2 teaspoon ground cinnamon

1/8 teaspoon ground cloves

1/3 cup packed brown sugar

Heat oven to 350°. Cut bananas crosswise in half; cut each half lengthwise in half. Place cut sides up in square baking dish, 9 × 9 × 2 inches.

Mix margarine, lemon juice, cinnamon and cloves; brush over bananas. Sprinkle with brown sugar. Bake uncovered about 15 minutes or until bananas are hot.

1 Serving: Calories 230 (Calories from Fat 55); Fat 6g (Saturated 1g); Cholesterol 0mg; Sodium 85mg; Carbohydrate 46g (Dietary Fiber 3g); Protein 1g
% Daily Value: Vitamin A 8%; Vitamin C 10%; Calcium 2%; Iron 4%
Diet Exchanges: 3 fruit, 1 fat

Creamy Frozen Apricot Bars

LO CAL / LO FAT / LO CHOL / LO SODIUM

PREP: 10 MIN; FREEZE: 2 HR

16 SERVINGS

Be as creative as you like when combining flavors of yogurt and fruit. How about frozen strawberry-banana or lemon-raspberry bars? Go for it!

1 cup vanilla fat-free yogurt

1/2 cup apricot spreadable fruit

1 package (8 ounces) light cream cheese (Neufchâtel), cubed

Line square pan, 8 × 8 × 2 inches, with plastic wrap. Place all ingredients in blender or food processor. Cover and blend on high speed, stopping occasionally to scrape sides, until smooth. Carefully spread in pan. Cover and freeze about 2 hours or until firm.

Remove frozen mixture from pan, using plastic wrap to lift. Cut into 4 squares; make 2 crisscross cuts in each square to form 4 triangles.

1 Serving: Calories 65 (Calories from Fat 30); Fat 3g (Saturated 2g); Cholesterol 10mg; Sodium 65mg; Carbohydrate 8g (Dietary Fiber 1g); Protein 2g
% Daily Value: Vitamin A 4%; Vitamin C 2%; Calcium 2%; Iron 0%
Diet Exchanges: 1/2 skim milk, 1/2 fat

Cantaloupe Sorbet

LO CAL / LO FAT / LO CHOL / LO SODIUM

PREP: 15 MIN; FREEZE: 3 HR 30 MIN;

STAND: 10 MIN

6 SERVINGS

Traditionally served between courses as a "palate refresher," sorbet is also the perfect ending to a filling meal.

1   medium cantaloupe, peeled and cut into 1-inch pieces (6 cups)

2   tablespoons sugar

2   tablespoons lemon juice

Fresh mint leaves

Place cantaloupe, sugar and lemon juice in blender or food processor. Cover and blend on high speed, stopping occasionally to scrape sides, until uniform consistency. Pour into square pan, 9 × 9 × 2 inches. Cover and freeze 1 to 1½ hours or until partially frozen.

Spoon partially frozen mixture into blender or food processor. Cover and blend on high speed until smooth. Pour into pan. Cover and freeze about 2 hours or until firm. (Or pour into 1-quart ice-cream freezer; freeze according to manufacturer's directions.)

Let stand 10 minutes at room temperature before spooning into dessert dishes. Garnish with mint leaves.

1 Serving: Calories 50 (Calories from Fat 0); Fat 0g (Saturated 0g); Cholesterol 0mg; Sodium 10mg; Carbohydrate 13g (Dietary Fiber 1g); Protein 1g
% Daily Value: Vitamin A 26%; Vitamin C 70%; Calcium 0%; Iron 0%
Diet Exchanges: 1 fruit

Pineapple Ice

LO CAL / LO FAT / LO CHOL / LO SODIUM

PREP: 15 MIN; FREEZE: 5 HR; STAND: 10 MIN

8 SERVINGS

Save yourself from chopping! Look for precut pineapple chunks, usually available in the produce section of your supermarket. Next time, you might want to try cantelope or watermelon for a fun flavor twist.

1   medium pineapple, cut into 1-inch pieces (4 cups)

½   cup light corn syrup

2   tablespoons lemon juice

Place all ingredients in blender or food processor. Cover and blend on high speed, stopping occasionally to scrape sides, until smooth. Pour into loaf pan, 9 × 5 × 3 inches. Cover and freeze about 2 hours or until firm around edges but soft in center.

Spoon partially frozen mixture into blender or food processor. Cover and blend on high speed until smooth. Pour back into pan. Cover and freeze about 3 hours or until firm. (Or pour into 1-quart ice-cream freezer; freeze according to manufacturer's directions.)

Let stand 10 minutes at room temperature before spooning into dessert dishes.

1 Serving: Calories 100 (Calories from Fat 0); Fat 0g (Saturated 0g); Cholesterol 0mg; Sodium 25mg; Carbohydrate 26g (Dietary Fiber 1g); Protein 0g
% Daily Value: Vitamin A 0%; Vitamin C 20%; Calcium 0%; Iron 2%
Diet Exchanges: 1 fruit

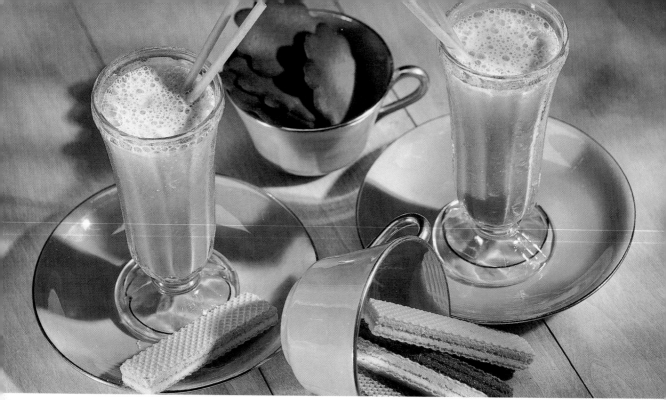

Frosty Mocha Cappuccino

Frosty Mocha Cappuccino

LO CAL / LO FAT / LO CHOL / LO SODIUM

PREP: 5 MIN

4 SERVINGS

Creamy and chocolatey, this milkshake for grown-ups is great with an added tablespoon of instant espresso coffee (dry).

1 cup cold very strong coffee

2 cups vanilla fat-free ice cream

2 tablespoons chocolate-flavored syrup

Place all ingredients in blender or food processor. Cover and blend on high speed until smooth.

1 Serving: Calories 95 (Calories from Fat 0); Fat 0g (Saturated 0g); Cholesterol 0mg; Sodium 55mg; Carbohydrate 24g (Dietary Fiber 0g); Protein 3g
% Daily Value: Vitamin A 8%; Vitamin C 0%; Calcium 10%; Iron 2%
Diet Exchanges: 1 starch, ½ fruit

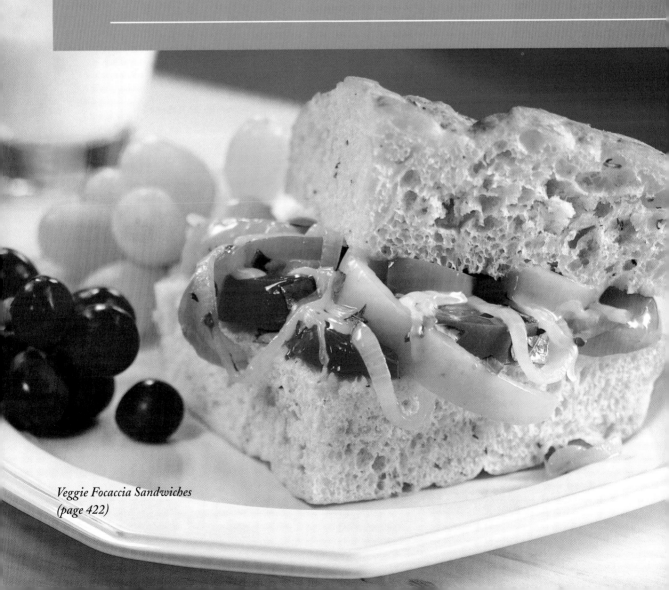

EAT AND LOSE WEIGHT: A WEEK'S WORTH OF SLIMMING MENUS

Veggie Focaccia Sandwiches
(page 422)

Maintaining a healthy weight is key to achieving good health, and one of the easiest ways to get there is with smart meal and menu planning. This isn't difficult or time consuming, even if you are trying to lose weight.

On the pages that follow you'll find plenty of ideas for healthy, quick meals that meet a reduced-calorie and reduced-fat eating plan. These menus vary from 1,300 to 1,600 calories and 17 to 40 grams of total fat per day. You don't have to follow these menus in any particular order; feel free to mix and match meals from different days to add variety to your eating plan. The recipes in this chapter will give you a terrific start, and when you decide to expand your repertoire in the kitchen, begin incorporating recipes from the other chapters in this book for even more delicious, healthy variety. Just keep track of your total calories and grams of fat to make sure you're not eating too much or too little.

The average recommended caloric intake for healthy adults is 2,000 calories and 65 grams of fat per day. Your needs may be higher or lower depending on your height, weight, gender and activity level. If you are trying to lose weight, you will want to decrease your calorie and fat intake and increase your activity level.

Menu 1

Breakfast

½ cup bran cereal
½ grapefruit
1 cup fat-free (skim) milk

Calories 195 • Total Fat 3g
• Saturated Fat 0g • Fiber 4g

Lunch

1 serving Veggie Focaccia
Sandwiches (page 422)
1 cup grapes
1 cup fat-free (skim) milk

Calories 440 • Total Fat 10g
• Saturated Fat 3g • Fiber 14g

Dinner

1 serving Marinated Tuna Steaks
with Cucumber Sauce
(page 436)
1 cup cooked frozen snap peas,
cauliflower and carrots
½ cup cooked brown rice

½ cup frozen fruit-flavored sorbet
or sherbet with ¼ cup blackberries

Calories 460 • Total Fat 7g
• Saturated Fat 2g • Fiber 8g

Snack

⅓ cup raisins
1 ounce peanuts

Calories 325 • Total Fat 14g
• Saturated Fat 2g • Fiber 5g

Total

Calories 1,420 • Total Fat 34g
• Saturated Fat 7g • Fiber 31g

Menu 2

Breakfast

2 shredded whole wheat
cereal biscuits
1 banana
1 cup fat-free (skim) milk

Calories 360 • Total Fat 2g
• Saturated Fat 1g • Fiber 6g

Lunch

1 serving Flank Steak Sandwiches (page 423)
1 medium pear
1 cup fat-free (skim) milk

Calories 500 • Total Fat 8g
• Saturated Fat 3g • Fiber 5g

Dinner

1 serving Seafood and Vegetables
with Rice (page 435)
½ cup oyster crackers
1 cup cooked frozen broccoli,
cauliflower and carrots
Romaine salad with
1 Tbsp reduced-fat Caesar dressing
1 Mini Pumpkin Cheesecake (page 443)

Calories 490 • Total Fat 10g
• Saturated Fat 2g • Fiber 6g

Snack

3 cups air-popped popcorn
1 medium orange

Calories 155 • Total Fat 2g
• Saturated Fat 0g • Fiber 8g

Total

Calories 1505 • Total Fat 22g
• Saturated Fat 6g • Fiber 25g

Menu 3

Breakfast

1 serving Cinnamon-Raisin French Toast
(page 438) sprinkled with 2 Tbsp wheat germ
1 Tbsp maple-flavored syrup
1 medium orange
1 cup fat-free (skim) milk

Calories 245 • Total Fat 4g
• Saturated Fat 1g • Fiber 6g

Lunch

1 serving Zesty Autumn
Pork Stew (page 430)
1 corn muffin with 1 tsp margarine
1 cup fat-free (skim) milk

Calories 495 • Total Fat 14g
• Saturated Fat 5g • Fiber 4g

Dinner

1 serving Pizza Casserole (page 427)
1 small dinner roll with 1 tsp margarine
1 cup cooked peas
Mixed-greens salad with
1 Tbsp reduced-fat dressing
1 tomato, sliced

Calories 595 • Total Fat 18g
• Saturated Fat 5g • Fiber 14g

Snack

1 serving Pear and Cherry Crisp
(page 444)

Calories 250 • Total Fat 4g
• Saturated Fat 2g • Fiber 4g

Total

Calories 1,585 • Total Fat 40g
• Saturated Fat 13g • Fiber 28g

Menu 4

Breakfast

1 scrambled egg
2 slices whole wheat bread,
toasted, with 1 Tbsp jam or jelly
½ grapefruit
1 cup fat-free
(skim) milk

Calories 400 • Total Fat 9g
• Saturated Fat 3g • Fiber 6g

Lunch

1 serving Turkey–Wild Rice
Salad (page 426)
1 small whole wheat dinner
roll with 1 tsp margarine
1 cup fat-free (skim) milk

Calories 530 • Total Fat 10g
• Saturated Fat 2g • Fiber 9g

Dinner

1 serving Vegetarian Paella
(page 432)
1 cup steamed green beans
1/2 cup melon cubes
1 serving Mocha Angel Cake
(page 442)

Calories 510 • Total Fat 3g
• Saturated Fat 0g • Fiber 15g

Snack

1/2 English muffin
with 1 tsp peanut butter
1/2 cup apple juice

Calories 160 • Total Fat 3g
• Saturated Fat 1g • Fiber 1g

Total

Calories 1,600 • Total Fat 25g
• Saturated Fat 6g • Fiber 31g

Menu 5

Breakfast

1 bagel with 1 Tbsp fat-free
cream cheese
1 cup orange juice

Calories 280 • Total Fat 2g
• Saturated Fat 0g • Fiber 2g

Lunch

1 serving Cuban Spicy Bean
Salad with Oranges and Cilantro
(page 425)
1 serving Lime Tortilla Chips
(page 420)
1 cup fat-free (skim) milk

Calories 515 • Total Fat 2g
• Saturated Fat 0g • Fiber 19g

Dinner

1 serving Creamy Ham
and Pasta (page 434)
1 slice French bread with 1 tsp margarine
Mixed-greens salad with
1 Tbsp reduced-fat dressing
1 cup sliced cucumbers and tomatoes
1/2 cup mixed fresh fruit

Calories 310 • Total Fat 6g
• Saturated Fat 2g • Fiber 4g

Snack

2 Ginger Gems Cookies (page 441)
1 cup fat-free (skim) milk

Calories 170 • Total Fat 1g
• Saturated Fat 0g • Fiber 0g

Total

Calories 1,275 • Total Fat 11g
• Saturated Fat 2g • Fiber 25g

Menu 6

Breakfast

1 Orange-Cranberry Scone (page 439)
1 cup raspberries
1 cup fat-free (skim) milk

Calories 245 • Total Fat 6g
• Saturated Fat 3g • Fiber 10g

Lunch

1 serving Barley-Burger Stew
(page 428)
1 slice whole wheat bread
with 1 tsp margarine
Celery sticks
1 cup fat-free (skim) milk

Calories 415 • Total Fat 7g
• Saturated Fat 2g • Fiber 8g

Dinner

1 serving Mediterranean Chicken
with Rosemary Orzo (page 431)
1 cup steamed broccoli
1 whole-grain dinner roll
with 1 tsp margarine
$\frac{1}{2}$ cup reduced-fat frozen yogurt with
1 Tbsp chocolate fudge fat-free topping

Calories 610 • Total Fat 11g
• Saturated Fat 3g • Fiber 11g

Snack

1 Savory Currant Wedge (page 440)
with 1 tsp margarine
$\frac{1}{2}$ cup cranberry juice

Calories 195 • Total Fat 4g
• Saturated Fat 2g • Fiber 1g

Total

Calories 1,465 • Total Fat 28g
• Saturated Fat 10g • Fiber 30g

Menu 7

Breakfast

1 serving Triple-Fruit Yogurt
Smoothie (page 421)

1 scrambled egg
1 cup fresh blueberries

Calories 335 • Total Fat 10g
• Saturated Fat 3g • Fiber 7g

Lunch

1 serving Turkey Burritos
(page 424)
10 reduced-fat potato chips
1 cup grapes
Carrot and celery sticks
1 cup fat-free (skim) milk

Calories 475 • Total Fat 7g
• Saturated Fat 2g • Fiber 7g

Dinner

1 serving Herbed Baked
Chicken Breasts (page 433)
1 serving Orzo Parmesan
(page 429)
Mixed-greens salad with
1 Tbsp reduced-fat dressing
1 medium tomato, sliced
1 cup steamed broccoli
$\frac{1}{2}$ cup fresh cherries

Calories 480 • Total Fat 10g
• Saturated Fat 3g • Fiber 9g

Snack

1 serving Chai Tea (page 420)
3 cups air-popped popcorn

Calories 190 • Total Fat 3g
• Saturated Fat 2g • Fiber 4g

Total

Calories 1,480 • Total Fat 20g
• Saturated Fat 10g • Fiber 27g

Lime Tortilla Chips

LO CAL / LO FAT / LO CHOL

PREP: 10 MIN; BAKE: 10 MIN

6 SERVINGS (8 CHIPS EACH)

1/2 teaspoon grated lime peel

Dash of salt

2 tablespoons lime juice

2 teaspoons olive or vegetable oil

2 teaspoons honey

4 fat-free flour tortillas (8 inches in diameter)

Heat oven to 350°. Spray large cookie sheet with cooking spray. Mix all ingredients except tortillas. Brush lime mixture on both sides of each tortilla. Cut each tortilla into 12 wedges. Place in single layer on cookie sheet.

Bake 8 to 10 minutes or until crisp and light golden brown; cool. Store in airtight container at room temperature.

1 Serving: Calories 100 (Calories from Fat 20); Fat 2g (Saturated 0g); Cholesterol 0mg; Sodium 230mg; Carbohydrate 18g (Dietary Fiber 0g); Protein 2g
% Daily Value: Vitamin A 0%; Vitamin C 0%; Calcium 0%; Iron 2%
Diet Exchanges: 1 starch

Eating Smart • Use the grated peel, or zest, of citrus fruits to bring fat-free flavor to spreads, marinades, dips, dressings, baked goods and sauces. For an additional fat-free flavor boost, combine grated peel with the juice of the same fruit.

Staying Active • Your mind is your most powerful piece of exercise equipment. If you believe there's no way you'll ever shed extra pounds, you won't. Believe you can achieve, and you will!

Chai Tea

LO CAL / LO FAT / LO CHOL / LO SODIUM

PREP: 5 MIN; COOK: 5 MIN

4 SERVINGS

2 cups water

4 tea bags black tea

2 cups milk

2 tablespoons honey

1/2 teaspoon ground ginger

1/2 teaspoon ground nutmeg

1/4 teaspoon ground cinnamon

Heat water to boiling. Add tea bags; reduce heat. Simmer 2 minutes. Remove tea bags.

Stir remaining ingredients into tea. Heat to boiling. Stir with wire whisk to foam milk. Pour into cups.

1 Serving: Calories 95 (Calories from Fat 20); Fat 2g (Saturated 1g); Cholesterol 10mg; Sodium 65mg; Carbohydrate 15g (Dietary Fiber 0g); Protein 4g
% Daily Value: Vitamin A 6%; Vitamin C 0%; Calcium 14%; Iron 0%
Diet Exchanges: 1/2 fruit, 1/2 skim milk, 1/2 fat

Eating Smart • Tea has long been linked to weight loss because of the feeling of fullness it provides. Chai, popular in India, is black tea mixed with a sweetener, milk and fragrant spices such as nutmeg and cinnamon. On cool mornings, this warming tea is especially comforting. It's also good served iced on warm days.

Staying Active • When exercising in hot weather, you can lose up to a quart of water each hour through sweat. Make sure you replenish this lost liquid by drinking a pint (2 cups) of fluid for each pound lost during your workout.

Triple-Fruit Yogurt Smoothie

LO CAL / LO FAT / LO CHOL / LO SODIUM / HI FIB

PREP: 5 MIN

4 SERVINGS

2   cups vanilla fat-free yogurt

1   cup fresh raspberries*

½   cup orange juice

1   medium banana, sliced (1 cup)

Place all ingredients in blender or food processor. Cover and blend on high speed about 30 seconds or until smooth. Pour into glasses. Serve immediately.

*1 package (10 ounces) frozen sweetened raspberries, partially thawed, can be substituted for the fresh raspberries.

1 Serving: Calories 145 (Calories from Fat 10); Fat 1g (Saturated 0g); Cholesterol 0mg; Sodium 50mg; Carbohydrate 31g (Dietary Fiber 3g); Protein 6g
% Daily Value: Vitamin A 12%; Vitamin C 18%; Calcium 16%; Iron 8%
Diet Exchanges: 1½ fruit, ½ skim milk

Eating Smart • Besides containing low-fat protein and calcium, yogurt—a cultured dairy product—is easy, convenient and versatile. Enjoy it as is, or use as an ingredient in breakfast smoothies, salad dressings, dips and sauces. Use low-fat and nonfat varieties to keep fat grams down without sacrificing flavor.

Staying Active • Looking for an exercise video? Before you buy, check your local library or video rental store for ones to sample. Make sure the workout is appropriate for your fitness level, and check for required equipment. Do you have enough room to do the routine safely, and is your workout surface carpeted to provide shock absorption? Research the instructor's reputation in the fitness industry. Finally, can you vary the routine as your fitness level increases?

Veggie Focaccia Sandwiches

LO CAL / LO CHOL

PREP: 15 MIN; COOK: 5 MIN

4 SERVINGS

Mozzarella is perfect with Italian focaccia bread, but if you like, you can vary the flavor by substituting reduced-fat Cheddar, Monterey Jack, or feta cheese (photo on page 415).

1	round focaccia bread (8 inches in diameter)
1/2	yellow bell pepper, cut into strips
1/2	green bell pepper, cut into strips
1	small onion, sliced
2	tablespoons fat-free Italian dressing
2	roma (plum) tomatoes, sliced
2	tablespoons chopped fresh basil leaves
1/2	cup shredded reduced-fat mozzarella cheese (2 ounces)

Heat oven to 350°. Place focaccia on oven rack. Bake 5 to 7 minutes or until warm.

Spray 8- or 10-inch skillet with cooking spray; heat over medium-high heat. Cook bell peppers, onion and dressing in skillet 4 to 5 minutes, stirring occasionally, until peppers are crisp-tender. Stir in remaining ingredients; remove from heat.

Cut focaccia into 4 wedges; split each wedge horizontally. Spoon one-fourth of vegetable mixture onto each bottom half; top with other half of bread wedge.

1 Serving: Calories 240 (Calories from Fat 70); Fat 8g (Saturated 2g); Cholesterol 5mg; Sodium 670mg; Carbohydrate 35g (Dietary Fiber 2g); Protein 9g
% Daily Value: Vitamin A 6%; Vitamin C 54%; Calcium 12%; Iron 12%
Diet Exchanges: 2 starch, 1 vegetable, 1 fat

Eating Smart • If you're a fast-food fanatic, you might want to think about replacing some of those high-calorie meals with easy-to-make, low-fat, tasty sandwiches. Compared with a quarter-pound burger (430 calories and 21 fat grams), this sandwich wins hands down in nutrition, appearance and taste!

Staying Active • Making a gym date with a friend can strengthen your commitment to exercise. Schedule your workout dates like you'd schedule any other meeting or appointment. Write it down on your calendar to reinforce the importance of your new lifestyle.

Flank Steak Sandwiches

LOW CALORIE

PREP: 10 MIN; MARINATE: 4 HR; GRILL: 12 MIN

8 SERVINGS

2   beef flank steaks (1 pound each)

¼   cup honey

2   tablespoons soy sauce

1   tablespoon grated gingerroot

1   can or bottle (12 ounces) regular or nonalcoholic beer

8   pita breads (6 inches in diameter), cut in half to form pockets

Sliced tomato, if desired

Grilled sliced onion, if desired

Remove fat from beef. Make cuts about ½ inch apart and ⅛ inch deep in diamond pattern on both sides of beef. Place in shallow glass dish. Mix honey, soy sauce, gingerroot and beer; pour over beef. Cover and refrigerate, turning occasionally, at least 4 hours but no longer than 24 hours.

Brush grill rack with vegetable oil. Heat coals or gas grill for direct heat. Remove beef from marinade; reserve marinade. Cover and grill beef 6 inches from medium heat about 12 minutes for medium doneness, turning after 6 minutes and brushing frequently with marinade. Discard any remaining marinade.

Cut beef diagonally into thin slices. Serve beef in pita bread halves with tomato and onion.

1 Serving: Calories 320 (Calories from Fat 70); Fat 8g (Saturated 3g); Cholesterol 60mg; Sodium 530mg; Carbohydrate 36g (Dietary Fiber 1g); Protein 27g
% Daily Value: Vitamin A 0%; Vitamin C 0%; Calcium 4%; Iron 18%
Diet Exchanges: 2 starch, 3 lean meat

Eating Smart • Lunching on an oversized deli sandwich can cost you anywhere from 600 to 800 calories. Instead, bring a healthy lunch from home. Pack sandwiches that feature lean meats or cheeses for a midday protein punch. Also include raw vegetable sticks and fresh fruit for fiber and nutrients.

Staying Active • Contrary to popular belief, drinking cold beverages during exercise doesn't cause cramps. Cold drinks are actually better choices than warm—they leave the stomach more rapidly and quickly supply the body with the fluid it needs.

Turkey Burritos

LO CAL / LO FAT / HI FIB

PREP: 10 MIN; COOK: 7 MIN

6 SERVINGS

½	pound ground turkey breast
2	cloves garlic, finely chopped
1	jalapeño chili, seeded and chopped
½	cup fat-free refried beans
2	tablespoons lime juice
6	fat-free flour tortillas (6 to 8 inches in diameter)
6	tablespoons fat-free sour cream
1	large tomato, chopped (1 cup)
¼	cup chopped fresh cilantro
	Salsa, if desired

Spray 8- to 10-inch skillet with cooking spray; heat over medium-high heat. Cook turkey, garlic and chili in skillet about 5 minutes, stirring constantly, until turkey is no longer pink. Stir in beans and lime juice. Cook about 2 minutes, stirring occasionally, until heated.

Place one-fourth of the turkey mixture on center of each tortilla. Top with sour cream, tomato and cilantro. Fold one end of tortilla up about 1 inch over filling; fold right and left sides over folded end, overlapping. Fold remaining end down. Place seam side down on serving platter or plate. Serve with salsa.

1 Serving: Calories 185 (Calories from Fat 20); Fat 2g (Saturated 1g); Cholesterol 25mg; Sodium 460mg; Carbohydrate 31g (Dietary Fiber 3g); Protein 14g
% Daily Value: Vitamin A 12% ; Vitamin C 18% ; Calcium 4%; Iron 10%
Diet Exchanges: 2 starch, 1 very lean meat

Eating Smart • Jazzing up your diet by serving a variety of fun, ethnic foods can actually help you lose weight. Variety is key for a couple of reasons. First, more variety means more types of food and, as a result, more types of nutrients. Treating yourself to a wide variety of many different foods is also more satisfying and encourages smaller portions of each single food.

Staying Active • The latest fitness craze, pilates, is a series of non-impact conditioning exercises to strengthen and stretch muscles and properly align the body. This technique, developed by Joseph Pilates in the 1920s, is used to develop the deep muscles of the trunk, abdomen and spine, and has long been practiced by professional dancers.

Cuban Spicy Bean Salad with Oranges and Cilantro

LO CAL / LO FAT / LO CHOL / HI FIB

PREP: 10 MIN; STAND: 30 MIN

4 SERVINGS

2 oranges, peeled and sliced, or 1 can (11 ounces) mandarin orange segments in light syrup, drained

2 cans (15 ounces each) black beans, rinsed and drained

3 medium carrots, shredded (2 cups)

²/₃ cup chopped fresh cilantro

½ cup balsamic or red wine vinegar

2 tablespoons sugar

2 teaspoons chopped fresh or canned jalapeño chilies

4 cups bite-size pieces curly endive or lettuce

Mix all ingredients except endive in glass or plastic bowl. Cover and let stand 30 minutes.

Divide endive among 4 salad plates. Top with bean mixture.

1 Serving: Calories 330 (Calories from Fat 10); Fat 1g (Saturated 0g); Cholesterol 0mg; Sodium 840mg; Carbohydrate 78g (Dietary Fiber 18g); Protein 20g
% Daily Value: Vitamin A 94%; Vitamin C 38%; Calcium 20%; Iron 34%
Diet Exchanges: 2 starch, 3 vegetable, 2 fruit

Eating Smart • With only about 65 calories, one orange supplies you with 100 percent of the RDA for vitamin C. Oranges are also good sources of fiber, containing nearly 7 grams. Studies have shown that oranges outrank other fruits, including bananas, in providing a feeling of fullness.

Staying Active • Want to add variety to your workout? Crank up the tunes, and dance around your house. An hour of fast dancing can burn more than 400 calories. The harder you dance, the more calories you burn. No partner? No problem. This is your chance to claim the dance floor as your own!

Turkey–Wild Rice Salad

LO CAL / HI FIB

PREP: 20 MIN; COOK: 6 MIN

4 SERVINGS

1	pound uncooked turkey breast slices, about ¼ inch thick
¼	teaspoon seasoned salt
¼	teaspoon dried marjoram leaves
3	cups cold cooked wild rice
¼	cup chopped walnuts
¼	cup dried cranberries
4	medium green onions, chopped (¼ cup)
¼	teaspoon salt
½	cup raspberries
	Leaf lettuce leaves
½	cup fat-free raspberry vinaigrette dressing

Sprinkle turkey with seasoned salt and marjoram. Spray skillet with cooking spray; heat over medium-high heat. Cook turkey in skillet 4 to 6 minutes, turning once, until no longer pink in center. Cut into 2-inch pieces.

Mix wild rice, walnuts, cranberries, onions and salt. Carefully stir in raspberries.

Arrange rice mixture on lettuce leaves on 4 plates. Arrange warm turkey on rice mixture. Drizzle with dressing.

1 Serving: Calories 345 (Calories from Fat 45); Fat 5g (Saturated 1g); Cholesterol 75mg; Sodium 440mg; Carbohydrate 50g (Dietary Fiber 7g); Protein 32g
% Daily Value: Vitamin A 6%; Vitamin C 32%; Calcium 4%; Iron 16%
Diet Exchanges: 2 starch, 3 very lean meat, 1 vegetable, 1 fruit

Eating Smart • On average, nuts weigh in at about 275 calories and 28 grams of fat per ⅓ cup, chopped. Sounds like a lot. But by sprinkling a small handful of nuts on a salad, stir-fry or veggie side dish, you balance out other low-fat, low-calorie ingredients with protein and a bit of heart-healthy fat.

Staying Active • If you're able to walk to work, make this a part of your daily exercise plan. For a more intense workout, give yourself less time than you know you'll need. For instance, if it takes you 15 minutes to walk to work, give yourself only 10. Unless you don't mind being late, you'll pick up your pace and burn more calories.

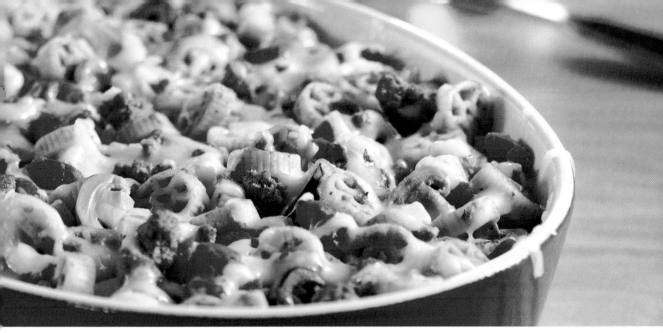

Pizza Casserole

LO CAL / HI FIB

PREP: 20 MIN; BAKE: 30 MIN; STAND: 5 MIN

6 SERVINGS

4 cups uncooked wagon wheel pasta (8 ounces)

$\frac{1}{2}$ pound diet-lean or extra-lean ground beef

$\frac{1}{4}$ cup sliced ripe olives

1 can (4 ounces) mushroom pieces and stems, drained

1 jar (26 to 28 ounces) fat-free tomato pasta sauce

1 cup shredded reduced-fat mozzarella cheese (4 ounces)

Heat oven to 350°. Cook and drain pasta as directed on package. While pasta is cooking, cook beef in 10-inch skillet over medium-high heat, stirring frequently, until brown; drain. Mix pasta, beef and remaining ingredients except cheese in ungreased 2$\frac{1}{2}$-quart casserole.

Cover and bake about 30 minutes or until hot. Sprinkle with cheese. Cover and let stand about 5 minutes or until cheese is melted.

1 Serving: Calories 310 (Calories from Fat 80); Fat 9g (Saturated 4g); Cholesterol 30mg; Sodium 630mg; Carbohydrate 41g (Dietary Fiber 3g); Protein 19g
% Daily Value: Vitamin A 8%; Vitamin C 4%; Calcium 16%; Iron 16%
Diet Exchanges: 2 starch, 1 lean meat, 2 vegetable, 1 fat

Eating Smart • Move over, macaroni! Using different pasta shapes and colors brings variety to your meals. Wagon wheel, radiatore, penne, farfalle and rigatoni are only a few of many fun pasta shapes available. Or treat yourself to spinach, lemon pepper or sun-dried tomato pasta. These pasta varieties add fat-free fun to your meal.

Staying Active • When you visit the grocery store or mall, walk around the periphery two or three times before you start shopping. You'll get an especially good workout at the mall. You might even feel less guilty about exercising your credit card if you've gotten *your* exercise first!

Barley-Burger Stew

LO CAL / HI FIB

PREP: 15 MIN; COOK: 1 HR 10 MIN

4 SERVINGS

1	pound diet-lean or extra-lean ground beef
2	medium onions, chopped (1 cup)
$^1\!/_2$	cup uncooked barley
1	cup water
2 to 3	teaspoons chili powder
$1^1\!/_2$	teaspoons salt
$^1\!/_2$	teaspoon pepper
1	medium stalk celery, chopped ($^1\!/_2$ cup)
4	cups tomato juice

Cook beef and onions in 4-quart Dutch oven over medium heat, stirring occasionally, until beef is brown; drain.

Stir in remaining ingredients. Heat to boiling; reduce heat. Cover and simmer about 1 hour or until barley is tender and stew is desired consistency.

1 Serving: Calories 320 (Calories from Fat 80); Fat 9g (Saturated 5g); Cholesterol 70mg; Sodium 1950mg; Carbohydrate 37g (Dietary Fiber 7g); Protein 30g
% Daily Value: Vitamin A 20%; Vitamin C 46%; Calcium 6%; Iron 28%
Diet Exchanges: 2 starch, 3 lean meat, 1 vegetable

Eating Smart • Just 1 cup of cooked barley packs about 6 grams of fiber. This virtually fat-free whole grain also contains complex carbohydrates, B vitamins and protein.

Staying Active • Exercise with encouraging friends to increase your confidence in your workout. Researchers have found that regardless of actual performance, women who were told they had done well felt better about their workouts than those who had been told they had performed poorly.

Orzo Parmesan

LO CAL / LO FAT / LO CHOL

PREP: 10 MIN; COOK: 15 MIN

6 SERVINGS

1   can (14½ ounces) fat-free chicken broth

½   cup water

¼   teaspoon salt

1⅓   cups uncooked rosamarina (orzo) pasta

2   cloves garlic, finely chopped

8   medium green onions, sliced (½ cup)

⅓   cup grated fat-free Parmesan cheese topping

1   tablespoon chopped fresh or 1 teaspoon
     dried basil leaves

⅛   teaspoon freshly ground pepper

Heat broth, water and salt to boiling in 2-quart saucepan. Stir in pasta, garlic and onions. Heat to boiling; reduce heat. Cover and simmer about 12 minutes, stirring occasionally, until most of the liquid is absorbed. Stir in remaining ingredients.

1 Serving: Calories 145 (Calories from Fat 20); Fat 2g (Saturated 1g); Cholesterol 0mg; Sodium 510mg; Carbohydrate 28g (Dietary Fiber 2g); Protein 6g
% Daily Value: Vitamin A 0%; Vitamin C 2%; Calcium 4%; Iron 8%
Diet Exchanges: 2 starch

Eating Smart • Italian for "barley," orzo is a tiny, rice-shaped pasta. Add variety to your meals by substituting this small, complex carbohydrate-rich pasta for rice in pilafs, salads, soups and casseroles.

Staying Active • When you start an exercise program, you'll be replacing fat with muscle. And because muscle weighs more than fat, your weight may not drop much at first. Rather than falsely discouraging yourself by using the scale, go by how well your clothes fit or how much more energy you have, or most importantly, by how you feel overall.

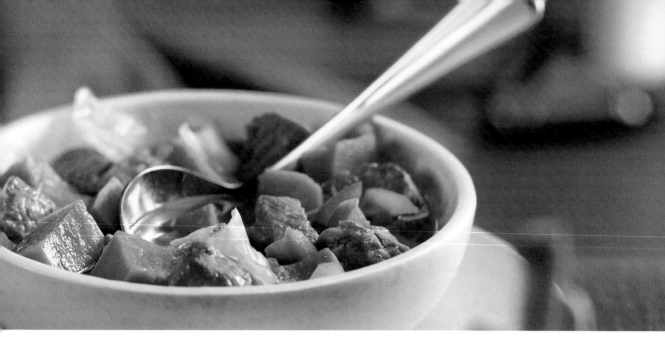

Zesty Autumn Pork Stew

Zesty Autumn Pork Stew

LO CAL / LO FAT / HI FIB

PREP: 10 MIN; COOK: 20 MIN

4 SERVINGS

1   pound pork tenderloin

2   cloves garlic, finely chopped

2   medium sweet potatoes, peeled and cubed
    (2 cups)

1   cup coarsely chopped cabbage

1   medium green bell pepper, chopped (1 cup)

1   can (14½ ounces) fat-free chicken broth

1   teaspoon Cajun seasoning

Remove fat from pork. Cut pork into 1-inch cubes. Spray 4-quart Dutch oven with cooking spray; heat over medium-high heat. Cook pork in Dutch oven, stirring occasionally, until brown.

Stir in remaining ingredients. Heat to boiling; reduce heat. Cover and simmer about 15 minutes, stirring once, until sweet potatoes are tender.

1 Serving: Calories 240 (Calories from Fat 45); Fat 5g (Saturated 2g); Cholesterol 70mg; Sodium 530mg; Carbohydrate 22g (Dietary Fiber 3g); Protein 30g
% Daily Value: Vitamin A 100%; Vitamin C 44%; Calcium 4%; Iron 12%
Diet Exchanges: 1 starch, 3 very lean meat, 1 vegetable, 1 fat

Eating Smart • Comfort foods, like stew, are really satisfying. Savor hearty stews, creamy mashed potatoes or any other food that brings you comfort. Enjoy every moment of your meal. You may just find yourself eating less than if you had forced yourself to eat food you don't enjoy.

Staying Active • Subscribing to a fitness-themed magazine or newsletter is a great motivator. Reading about the latest fitness research and trends can be very informative. And the regular delivery of an exercise-based publication to your doorstep will serve as an ongoing reminder of your fitness goals.

Mediterranean Chicken with Rosemary Orzo

LO CAL / LO FAT / HI FIB

PREP: 10 MIN; COOK: 20 MIN

4 SERVINGS

1   pound chicken breast tenders

2   cloves garlic, finely chopped

1⅓ cups uncooked rosamarina (orzo) pasta

1   can (14½ ounces) fat-free chicken broth

½   cup water

1   tablespoon chopped fresh or 1 teaspoon dried rosemary leaves

½   teaspoon salt

2   medium zucchini, cut lengthwise into fourths, then cut crosswise into slices (1½ cups)

3   roma (plum) tomatoes, cut into fourths and sliced (1½ cups)

1   medium green bell pepper, chopped (1 cup)

Spray 10-inch skillet with cooking spray; heat over medium-high heat. Add chicken; stir-fry about 5 minutes or until brown. Stir in garlic, pasta and broth. Heat to boiling; reduce heat. Cover and simmer about 8 minutes or until most of the liquid is absorbed.

Stir in remaining ingredients. Heat to boiling; reduce heat. Cover and simmer about 5 minutes, stirring once, until bell pepper is crisp-tender and pasta is tender.

1 Serving: Calories 300 (Calories from Fat 35); Fat 4g (Saturated 1g); Cholesterol 50mg; Sodium 820mg; Carbohydrate 42g (Dietary Fiber 4g); Protein 28g
% Daily Value: Vitamin A 8%; Vitamin C 42%; Calcium 4%; Iron 18%
Diet Exchanges: 2 starch, 3 very lean meat, 2 vegetable

Eating Smart • Although people in the Mediterranean region consume as much as 40 percent of their calories from fat, they have nowhere near the health and weight problems that exist in the United States. Researchers say this may be due, in part, to the plentiful supply of fresh vegetables in the Mediterranean diet.

Staying Active • Metabolism is the term for how our bodies convert food into energy. These rates vary from person to person. Someone with a fast metabolism burns more fat at rest than someone with a slow metabolism. Heredity is partially responsible for metabolism, but you can counteract an inherited slow metabolism with regular aerobic exercise and weight lifting.

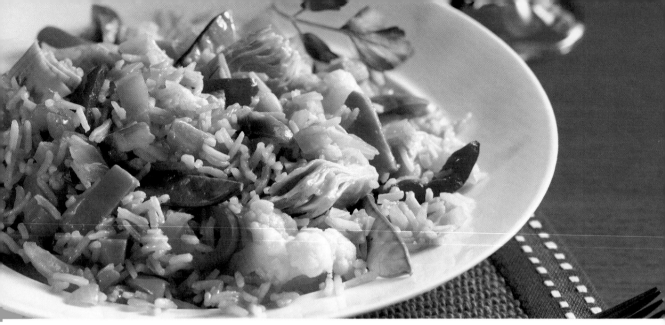

Vegetarian Paella

Vegetarian Paella

LO CAL / LO FAT / LO CHOL / HI FIB

PREP: 10 MIN; COOK: 25 MIN

4 SERVINGS

2 large onions, chopped (2 cups)

5 cloves garlic, finely chopped

1 cup uncooked basmati or regular long-grain rice

1 can (14 ounces) quartered artichoke hearts, drained

2 cups dry white wine or fat-free vegetable broth

1 teaspoon salt

1 bag (1 pound) cauliflower, carrots and snow pea pods (or other combination), thawed

1 cup frozen sliced bell peppers (from 16-ounce bag)

Spray 10-inch nonstick skillet with cooking spray; heat over medium-high heat. Cook onions and garlic in skillet about 5 minutes, stirring occasionally, until onions are tender.

Stir in rice and artichoke hearts. Cook 3 minutes, stirring occasionally. Stir in wine and salt. Heat to boiling; reduce heat. Cover and simmer about 10 minutes. Stir in vegetables. Cover and cook about 5 minutes or until liquid is absorbed.

1 Serving: Calories 285 (Calories from Fat 10); Fat 1g (Saturated 0g); Cholesterol 0mg; Sodium 640mg; Carbohydrate 68g (Dietary Fiber 11g); Protein 12g
% Daily Value: Vitamin A 40%; Vitamin C 72%; Calcium 12%; Iron 24%
Diet Exchanges: 3 starch, 4 vegetable

Eating Smart • A Spanish dish of rice, meat, shellfish and vegetables, paella can be high in saturated fat and calories. Eliminating the meat and relying on fiber-rich complex carbohydrates make our adaptation of paella a flavorful, low-fat feast.

Staying Active • Ask your coworkers to join you for a walking business meeting. Besides the exercise and fresh air you'll be getting, you'll also boost your creative powers with the feel-good chemicals that come from exercise.

Herbed Baked Chicken Breasts

LO CAL / LO FAT / LO CHOL

PREP: 15 MIN; BAKE: 35 MIN

6 SERVINGS

6	boneless, skinless chicken breast halves (about 1¾ pounds)
½	cup fat-free mayonnaise or salad dressing
1	teaspoon garlic salt
1	tablespoon chopped fresh or 1 teaspoon dried marjoram leaves
2	teaspoons chopped fresh or ½ teaspoon dried rosemary leaves
2	teaspoons chopped fresh or ½ teaspoon dried thyme leaves
1	cup cornflakes cereal, crushed (½ cup)
½	teaspoon paprika

Heat oven to 375°. Spray rectangular pan, 13 × 9 × 2 inches, with cooking spray. Remove fat from chicken.

Mix mayonnaise, garlic salt, marjoram, rosemary and thyme; set aside. Mix cereal and paprika. Spread rounded tablespoon of mayonnaise mixture over both sides of each chicken breast half; coat evenly with cereal mixture. Place chicken in pan.

Bake uncovered 30 to 35 minutes or until juice of chicken is no longer pink when centers of thickest pieces are cut.

1 Serving: Calories 175 (Calories from Fat 35); Fat 4g (Saturated 1g); Cholesterol 5mg; Sodium 650mg; Carbohydrate 8g (Dietary Fiber 0g); Protein 27g
% Daily Value: Vitamin A 4%; Vitamin C 2%; Calcium 2%; Iron 14%
Diet Exchanges: ½ starch, 4 very lean meat

Eating Smart • By relying on flavor-intense herb coatings instead of fat-laden batters, you maximize flavor and minimize fat and calories. After you get the hang of it, experiment with your own herb combinations. You may never have the same dish twice!

Staying Active • Several brief bouts of exercise may burn more calories than one long exercise session. Some studies have shown that short-session exercisers drop a few more pounds than their longer-session counterparts. Short bursts of exercise boost metabolism regularly throughout the day, meaning calories are burned at a steady rate over a longer period of time.

Creamy Ham and Pasta

LO CAL / LO FAT

PREP: 15 MIN; COOK: 20 MIN

4 SERVINGS

1 cup uncooked penne pasta (3 ounces)

1 cup baby-cut carrots, cut lengthwise in half

8 medium green onions, sliced ($^{1}/_{2}$ cup)

12 ounces fully cooked lean ham, cut into thin strips ($1^{1}/_{2}$ cups)

$^{3}/_{4}$ cup fat-free half-and-half

2 ounces fat-free cream cheese

1 teaspoon Dijon mustard

$^{1}/_{4}$ teaspoon dried tarragon leaves

$^{1}/_{8}$ teaspoon white pepper

Cook pasta as directed on package, adding carrots during last 4 minutes of cooking. Cook until carrots are crisp-tender; drain.

Spray 12-inch nonstick skillet with cooking spray; heat over medium heat. Cook onions in skillet 1 minute. Stir in ham. Cook 2 to 3 minutes, stirring frequently, until thoroughly heated. Stir in remaining ingredients until cheese is melted and mixture is smooth. Stir in pasta and carrots.

1 Serving: Calories 265 (Calories from Fat 55); Fat 6g (Saturated 2g); Cholesterol 45mg; Sodium 1170mg; Carbohydrate 30g (Dietary Fiber 2g); Protein 25g
% Daily Value: Vitamin A 58%; Vitamin C 6%; Calcium 10%; Iron 14%
Diet Exchanges: 2 starch, 3 very lean meat

Eating Smart • Not all low-fat dairy products are created equal. One cup of 2 percent milk has 5 grams of fat and gets 25 percent of its calories from fat. Better bets include 1 percent milk (less than 3 grams of fat per cup) or fat-free (skim) milk. Other fat-free dairy products to try include fat-free half-and-half and evaporated fat-free milk.

Staying Active • Don't have 10 minutes to exercise? Take 2! Briskly walk around the block (or in your office building or at the store) for 2 minutes. You'll be surprised at how quickly time passes and by the distance you cover. Fit as many 2-minute walks in your day as possible. It's amazing how quickly the time will add up.

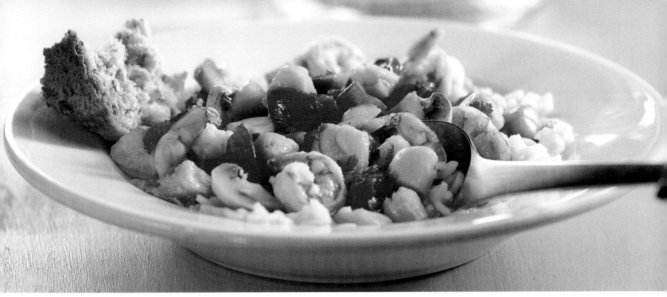

Seafood and Vegetables with Rice

Seafood and Vegetables with Rice

LO CAL / LO FAT

PREP: 15 MIN; COOK: 10 MIN

6 SERVINGS

1	package (8 ounces) sliced mushrooms
1	can (14$\frac{1}{2}$ ounces) fat-free chicken broth
3	roma (plum) tomatoes, cut into fourths and sliced (1$\frac{1}{2}$ cups)
$\frac{1}{2}$	cup sliced drained roasted red bell peppers
$\frac{1}{2}$	pound uncooked peeled deveined small shrimp, thawed if frozen
$\frac{1}{2}$	pound cod fillets, cubed
6	ounces bay scallops
$\frac{1}{2}$	cup white wine or chicken broth
$\frac{1}{2}$	teaspoon salt
$\frac{1}{4}$ to $\frac{1}{2}$	teaspoon red pepper sauce
$\frac{1}{4}$	cup chopped fresh cilantro
4	cups hot cooked rice

Heat mushrooms and broth to boiling in 3-quart saucepan. Stir in remaining ingredients except cilantro and rice. Heat to boiling; reduce heat. Cover and simmer 5 to 7 minutes or until shrimp are pink and firm. Stir in cilantro. Serve in bowls over rice.

1 Serving: Calories 225 (Calories from Fat 20); Fat 2g (Saturated 0g); Cholesterol 55mg; Sodium 710mg; Carbohydrate 31g (Dietary Fiber 1g); Protein 19g
% Daily Value: Vitamin A 8%; Vitamin C 22%; Calcium 4%; Iron 18%
Diet Exchanges: 2 starch, 1$\frac{1}{2}$ very lean meat, 1 vegetable

Eating Smart • Enliven sauces, sandwiches, soups and salads by adding a handful of chopped roasted red bell peppers. These nutrient-rich gems are also rich in fat-free flavor. One-half cup contains less than 10 calories.

Staying Active • Varying the intensity of your workouts keeps them interesting and may even help burn calories. Your metabolism idles when you repeatedly do the same activities at the same intensity. By working at a higher target heart rate, cutting back during your next session and revving up again later, you increase your calorie burn.

Marinated Tuna Steaks with Cucumber Sauce

LO CAL / LO FAT

PREP: 10 MIN; MARINATE: 1 HR; BROIL: 10 MIN

4 SERVINGS

- 3 tablespoons lime juice
- 2 tablespoons chopped fresh cilantro
- 1 clove garlic, finely chopped
- 1/4 teaspoon salt
- 1 pound tuna steaks
   Cucumber Sauce (right)

Mix lime juice, cilantro, garlic and salt in pie plate, 9 × 1¼ inches. Cut fish steaks into 4 serving pieces. Add fish to lime mixture, turning several times to coat with marinade. Cover and refrigerate 1 hour, turning once.

Set oven control to broil. Spray broiler pan rack with cooking spray. Remove fish from marinade; discard marinade. Place fish on rack in broiler pan. Broil with tops 4 inches from heat 7 to 10 minutes, turning once, until fish flakes easily with fork. Serve with Cucumber Sauce.

Cucumber Sauce

- 1/2 cup chopped cucumber
- 1/4 cup plain yogurt
- 2 tablespoons chopped fresh cilantro
- 1 tablespoon fat-free mayonnaise or salad dressing

Mix all ingredients.

1 Serving: Calories 140 (Calories from Fat 45); Fat 5g (Saturated 2g); Cholesterol 60mg; Sodium 240mg; Carbohydrate 3g (Dietary Fiber 0g); Protein 20g
% Daily Value: Vitamin A 2%; Vitamin C 4%; Calcium 4%; Iron 4%
Diet Exchanges: 3 very lean meat, 1 fat

Eating Smart • Studies show that eating fatty fish, such as tuna and salmon, once or twice a week is good for the heart and waistline. The omega-3 fatty acids found in fish oil may protect against heart disease. Eating fatty fish will also help you feel full faster, meaning you'll eat less overall.

Staying Active • Warm-ups and cool-downs are important parts of any exercise program. By gently stretching before you work out, you tell your muscles that they'll soon be needed. Cooling down with light calisthenics and more gentle stretching will help return your heart rate to normal, and help reduce post-workout soreness.

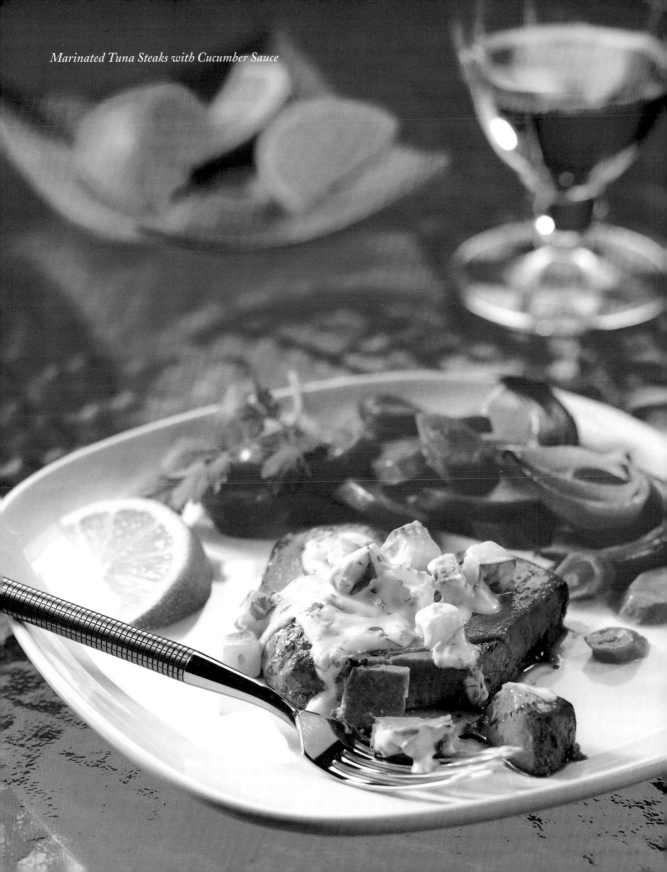

Marinated Tuna Steaks with Cucumber Sauce

Cinnamon-Raisin French Toast

LO CAL / LO FAT / LO CHOL

PREP: 5 MIN; COOK: 16 MIN

4 SERVINGS

¾ cup fat-free cholesterol-free egg product or 2 eggs plus 1 egg white

¾ cup fat-free (skim) milk

1 tablespoon sugar

¼ teaspoon vanilla

⅛ teaspoon salt

8 slices cinnamon-raisin bread

Beat egg product, milk, sugar, vanilla and salt with hand beater until smooth.

Spray griddle or 10-inch skillet with cooking spray. Heat griddle to 375° or heat skillet over medium heat. (To test, sprinkle with a few drops of water. If bubbles jump around, heat is just right.)

Dip bread into egg mixture, coating both sides. Place on griddle. Cook about 4 minutes on each side or until golden brown.

1 Serving: Calories 180 (Calories from Fat 20); Fat 2g (Saturated 0g); Cholesterol 0mg; Sodium 440mg; Carbohydrate 32g (Dietary Fiber 2g); Protein 10g
% Daily Value: Vitamin A 4%; Vitamin C 0%; Calcium 12%; Iron 12%
Diet Exchanges: 2 starch

Eating Smart • To save fat and calories, skip the butter and margarine. Top waffles, pancakes and French toast with modest amounts of syrup, molasses, applesauce, fruit preserves or fresh fruit slices.

Staying Active • If you're new to exercising, check with your doctor first. Checking with a physician is especially important if you're over 35, you're at least 25 pounds overweight, you have a personal or family history of high blood pressure or heart disease, and/or you haven't had a medical checkup recently.

Orange-Cranberry Scones

LO CAL / HI FIB

PREP: 20 MIN; BAKE: 9 MIN; COOL: 5 MIN

12 SCONES

- 2 cups Basic 4® cereal or other whole wheat flake cereal with cranberries, slightly crushed
- 1 cup all-purpose flour
- $1/4$ cup packed brown sugar
- 2 teaspoons baking powder
- 1 teaspoon grated orange peel
- $1/4$ teaspoon salt
- $1/4$ cup firm margarine or butter
- $1/2$ cup dried cranberries
- $1/4$ cup fat-free cholesterol-free egg product or 1 egg, slightly beaten
- $1/4$ cup orange low-fat yogurt

   Orange Glaze (right)

Heat oven to 400°. Slightly crush cereal; set aside.

Mix flour, brown sugar, baking powder, orange peel and salt in medium bowl. Cut in margarine, using pastry blender or crisscrossing 2 knives, until mixture looks like coarse crumbs. Stir in cereal, cranberries, egg product and yogurt until soft dough forms.

Place dough on lightly floured surface. Gently roll in flour to coat; shape into ball. Pat dough into 8-inch circle with floured hands. Cut circle into 12 wedges with sharp knife dipped in flour. Place wedges about 1 inch apart on ungreased cookie sheet.

Bake 7 to 9 minutes or until edges are light brown. Immediately remove from cookie sheet to wire rack. Cool 5 minutes; drizzle with Orange Glaze. After glaze is set, store tightly covered.

Orange Glaze

- $1/2$ cup powdered sugar
- $1/4$ teaspoon grated orange peel
- 2 to 3 teaspoons orange juice

Mix all ingredients until thin enough to drizzle.

1 Scone: Calories 170 (Calories from Fat 45); Fat 5g (Saturated 3g); Cholesterol 30mg; Sodium 220mg; Carbohydrate 31g (Dietary Fiber 3g); Protein 3g
% Daily Value: Vitamin A 10%; Vitamin C 6% ; Calcium 12%; Iron 8%
Diet Exchanges: 1 starch, 1 fruit, $1/2$ fat

Eating Smart • For a breakfast that stays with you through the morning, try a well-rounded meal of 300 to 400 calories that is high in complex carbohydrates and contains some protein and fat.

Staying Active • To get the most out of sit-ups, keep your knees bent, your feet flat on the floor and come up to only a 30-degree angle. Forget about the old-fashioned straight-leg sit-ups, which can make you overarch and strain your lower back.

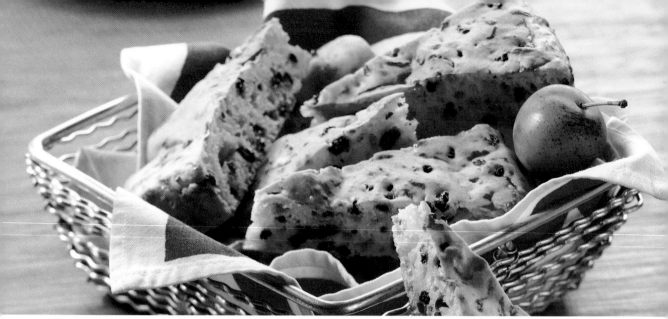

Savory Currant Wedges

Savory Currant Wedges

LO CAL / LO CHOL

PREP: 10 MIN; BAKE: 35 MIN; COOL: 10 MIN

12 WEDGES

1½   cups all-purpose flour

½   cup currants or raisins

1   teaspoon baking powder

½   teaspoon salt

¼   teaspoon baking soda

1   cup shredded reduced-fat mozzarella cheese (4 ounces)

¾   cup buttermilk

¼   cup fat-free cholesterol-free egg product or 1 egg

2   tablespoons olive or vegetable oil

Heat oven to 375°. Spray round pan, 9 × 1½ inches, with cooking spray.

Mix flour, currants, baking powder, salt and baking soda in large bowl. Stir in remaining ingredients. Spread in pan.

Bake 30 to 35 minutes or until golden brown. Cool 10 minutes. Cut into wedges. Serve warm.

1 Wedge: Calories 125 (Calories from Fat 35); Fat 4g (Saturated 1g); Cholesterol 5mg; Sodium 240mg; Carbohydrate 18g (Dietary Fiber 1g); Protein 5g
% Daily Value: Vitamin A 2%; Vitamin C 0%; Calcium 12%; Iron 6%
Diet Exchanges: 1 starch, 1 fat

Eating Smart • Even though they look like baby raisins, currants are actually a different variety of dried fruit. Currants are dried Zante grapes—most raisins are dried from Thompson or Muscat grapes. Dried fruits are concentrated sources of many nutrients. Include them in baked goods for a sweet, low-fat burst of flavor.

Staying Active • The next time you pass a playground, steal a few seconds for yourself. Return to your childhood by swinging, sliding and climbing. When you're playing and having fun, you don't even realize that you're also working out and burning calories.

Ginger Gems Cookies

LO CAL / LO FAT / LO CHOL / LO SODIUM

PREP: 15 MIN; CHILL: 2 HR;

BAKE: 10 MIN PER SHEET; COOL: 30 MIN

ABOUT 5 DOZEN COOKIES

1	cup sugar
1/4	cup margarine or butter, softened
1/4	cup fat-free cholesterol-free egg product or 1 egg
1/4	cup molasses
1 3/4	cups all-purpose flour
1	teaspoon baking soda
1/2	teaspoon ground cinnamon
1/2	teaspoon ground ginger
1/4	teaspoon ground cloves
1/4	teaspoon salt
5	tablespoons orange marmalade
5	tablespoons finely chopped crystallized ginger

Beat 3/4 cup of the sugar, the margarine, egg product and molasses in medium bowl with electric mixer on medium speed, or mix with spoon. Stir in flour, baking soda, cinnamon, ground ginger, cloves and salt. Cover and refrigerate at least 2 hours until firm.

Heat oven to 350°. Lightly spray cookie sheet with cooking spray. Shape dough into 3/4-inch balls; roll in remaining 1/4 cup sugar. Place about 2 inches apart on cookie sheet. Make indentation in center of each ball, using finger. Fill each indentation with about 1/4 teaspoon of the marmalade. Sprinkle with about 1/4 teaspoon of the crystallized ginger.

Bake 8 to 10 minutes or until set. Immediately re-move from cookie sheet to wire rack. Cool com-pletely, about 30 minutes.

1 Cookie: Calories 40 (Calories from Fat 10); Fat 1g (Saturated 0g); Cholesterol 0mg; Sodium 45mg; Carbo-hydrate 8g (Dietary Fiber 0g); Protein 0g
% Daily Value: Vitamin A 0% ; Vitamin C 0% ; Calcium 0%; Iron 2%
Diet Exchanges: 1/2 fruit

Eating Smart • If you haven't switched from 2 percent milk to the fat-free variety because you think it tastes watery, add a tablespoon of nonfat dried milk to each cup of fat-free milk. The milk will taste thicker and richer, and you'll get an extra protein and calcium boost.

Staying Active • Don't make exercise out to be the bad guy. Our bodies are designed to move and be active. By becoming a couch potato, we defy nature. Think of exercise as play, and cele-brate your body as it continues to get slimmer, stronger and healthier.

Mocha Angel Cake

LO CAL / LO FAT / LO CHOL

PREP: 15 MIN; BAKE: 45 MIN; COOL: 1 HR

12 SERVINGS

1 package (1 pound) one-step white angel food cake mix

1 tablespoon baking cocoa

1¼ cups cold coffee

Mocha Topping (below)

Chocolate shot, if desired

Bake and cool cake as directed on package for two 9-inch loaf pans—except stir cocoa into cake mix (dry) and substitute cold coffee for the water.

Serve cake with Mocha Topping. Sprinkle with chocolate shot. Store covered in refrigerator.

Mocha Topping

½ package (2.8-ounce size) whipped topping mix (1 envelope)

½ cup cold fat-free (skim) milk

½ teaspoon vanilla

2 tablespoons powdered sugar

2 teaspoons baking cocoa

Make topping mix as directed on package, using fat-free milk and vanilla; add powdered sugar and cocoa for the last minute of beating.

1 Serving: Calories 165 (Calories from Fat 10); Fat 1g (Saturated 0g); Cholesterol 0mg; Sodium 260mg; Carbohydrate 35g (Dietary Fiber 0g); Protein 4g
% Daily Value: Vitamin A 0%; Vitamin C 0%; Calcium 0%; Iron 4%
Diet Exchanges: 2 starch

Eating Smart • Made with egg whites, angel food cake is lower in fat than other sweets. Why? Egg whites contain only about 20 of an egg's 75 calories. The white is also fat and cholesterol free. Two whites can often be substituted for one whole egg in baking recipes.

Staying Active • Research has found that exercise is one of the most effective ways to lift poor spirits. Instead of reaching for chocolate next time you're down, try a 10-minute walk or bike ride.

Mini Pumpkin Cheesecakes

LO CAL / LO FAT / LO CHOL

PREP: 15 MIN; BAKE: 35 MIN; COOL: 15 MIN;

CHILL: 1 HR

8 SERVINGS

2   soft molasses cookies (3 inches in diameter)

1   package (8 ounces) fat-free cream cheese, softened

$1/3$ cup packed brown sugar

$1/2$ cup fat-free cholesterol-free egg product or 2 eggs

$1/2$ teaspoon vanilla

$2/3$ cup canned pumpkin (not pumpkin pie mix)

$1/2$ teaspoon pumpkin pie spice

1   cup frozen (thawed) reduced-fat whipped topping

Heat oven to 350°. Line 8 medium muffin cups, $2^1/2 \times 1^1/4$ inches, with aluminum foil or paper baking cups. Break cookies into fine crumbs. Reserve 2 teaspoons cookie crumbs for topping. Divide remaining crumbs among muffin cups.

Beat cream cheese and brown sugar in medium bowl with electric mixer on medium speed until smooth. Stir in egg product and vanilla just until blended. Stir in pumpkin and pumpkin pie spice. Spoon evenly into muffin cups.

Bake 30 to 35 minutes or until edges are set; cool 15 minutes. Remove cheesecakes from pan. Refrigerate about 1 hour or until completely chilled. Serve each cheesecake topped with 2 tablespoons whipped topping. Sprinkle with reserved cookie crumbs. Store covered in refrigerator.

1 Serving: Calories 110 (Calories from Fat 20); Fat 2g (Saturated 1g); Cholesterol 0mg; Sodium 190mg; Carbohydrate 18g (Dietary Fiber 1g); Protein 6g
% Daily Value: Vitamin A 60%; Vitamin C 0%; Calcium 10%; Iron 4%
Diet Exchanges: 1 starch, $1/2$ fat

Eating Smart • Canned pumpkin is just as nutritious as its fresh counterpart. One-half cup contains about 40 calories and is free of fat, sodium and cholesterol. The same $1/2$ cup also contains 100% of the RDA for Vitamin A, along with a good amount of fiber, iron and other minerals.

Staying Active • Do you want to burn 450 calories? You can: a) swim for an hour; or b) float on a pool chair for 8 hours. Anyone with a schedule to keep knows that option "a" is the best bet.

Pear and Cherry Crisp

LO CAL / LO CHOL / LO SODIUM / HI FIB

PREP: 30 MIN; BAKE: 35 MIN; COOL: 15 MIN

8 SERVINGS

¾   cup quick-cooking oats

¼   cup packed brown sugar

3   tablespoons all-purpose flour

2   tablespoons margarine or butter, melted

2   tablespoons dried cherries

4   medium pears, peeled, cored and sliced
    (4 cups)

1   cup frozen pitted tart cherries

⅓   cup granulated sugar

3   tablespoons all-purpose flour

½   teaspoon almond extract
    Almond Custard Sauce (right)

Heat oven to 375°. Mix oats, brown sugar, 3 table-spoons flour and the margarine until crumbly. Stir in dried cherries; set aside.

Mix remaining ingredients except Almond Custard Sauce in square baking dish, 8 × 8 × 2 inches. Sprinkle oat mixture over filling; press slightly.

Bake 30 to 35 minutes or until topping is golden brown and mixture is bubbly. Cool 15 minutes. Serve with Almond Custard Sauce.

Almond Custard Sauce

2   containers (3 to 4 ounces each)
    refrigerated vanilla fat-free pudding

¼   cup fat-free half-and-half

¼   teaspoon almond extract

Mix all ingredients.

1 Serving: Calories 250 (Calories from Fat 35); Fat 4g (Saturated 1g); Cholesterol 0mg; Sodium 90mg; Carbohydrate 54g (Dietary Fiber 4g); Protein 4g
% Daily Value: Vitamin A 6%; Vitamin C 6%; Calcium 6%; Iron 6%
Diet Exchanges: 1 starch, 2½ fruit, ½ fat

Eating Smart • Fruit is the perfect portable snack! Few foods are easier to throw into a backpack or briefcase than apples, pears, oranges and bananas. Fruit is also low in calories and high in fiber, vitamins and carbohydrates.

Staying Active • Make spring cleaning a full-fledged workout. Mix and match the following activities: rearranging your wardrobe (2.3 calories per minute), cleaning out the attic (3.4 calories per minute), washing windows (4.4 calories per minute) and scrubbing floors (5.4 calories per minute).

REFERENCES

What Are Diet Exchanges?

Exchanges are measured choices of foods. *Exchange Lists for Meal Planning,* first published by the American Dietetic Association and the American Diabetes Association, places foods into three main groups, *Carbohydrate Group, Protein Group* and *Fat Group,* which are divided into lists on the basis of their nutritional content.

How the Exchanges Measure Up

Exchange Groups/Lists	*Carbohydrate (grams)*	*Protein (grams)*	*Fat (grams)*	*Calories*
Carbohydrate Group				
1 starch	15	3	trace	80
1 fruit	15	—	—	60
1 milk (skim)	12	8	trace	90
1 vegetable	5	2	—	25
Protein Group				
1 very lean meat	—	7	0–1	35
1 lean meat	—	7	3	55
1 medium-fat meat	—	7	5	75
1 high-fat meat	—	7	8	100
Fat Group				
1 fat	—	—	5	45

Source: The American Dietetic Association, 1995.

The *Carbohydrate Group* is broken down into exchange lists: *starch, fruit, milk* and *vegetables*. The *Protein Group* is divided into four lists: *very lean meat, lean meat, medium-fat meat* and *high-fat meat*. The *Fat Group* is just that—fat.

Foods in each exchange list have about the same number of calories and amounts of nutrients as other foods in the same list (see chart on page 445). Within any list, foods can be traded for one another.

The exchange system also includes *free foods,* those foods and beverages with fewer than 20 calories per serving that can be eaten freely throughout the day. Foods such as pizza and casseroles actually are combinations of foods and have several exchanges to represent the ingredients.

Check side panels of product packages and in cookbooks and magazines for exchanges. To find a registered dietitian in your area to help you work with exchanges, ask your doctor, call a local hospital or call The American Dietetic Association at (800) 366-1655.

Nutrition Glossary

Ever wonder what those nutrition and health experts are saying? Here's a quick reference list that explains some important key words.

ADDITIVE   Substance added to food to perform certain useful functions, such as to add color or flavor, prevent spoilage, add nutritional value or improve texture or consistency.

CARBOHYDRATES   Key human energy source. All simple sugars and complex carbohydrates (starches) fit into this category.

CHOLESTEROL   Essential fatlike substance, found in animal foods, that is needed by the body in order for hormones to function properly. Our bodies make cholesterol, as well.

CHOLESTEROL, HDL   High-density lipoprotein (HDL) cholesterol that helps to remove cholesterol from body tissues and blood and return the cholesterol to the liver to be used again. This recycling process has earned it a "good" reputation.

CHOLESTEROL, LDL   Low-density lipoprotein (LDL) cholesterol that travels through the bloodstream making cholesterol available for cell structures, hormones and nerve coverings. Often tagged the "bad" cholesterol because it deposits cholesterol on artery walls.

DIET EXCHANGES   Developed by The American Dietetic Association and The American Diabetes Association, Diet Exchanges place foods into groups and lists based on their nutritional content. Foods grouped together have about the same number of calories and amounts of nutrients as other foods in the same list. See page 445 for more information.

FAT   Provides energy—more than twice the amount supplied by carbohydrates or protein. Also provides essential nutrients and the insulation and protection of body organs.

FAT, SATURATED   Found primarily in animal foods, this type of fat is solid at room temperature. Diets high in saturated fats have been linked to higher blood-cholesterol levels, but not all saturated fats have the same cholesterol-raising potential.

FAT, UNSATURATED   Found most commonly in plant foods, this type of fat usually is liquid at room temperature. Unsaturated fats are often found as monounsaturated or polyunsaturated fats. A laboratory process called *hydrogenation* is used to alter the chemical structure of unsaturated fats, making them saturated and more shelf stable.

FIBER, DIETARY   Often described as the components of plant foods that are not broken down or absorbed by the human digestive tract. Fiber is a complex carbohydrate, based on its chemical structure.

FIBER, INSOLUBLE   This form of fiber does not dissolve in water and is best known for its water-holding capacity. Often referred to as *roughage*, insoluble fiber helps digestion by absorbing water and keeping things moving through the digestive tract.

FIBER, SOLUBLE   A form of fiber that dissolves in watery solutions and helps with digestion and absorption processes. Soluble fiber may help to lower blood cholesterol.

FOOD GUIDE PYRAMID   A nutrition education guide used to help people learn about the foods they should eat and the recommended number of servings from each food group for a balanced and healthy diet. It replaces the former Four Basic Food Groups. See page 16 for illustration.

MINERALS   Essential elements (except carbon, hydrogen, oxygen and nitrogen) needed by the body in very small amounts. Minerals are inorganic elements, such as calcium and iron, and are found in our foods and water. See charts on pages 11 and 15.

NUTRIENTS   Substances necessary for life and to build, repair and maintain body cells. Includes protein, carbohydrate, fat, water, vitamins and minerals.

PERCENT DAILY VALUE   Developed as a relative standard for nutrition labeling of foods based on a 2,000-calorie diet. It is based on the needs of healthy people of various ages and is generally the highest recommended level of each nutrient for all age groups. In replaces Percent of U.S. Recommended Daily Allowance.

PROTEIN   Vital for life, protein provides energy and the structural support of body cells and is important for growth. Made from amino-acid building blocks that contain nitrogen.

VITAMINS   Essential substances, found in small amounts in many foods that are necessary for controlling body processes. Different from minerals in that vitamins are organic compounds containing carbon. They include vitamin A, B vitamins (such as niacin and riboflavin), vitamin C and more. See chart on page 12.

Nutrition Criteria for Flags

Each recipe in this book meets at least one of the five nutrition criteria described below; many recipes meet several criteria. The nutrition information that accompanies each recipe, along with the special nutrition criteria flags and Diet Exchanges, will help you make healthy new choices for you and your family. Keep in mind that no one recipe, or even one meal, will meet all your nutrition needs. Eat a variety of foods for a healthy, well-balanced diet.

Low Calorie (LO CAL): Recipes have 350 or fewer calories per serving with the exception of desserts. Low-calorie dessert recipes have 250 or fewer calories per serving.

Low Fat (LO FAT): Recipes have 3 or fewer grams of fat per serving for most foods; 6 or fewer grams of fat per serving for main-dish items.

Low Cholesterol (LO CHOL): Recipes have 20 or fewer milligrams of cholesterol per serving.

Low Sodium (LO SODIUM): Recipes have 140 or fewer milligrams of sodium per serving.

High Fiber (HI FIB): Recipes have 3 or more grams of fiber per serving.

Substitution Chart

CHOOSE THESE	INSTEAD OF THESE	SAVINGS/BENEFIT
CALORIES		
Frozen fruit-juice bar	Ice-cream bar	150 calories
Graham cracker, 3 squares	Chocolate sandwich cookies, 3	80 calories
Hard candy, 1 oz	Chocolate candy	50 calories
Low-fat yogurt, ½ cup	Sour cream	150 calories
Pretzels, 1 oz	Potato chips	60 calories
Salsa, ¼ cup	Cheese sauce	100 calories
Sparkling water (any flavor) or sugar-free soda pop, 12 oz	Soda pop (any flavor)	150 calories
Nonstick cooking spray, 1 spray	Vegetable oil, 1 Tbsp	120 calories
FAT		
Fat-free mayonnaise, 1 Tbsp	Mayonnaise	10g fat
Fat-free sour cream, ½ cup	Sour cream	20g fat
Ground turkey breast cooked, 3 oz	Hamburger (lean), cooked	10g fat
Neufchâtel (reduced-fat cream cheese), 1 Tbsp	Cream cheese	2g fat
Nonfat frozen yogurt, 1 cup	Ice cream, 16% fat	24g fat
Pretzels, 1 oz	Potato chips	10g fat
Reduced-fat Cheddar cheese, 1 oz	Cheddar cheese	5g fat
Reduced-fat whipped topping, 2 Tbsp	Whipped cream	10g fat
CHOLESTEROL		
Cholesterol-free egg substitute, ¼ cup	Whole egg, 1	210mg cholesterol
Cholesterol-free noodles, uncooked, 2 oz	Egg noodles	70mg cholesterol
Egg whites, 2	Whole egg, 1	205mg cholesterol
Fat-free cottage cheese, ½ cup	Ricotta cheese	60mg cholesterol
Imitation crabmeat sticks, cooked, 3 oz	Crabmeat	60mg cholesterol
Low-fat yogurt, ½ cup	Sour cream	70mg cholesterol
Margarine, 1 Tbsp	Butter	30mg cholesterol
Nonfat frozen yogurt, 1 cup	Ice cream, 16% fat	90mg cholesterol
Skim milk, 1 cup	Whole milk	30mg cholesterol
SODIUM		
Apple juice, ½ cup	Chicken broth	510mg sodium
Balsamic vinegar, 1 tsp	Salt	2300mg sodium
Basil, dried, 1 tsp	Season salt	1350mg sodium
Corn, fresh or frozen, ½ cup	Corn, canned	250mg sodium
Lemon juice, 1 tsp	Salt	2000mg sodium
Reduced-sodium soy sauce, 1 Tbsp	Soy sauce	500mg sodium
Reduced-sodium chicken broth, 1 cup	Chicken broth	700mg sodium
FIBER		
Apple	Apple juice, ½ cup	4g fiber added
Bean or lentil soup, 1 cup	Cream of mushroom soup	4g fiber added
Bran cereal with dried fruit, 1 oz	Corn flake cereal	6g fiber added
Brown rice, cooked, 1 cup	White rice	2g fiber added
Cabbage, raw, 1 cup	Iceberg lettuce	3g fiber added
Fiber One® cereal, 1 oz	Raisin bran cereal	10g fiber added
Mango, ½ cup	Orange juice, ½ cup	4g fiber added
Popcorn, popped, 4 cups (1 oz)	Chips, 1 oz	3g fiber added
Whole wheat bread, 1 slice	White bread	2g fiber added

Top Twenty Sources of Calcium

	FOOD	AMOUNT	CALCIUM (MG)
DAIRY PRODUCTS	Milk	1 cup	300
	Yogurt, Colombo®, light	8 ounces	260
	Yogurt, Yoplait®, low-fat	6 ounces	190–230
	Cheese	1 ounce	150–225
	Pudding, cooked	1/2 cup	150
	Frozen yogurt, nonfat	1/2 cup	110
	Ice cream or ice milk	1/2 cup	100
	Cottage cheese	1/2 cup	75
FRUITS AND VEGETABLES	Orange juice, calcium-fortified	1 cup	300
	Rhubarb (cooked with sugar)	1/2 cup	175
	Turnip greens, cooked	1/2 cup	125
	Spinach, cooked	1/2 cup	120
	Broccoli, cooked	1/2 cup	90
	Orange	1 medium	50
GRAINS AND OTHER FOODS	Rice, calcium-fortified	1/2 cup	300
	Whole grain Total® cereal	3/4 cup	250
	Molasses, blackstrap	1 Tbsp	170
	Oatmeal, fortified, instant	3/4 cup	165
	Tofu	1/2 cup	130
	Almonds	1/4 cup	95

Top Twenty Sources of Folic Acid

	FOOD	AMOUNT	FOLIC ACID (μG)
GRAINS	Total® cereal	1 cup	400
	Cereal, ready-to-eat	3/4 to 1 cup	100
	Wheat germ	1/4 cup	80
	Bread, enriched	1 slice	40
FRUITS AND VEGETABLES	Asparagus	1/2 cup	130
	Spinach	1/2 cup	130
	Avocado	1/2 medium	70
	Tomato juice	1 cup	50
	Broccoli	1/2 cup	40
	Strawberries, frozen	1 cup	40
NUTS AND LEGUMES	Lentils	1/2 cup	180
	Garbanzo beans	1/2 cup	140
	Black beans	1/2 cup	130
	Soybean nuts, roasted	1/3 cup	120
	Kidney beans	1/2 cup	115
	Peanuts, dry roasted	1/3 cup	110
	Pistachios	1 ounce	100
	Baked beans with pork	1 cup	90
	Filberts	1 ounce	70
	Almonds	1/3 cup	50

Nutrition and Recipe Testing Guidelines

NUTRITION GUIDELINES

Daily Values are set by the Food and Drug Administration and are based on the needs of most healthy adults. Percent Daily Values are based on an average diet of 2,000 calories per day. Your daily values may be higher or lower depending on your calorie needs.

Recommended intake for a daily diet of 2,000 calories:

Total Fat	*Less than 65g*
Saturated Fat	*Less than 20g*
Cholesterol	*Less than 300 mg*
Sodium	*Less than 2,400 mg*
Total Carbohydrate	*300g*
Dietary Fiber	*25g*

Diet Exchanges are based on criteria set by the American Dietetic Association and the American Diabetes Association.

CALCULATING NUTRITION INFORMATION GUIDELINES

➤ The first ingredient is used wherever a choice is given (such as ⅓ cup sour cream or plain yogurt).

➤ The first ingredient amount is used wherever a range is given (such as 2 to 3 teaspoons).

➤ The first serving number is used wherever a range is given (such as 4 to 6 servings).

➤ "If desired" ingredients are not included, whether mentioned in the ingredient list or in the recipe directions as a suggestion (such as sprinkle with brown sugar, if desired).

➤ Only the amount of a marinade or frying oil that is absorbed during preparation is calculated.

Cooking Terms Glossary

BEAT: Mix ingredients vigorously with spoon, fork, wire whisk, hand beater or electric mixer until smooth and uniform.

BOIL: Heat liquid until bubbles rise continuously and break on the surface and steam is given off. For rolling boil, the bubbles form rapidly.

CHOP: Cut into coarse or fine irregular pieces with a knife, food chopper, blender or food processor.

CUBE: Cut into squares 1/2 inch or larger.

DICE: Cut into squares smaller than 1/2 inch.

GRATE: Cut into tiny particles using small rough holes of grater (citrus peel or chocolate).

GREASE: Rub the inside surface of a pan with shortening, using pastry brush, piece of waxed paper or paper towel, to prevent food from sticking during baking (as for some casseroles).

JULIENNE: Cut into thin, matchlike strips, using knife or food processor (vegetables, fruits, meats).

MIX: Combine ingredients in any way that distributes them evenly.

SAUTÉ: Cook foods in hot oil or margarine over medium-high heat with frequent tossing and turning motion.

SHRED: Cut into long thin pieces by rubbing food across the holes of a shredder, as for cheese, or by using a knife to slice very thinly, as for cabbage.

SIMMER: Cook in liquid just below the boiling point on top of the stove; usually after reducing heat from a boil. Bubbles will rise slowly and break just below the surface.

STIR: Mix ingredients until uniform consistency. Stir once in a while for "stirring occasionally," often for "stirring frequently" and continuously for "stirring constantly."

TOSS: Tumble ingredients lightly with a lifting motion (such as green salad), usually to coat evenly or mix with another food.

Ingredients Used in Recipe Testing and Nutrition Calculations

➤ Ingredients used for testing represent those that the majority of consumers use in their homes: large eggs, 2% milk, 80 percent lean ground beef, canned ready-to-use chicken broth, and vegetable oil spread containing not less than 65 percent fat.

➤ Fat-free, low-fat or low-sodium products are not used, unless otherwise indicated.

➤ Solid vegetable shortening (not butter, margarine, nonstick cooking sprays or vegetable oil spread, as they can cause sticking problems) is used to grease pans, unless otherwise indicated.

Equipment Used in Recipe Testing

We use equipment for testing that the majority of consumers use in their homes. If a specific piece of equipment (such as a wire whisk) is necessary for recipe success, it will be listed in the recipe.

➤ Cookware and bakeware **without** nonstick coatings were used, unless otherwise indicated.

➤ No dark colored, black or insulated bakeware was used.

➤ When a baking pan is specified in a recipe, a metal pan was used; a baking dish or pie plate means oven-proof glass was used.

➤ An electric hand mixer was used for mixing only when mixer speeds are specified in the recipe directions. When a mixer speed is not given, a spoon or fork was used.

Metric Conversion Guide

Volume

U.S. Units	Canadian Metric	Australian Metric
1/4 teaspoon	1 mL	1 ml
1/2 teaspoon	2mL	2 ml
1 teaspoon	5 mL	5 ml
1 tablespoon	15 mL	20 ml
1/4 cup	50 mL	60 ml
1/3 cup	75 mL	80 ml
1/2 cup	125 mL	125 ml
2/3 cup	150 mL	170 ml
3/4 cup	175 mL	190 ml
1 cup	250 mL	250 ml
1 quart	1 liter	1 liter
1 1/2 quarts	1.5 liters	1.5 liters
2 quarts	2 liters	2 liters
2 1/2 quarts	2.5 liters	2.5 liters
3 quarts	3 liters	3 liters
4 quarts	4 liters	4 liters

Weight

U.S. Units	Canadian Metric	Australian Metric
1 ounce	30 grams	30 grams
2 ounces	55 grams	60 grams
3 ounces	85 grams	90 grams
4 ounces (1/4 pound)	115 grams	125 grams
8 ounces (1/2 pound)	225 grams	225 grams
16 ounces (1 pound)	455 grams	500 grams
1 pound	455 grams	1/2 kilogram

Measurements

Inches	Centimeters
1	2.5
2	5.0
3	7.5
4	10.0
5	12.5
6	15.0
7	17.5
8	20.5
9	23.0
10	25.5
11	28.0
12	30.5
13	33.0

Temperatures

Fahrenheit	Celsius
32°	0
212°	100°
250°	120°
275°	140°
300°	150°
325°	160°
350°	180°
375°	190°
400°	200°
425°	220°
450°	230°
475°	240°
500°	260°

Note: The recipes in this cookbook have not been developed or tested using metric measures. When converting recipes to metric, variations in quality may be noted.

INDEX